A·N·N·U·A·L E·D·I·T·I·O·N·S

Drugs, Society, and Behavior

04/05

Nineteenth Edition

EDITOR

Hugh T. Wilson

California State University-Sacramento

Hugh Wilson received his Bachelor of Arts degree from California State University, Sacramento, and a Master of Arts degree in Justice Administration and a Doctorate in Public Administration from Golden Gate University in San Francisco. Dr. Wilson is currently a professor of criminal justice at California State University, Sacramento. He has taught drug abuse recognition, enforcement, and policy to police officers and students of criminal justice for more than 20 years.

McGraw-Hill/Dushkin

530 Old Whitfield Street, Guilford, Connecticut 06437

Visit us on the Internet
http://www.dushkin.com

Credits

1. **Living With Drugs**
   Unit photo—© 2004 by PhotoDisc, Inc.
2. **Understanding How Drugs Work—Use, Dependency, and Addiction**
   Unit photo—United Nations photo.
3. **The Major Drugs of Use and Abuse**
   Unit photo—United Nations photo.
4. **Other Trends in Drug Use**
   Unit photo—© 2004 by PhotoDisc, Inc.
5. **Drugs and Crime**
   Unit photo—© 2004 by PhotoDisc, Inc.
6. **Measuring the Social Cost of Drugs**
   Unit photo—© 2004 by Cleo Freelance Photography.
7. **Creating and Sustaining Effective Drug Control Policy**
   Unit photo—Courtesy of the Drug Enforcement Agency.
8. **Prevention, Treatment, and Education**
   Unit photo—© 2004 by Sweet By & By/Cindy Brown.

Copyright

Cataloging in Publication Data
Main entry under title: Annual Editions: Drugs, Society, and Behavior. 2004/2005.
1. Drugs, Society, and Behavior—Periodicals. I. Wilson, Hugh T., *comp.* II. Title: Drugs, Society, and Behavior.
ISBN 0–07–286073–1   658'.05   ISSN 1091–9945

Nineteenth Edition

Cover image © 2004 PhotoDisc, Inc.
Printed in the United States of America   1234567890BAHBAH54   Printed on Recycled Paper

Editors/Advisory Board

Members of the Advisory Board are instrumental in the final selection of articles for each edition of ANNUAL EDITIONS. Their review of articles for content, level, currentness, and appropriateness provides critical direction to the editor and staff. We think that you will find their careful consideration well reflected in this volume.

To the Reader

In publishing ANNUAL EDITIONS we recognize the enormous role played by the magazines, newspapers, and journals of the public press in providing current, first-rate educational information in a broad spectrum of interest areas. Many of these articles are appropriate for students, researchers, and professionals seeking accurate, current material to help bridge the gap between principles and theories and the real world. These articles, however, become more useful for study when those of lasting value are carefully collected, organized, indexed, and reproduced in a low-cost format, which provides easy and permanent access when the material is needed. That is the role played by ANNUAL EDITIONS.

It is difficult to define the framework by which Americans make decisions and develop perspectives on the use of drugs. There is no predictable expression of ideology. A wide range of individual and collective experience defines our national will toward drugs.

Despite drug prevention efforts, 16 million Americans use drugs on a monthly basis; 6 million meet the clinical criteria for needing drug-abuse treatment. Social costs from drugs are measured in the billions. Drugs impact almost every aspect of public and private life. Drugs are the subjects of presidential elections, congressional appointments, and military interventions. Financial transactions from smuggling help sustain terrorist organizations that in turn cause war and killing and destruction to return to fields where poppies grew. Drugs impact families, schools, health care systems, and governments, in more places and in more ways than many believe imaginable.

Although it takes little effort to expose evil manifested by the abuse of drugs, there are tiny victories through which harm from drug abuse can be reduced. Scientific discovery relative to creating a new understanding of the processes of addiction is one. New treatment modalities, the successful use of drug courts, and the political support to expand these concepts have reduced drug related impacts. Good evidence suggests that many of the most egregious forms of drug abuse have leveled off and, in some important cases, been reduced. Reducing harm is probably all that is possible. The multitude of life's processes and influences and their enduring linkages with drugs will persist, as they have for thousands of years. It is a multifaceted problem, requiring a multifaceted response. Hope, literacy, and understanding have always been some of the most powerful tools of progress.

The articles contained in *Annual Editions: Drugs, Society, and Behavior 04/05* are a collection of facts, issues, and perspectives designed to provide the reader with a framework for examining current drug-related issues. The book is designed to offer students something to think about and something with which to think. It is a unique collection of materials of interest to the casual as well as the serious student of drug-related social phenomena. Unit 1 addresses the significance that drugs have played in early as well as contemporary American history. It emphasizes the often-overlooked reality that drugs, legal and illegal, have remained a pervasive dimension of past as well as present American history. Unit 2 examines the ways that drugs affect the mind and body that result in dependence and addiction. Unit 3 examines the major drugs of use and abuse, along with issues relative to understanding the individual impacts of these drugs on society. This unit also illustrates the necessity to perceive the differences and similarities produced by the use of legal and illegal drugs. Unit 4 reviews the dynamic nature of drugs as it relates to changing patterns and trends of use. Unit 5 analyzes the link between drugs and crime. Implications of individual criminal behavior as well as organized, syndicated drug trafficking are discussed. Unit 6 focuses on the social costs of drug abuse and why the costs overwhelm many American institutions. Unit 7 illustrates the complexity and controversy in creating and implementing drug policy. Unit 8 concludes the book with discussions of current strategies for preventing and treating drug abuse. Can we deter people from harming themselves with drugs, and can we cure people addicted to drugs? What does work and what does not?

Annual Editions: Drugs, Society, and Behavior 04/05 contain a number of features that are designed to make the volume "user friendly." These include a *table of contents* with *abstracts* that summarize each article and key concepts in boldface, a *topic guide* to help locate articles on specific individuals or subjects, World Wide Web links that can be used to further explore the topics, and a comprehensive *index*.

We encourage your comments and criticisms on the articles provided and kindly ask for your review on the postage-paid *article rating form* at the end of the book.

Hugh T. Wilson

Hugh T. Wilson
Editor

Contents

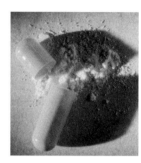

UNIT 1
Living With Drugs

Six articles in this unit examine the past and present historical evolution of drugs in the United States

The concepts in bold italics are developed in the article. For further expansion, please refer to the Topic Guide and the Index.

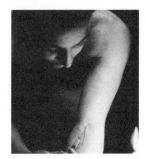

UNIT 2
Understanding How Drugs Work—Use, Dependency, and Addiction

Eight articles in this section examine the ways that drugs affect the mind and body. The relationship of pharmacology with dependence and addiction is described.

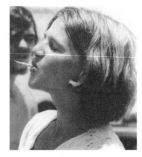

UNIT 3
The Major Drugs of Use and Abuse

In 11 articles, this unit addresses some major drugs of use and abuse. Cocaine, heroin, marijuana, and alcohol are discussed, along with prescription medicines.

The concepts in bold italics are developed in the article. For further expansion, please refer to the Topic Guide and the Index.

The concepts in bold italics are developed in the article. For further expansion, please refer to the Topic Guide and the Index.

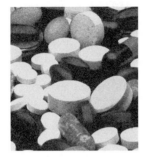

UNIT 4
Other Trends in Drug Use

The eleven articles in the unit discuss some developing patterns of drug use along with their subsequent implications for society.

The concepts in bold italics are developed in the article. For further expansion, please refer to the Topic Guide and the Index.

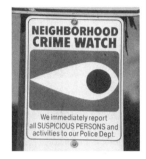

UNIT 5
Drugs and Crime

Six articles review the numbing social malady caused by criminal behavior that is created, sustained, and perpetuated by the use of drugs.

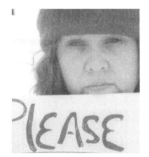

UNIT 6
Measuring the Social Cost of Drugs

Five articles speak to the diverse ways in which the impact of drugs affects and overwhelms numerous public and private American institutions.

The concepts in bold italics are developed in the article. For further expansion, please refer to the Topic Guide and the Index.

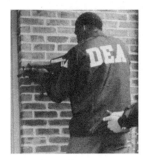

UNIT 7
Creating and Sustaining Effective Drug Control Policy

The five essays in this unit illustrate the complexity of creating effective drug policy.

The concepts in bold italics are developed in the article. For further expansion, please refer to the Topic Guide and the Index.

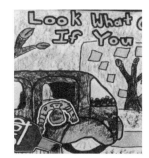

UNIT 8
Prevention, Treatment, and Education

Addressing some tough questions concerning previously accepted ideas about drug treatment, the eight unit articles review effectiveness, financial costs, education, and controversial new treatments.

The concepts in bold italics are developed in the article. For further expansion, please refer to the Topic Guide and the Index.

Topic Guide

This topic guide suggests how the selections in this book relate to the subjects covered in your course. You may want to use the topics listed on these pages to search the Web more easily.

On the following pages a number of Web sites have been gathered specifically for this book. They are arranged to reflect the units of this *Annual Edition*. You can link to these sites by going to the DUSHKIN ONLINE support site at *http://www.dushkin.com/online/*.

ALL THE ARTICLES THAT RELATE TO EACH TOPIC ARE LISTED BELOW THE BOLD-FACED TERM.

World Wide Web Sites

The following World Wide Web sites have been carefully researched and selected to support the articles found in this reader. The easiest way to access these selected sites is to go to our DUSHKIN ONLINE support site at *http://www.dushkin.com/online/*.

AE: Drugs, Society, and Behavior 04/05

The following sites were available at the time of publication. Visit our Web site—we update DUSHKIN ONLINE regularly to reflect any changes.

General Sources

Alcohol and Drug Links

http://www.realsolutions.org/druglink.htm

This set of Internet links provides information on Alcohol and Drug Use and Abuse. These links have been gathered by Real Solutions, a nonprofit organization dedicated to the needs of family and community.

Higher Education Center for Alcohol and Other Drug Prevention

http://www.edc.org/hec/

The U.S. Department of Education established the Higher Education Center for Alcohol and Other Drug Prevention to provide nationwide support for campus alcohol and other drug prevention efforts. The Center is working with colleges, universities, and preparatory schools throughout the country to develop strategies for changing campus culture, to foster environments that promote healthy lifestyles, and to prevent illegal alcohol and other drug use among students.

National Clearinghouse for Alcohol and Drug Information

http://www.health.org

This site provides information to teens about the problems and ramifications of drug use and abuse. There are numerous links to drug-related informational sites.

UNIT 1: Living With Drugs

National Council on Alcoholism and Drug Dependence, Inc.

http://www.ncadd.org

According to its Web site, The National Council on Alcoholism and Drug Dependence provides education, information, help, and hope in the fight against the chronic, and sometimes fatal, disease of alcoholism and other drug addictions.

UNIT 2: Understanding How Drugs Work—Use, Dependency, and Addiction

AMERSA

http://center.butler.brown.edu

AMERSA is an association of multidisciplinary health care professionals in the field of substance abuse. They are dedicated to improving education about alcohol, tobacco, and other drugs.

Centre for Addiction and Mental Health (CAMH)

http://www.camh.net

One of the largest addictions facilities in Canada, CAMH advances an understanding of addiction and translates this knowledge into resources that can be used to prevent problems and to provide effective treatments.

The National Center on Addiction and Substance Abuse at Columbia University

http://www.casacolumbia.org

The National Center on Addiction and Substance Abuse at Columbia University is a unique think/action tank that brings together all of the professional disciplines (health policy, medicine and nursing, communications, economics, sociology and anthropology, law and law enforcement, business, religion, and education) needed to study and combat all forms of substance abuse—illegal drugs, pills, alcohol, and tobacco—as they affect all aspects of society.

National Institute on Drug Abuse (NIDA)

http://www.nida.nih.gov

NIDA's mission is to lead the nation in bringing the power of science to bear on drug abuse and addiction.

UNIT 3: The Major Drugs of Use and Abuse

Drugs, Solvents and Intoxicants

http://www.termisoc.org/~harl/

This United Kingdom Web site presents the history, effects, dangers, and legal issues surrounding most legal and illegal drugs.

QuitNet

http://www.quitnet.org

The QuitNet helps smokers control their nicotine addiction. This site operates in association with the Boston University School of Public Health.

UNIT 4: Other Trends in Drug Use

Marijuana as a Medicine

http://mojo.calyx.net/~olsen/

This site promotes the concept of marijuana as medicine. This is a controversial issue that has been in the news quite a bit over the past few years. At this site, you will find numerous links to other sites that support this idea, as well as information developed specifically for this site.

UNIT 5: Drugs and Crime

Drug Enforcement Administration

http://www.usdoj.gov/dea/

The mission of the Drug Enforcement Administration is to enforce the controlled substances laws and regulations of the United States.

The November Coalition

http://www.november.org

The November Coalition is a growing body of citizens whose lives have been gravely affected by the present drug policy. This group represents convicted prisoners, their loved ones, and others who believe that U.S. drug policies are unfair and unjust.

TRAC DEA Site

http://trac.syr.edu/tracdea/index.html

The Transactional Records Access Clearinghouse (TRAC) is a data gathering, data research, and data distribution organization

www.dushkin.com/online/

associated with Syracuse University. According to its Web site, the purpose of TRAC is to provide the American people—and institutions of oversight such as Congress, news organizations, public interest groups, businesses, scholars, and lawyers—with comprehensive information about the activities of federal enforcement and regulatory agencies and the communities in which they take place.

UNIT 6: Measuring the Social Cost of Drugs

DrugText
http://www.drugtext.org

The DrugText library consists of individual drug-related libraries with independent search capabilities.

The National Organization on Fetal Alcohol Syndrome (NOFAS)
http://www.nofas.org

NOFAS is a nonprofit organization founded in 1990 dedicated to eliminating birth defects caused by alcohol consumption during pregnancy and improving the quality of life for those individuals and families affected. NOFAS is the only national organization focusing solely on fetal alcohol syndrome (FAS), the leading known cause of mental retardation.

National NORML Homepage
http://www.norml.org/

This is the home page for the National Organization for the Reform of Marijuana Laws.

UNIT 7: Creating and Sustaining Effective Drug Control Policy

The Drug Reform Coordination Network (DRC)
http://www.drcnet.org

According to its home page, the DRC Network is committed to reforming current drug laws in the United States.

Drug Watch International
http://www.drugwatch.org

Drug Watch International is a volunteer nonprofit information network and advocacy organization that promotes the creation of healthy drug-free cultures in the world and opposes the legalization of drugs. The organization upholds a comprehensive approach to drug issues involving prevention, education, intervention/treatment, and law enforcement/interdiction.

United Nations International Drug Control Program (UNDCP)
http://www.undcp.org

The mission of UNDCP is to work with the nations and the people of the world to tackle the global drug problem and its consequences.

Marijuana Policy Project
http://www.mpp.org

The purpose of the Marijuana Policy Project is to develop and promote policies to minimize the harm associated with marijuana.

Office of National Drug Control Policy (ONDCP)
http://www.whitehousedrugpolicy.gov

The principal purpose of ONDCP is to establish policies, priorities, and objectives for the nation's drug control program, the goals of which are to reduce illicit drug use, manufacturing, and trafficking; drug-related crime and violence; and drug-related health consequences.

UNIT 8: Prevention, Treatment, and Education

Creative Partnerships for Prevention
http://arts.endow.gov/partner/Creative.html

The goal of this national initiative is to provide current information, ideas, and resources on how to use the arts and humanities to enhance drug and violence prevention programming, foster resiliency in youth, and implement collaborations within communities to strengthen prevention programs for youth. The materials developed for this initiative have been designed with the guidance of educators, prevention specialists, youth workers, and professionals from cultural institutions (arts and humanities organizations, museums, libraries, etc.).

D.A.R.E.
http://www.dare-america.com

This year 33 million schoolchildren around the world—25 million in the United States—will benefit from D.A.R.E. (Drug Abuse Resistance Education), the highly acclaimed program that gives kids the skills they need to avoid involvement in drugs, gangs, or violence. D.A.R.E. was founded in 1983 in Los Angeles.

Hazelden
http://www.hazelden.org

Hazelden is a nonprofit organization providing high quality, affordable rehabilitation, education, prevention, and professional services and publications in chemical dependency and related disorders.

Indiana Prevention Resource Center
http://www.drugs.indiana.edu/home.html

The Indiana Prevention Resource Center at Indiana University is a statewide clearinghouse for prevention, technical assistance, and information about alcohol, tobacco, and other drugs.

We highly recommend that you review our Web site for expanded information and our other product lines. We are continually updating and adding links to our Web site in order to offer you the most usable and useful information that will support and expand the value of your Annual Editions. You can reach us at: *http://www.dushkin.com/annualeditions/*.

UNIT 1
Living With Drugs

Unit Selections

Key Points to Consider

- Why is history important when attempting to understand contemporary drug-related events?

- What historical trends are expressed by the use of legal drugs versus illegal drugs?

- What are the historical drug-related landmarks of drug prohibition and control?

- How is the evolution of drug-related influence on American society like and unlike that occurring in other countries?

- What can we learn from these comparisons?

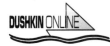 **Links: www.dushkin.com/online/**
These sites are annotated in the World Wide Web pages.

National Council on Alcoholism and Drug Dependence, Inc.
http://www.ncadd.org

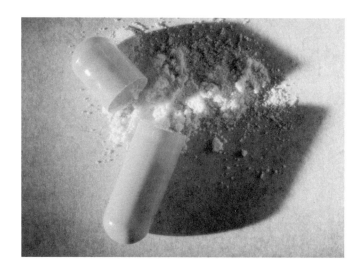

When attempting to define the American drug experience, one must examine the past as well as the present. Too often drug use and its associated phenomena are viewed through a contemporary looking glass relative to our personal views, biases, and perspectives. Although today's drug scene is definitely a product of the counterculture of the 1960s and 1970s, the crack trade of the 1980s, and the sophisticated, criminally syndicated, technologically efficient influence of the late 1980s and early 1990s, it is also a product of the past. This past and the lessons it has generated, although largely unknown, forgotten, or ignored, provide one important perspective from which to assess our current status and to guide our future in terms of optimizing our efforts to manage the benefits and control the harm from legal and illegal drugs.

The American drug experience is often defined in terms of a million individual realities, all meaningful and all different. In fact, these realities often originated as pieces of our national, cultural, racial, religious, and personal past that combine to influence present-day drug-related phenomena significantly.

The contemporary American drug experience is the product of centuries of human attempts to alter or sustain consciousness through the use of mind-altering drugs. Early American history is replete with accounts of the exorbitant use of alcohol, opium, morphine, and cocaine.

A review of this history clearly suggests the precedents for Americans' continuing pursuit of a vast variety of stimulant, depressant, and hallucinogenic drugs. Presently, 51 percent of Americans over the age of 12 are drinkers of alcohol and approximately 30 percent of Americans use tobacco. Approximately 22 million people, or 9.4 percent of the population, are believed to be drug-dependent on alcohol or illicit drugs. Americans spent more than $70 billion last year on illegal drugs alone.

Drug use in America is a dynamic phenomenon expressed within a multitude of social pathologies. One such pathology now being addressed at greater length in current research is the association between substance abuse and serious mental illness. Approximately 8.3 percent of all adults are believed to suffer from a serious mental illness (SMI). Of this group, over 22.2 percent are dependent on alcohol or illicit drugs. The rate of drug dependence among adults without SMI is 7 percent. Subsequently, the implications for treating such dually diagnosed persons are much larger than previously thought. Further complicating the issue is that too many drug-dependent persons, an estimated 4.6 million, do not recognize they have a problem with drugs.

Drugs impact our most powerful public institutions on many fronts. Drugs are the business of our criminal justice system, and drugs compete with terrorism, war, and other major national security concerns as demanding military issues. Many argue eloquently that drugs pose a "clear and present danger." Additional millions of dollars to fight drugs were pledged to South American countries this past year. Only terrorism and war distract the continuing military emphasis on drug fighting. As you read through the pages of this book, the pervasive nature of drug-related influences will become more apparent. Unfortunately, one of the most salient observations one can make is that drug use in our society is a topic about which many Americans have too little knowledge. History suggests that we have continually struggled to respond and react to the influence of drug use in our society. The lessons of our drug legacy are harsh, whether they are the subjects of public health or public policy. Turning an uninformed mind toward a social condition of such importance will only further our inability to address the dynamics of changing drug-related issues and problems.

Interestingly, since the September 11, 2001, terrorist bombings and the subsequent U.S. invasion of Iraq, research has identified certain drug trends also observed during previous national crises. The availability of illegal drugs, particularly heroin, declined in numerous reporting sites, apparently owing to heightened security at U.S. airports and the borders. Heroin is now recognized as having surpassed crack as the drug associated with the most serious consequences. Oxycodone abuse, apparently influenced by heroin shortages, especially on the East Coast, has surged. Oxycodone abuse is the most widely cited emerging drug problem. And since September 11, treatment admissions and demand in New York City and Washington, D.C., have increased markedly.

The articles and graphics contained in this unit illustrate the multitude of issues influenced by the historical evolution of legal and illegal drug use in America. The historical development of drug-related phenomena is reflected within the character of all issues and controversies addressed by this book. Drug-related events of yesterday provide important meaning for understanding and addressing drug-related events of today and the future. Creating public policy and controlling crime surface immediately as examples with long-standing historical influences. As you read this and other literature on drug-related events, the dynamics of drug-related historical linkages will become apparent. As you read further, try to identify these historical linkages as they help define the focus at hand. For example, what are the implications for public health resulting from a historical lack of drug-related educational emphasis? What will history reflect 20 years from now? Is there a historical pattern of drug-related educational shortcomings that we should change?

Drug Research and Children

Recent studies are providing important new information about drug safety and effectiveness for children. Pediatricians say it's about time.

By Michelle Meadows

Most drugs prescribed for children have not been tested in children. Only 20 percent to 30 percent of drugs approved by the Food and Drug Administration are labeled for pediatric use. So by necessity, doctors have routinely given drugs to children "off label," which means the drug hasn't been studied in children in adequate, well-controlled clinical trials approved by the agency.

To be well-controlled, a study should have an adequate number of people and a control group—people who are similar to the group taking the drug being studied, but who are receiving some different type of treatment, such as another drug or an inactive pill (placebo).

Experts say the historical lack of pediatric drug testing is due to a combination of reasons. The primary reason is that pharmaceutical companies generally have viewed children as a market that would only bring small financial benefits. The drugs that have been adequately studied in children—vaccines, some antibiotics, and some cough and cold medicines—have a large market.

"It's also harder to carry out studies in children," says Dianne Murphy, M.D., director of the FDA's Office of Pediatric Therapeutics. "You need child-friendly environments in every sense, from age-appropriate equipment and medical techniques to pediatric specialists who are sensitive to a child's fear."

Jeffrey Blumer, M.D., Ph.D., chief of pediatric pharmacology at Case Western Reserve University in Cleveland, says technical procedures that seem simple for adults, such as drawing blood or getting a urine sample, can be difficult with children.

The ethical issues are also stickier. For example, while adults can give informed consent to participate in a clinical trial, children can't because "consent" implies full understanding of potential risks and other considerations. Parents are involved in the decision to enroll children in a study, and children ages 7 or older can "assent" or "dissent," meaning they can agree or disagree to participate in a study.

Blumer says, "I've had parents who are enthusiastic about a study and then a 7-year-old who hears everything involved and says, 'No way!'"

Children Aren't Small Adults

But rather than avoiding pediatric research because of the challenges, experts say it's more important to build the foundation and resources needed to conduct the studies. Without them, children face significant risks.

In the absence of data, doctors use their medical judgment to decide on a particular drug and dose for children. "Some doctors stay away from drugs, which could deny needed treatment," Blumer says. "Generally, we take our best guess based on what's been done before."

A common approach has been to use data from adults and adjust the dose according to a child's weight. Experimenting over the years has taught doctors to use many drugs in children safely and effectively. But this trial-and-error approach has also resulted in tragedy, indicating that adult experiences with a drug aren't always a reliable predictor of how children will react.

For example, in the 1950s, the antibiotic chloramphenicol was widely used in adults to treat infections resistant to penicillin. But many newborn babies died after receiving the drug because their immature livers couldn't break down the antibiotic.

"Experience has shown us that we need to study drugs in children because they aren't small adults," says Ralph Kauffman, M.D., director of medical research at Children's Mercy Hospital in Kansas City, Mo. "It's not just about smaller weight," he says. "There are dynamics of growth and maturation of organs, changes in metabolism throughout infancy and childhood, changes in body proportion, and other developmental changes that affect how drugs are metabolized."

Proof Is in the Data

Fortunately, recent regulatory and legislative changes that give drug companies financial incentives to conduct drug studies in children have resulted in a dramatic increase in pediatric drug studies. "There have been more studies conducted in children in the last five years than in the previous 30 years combined," Kauffman says.

The information coming out of those studies has added pediatric information to the drug labeling for more than 40 drugs, and more changes are coming. Drug labeling is the guidance to doctors and other health-care providers on how to use a drug. "We knew that we needed science to determine proper dosing for children the same way we do with adults," says Dianne Murphy. "Now, we have confirmed it."

New discoveries have revealed underdosing, overdosing, ineffectiveness, and safety problems.

Ibuprofen, one of the most common over-the-counter drugs that parents rely on to reduce children's fevers, carried no dosing information for children younger than 2 years old until recently. Now, because of studies in thousands of young infants, the dose considered to be safe and effective for over-the-counter use has been established for children ages 6 months to 2 years.

The labeling has also been changed for Zantac (ranitidine), a drug used to treat gastroesophageal reflux. This condition can be life-threatening in infants. When reflux occurs, the stomach contents can flow up the esophagus and be aspirated into the lungs. This can harm the lungs of infants and result in breathing problems.

Studies have given doctors accurate dosing information for safer and more effective use of the drug to manage reflux in seriously ill infants. Richard Gorman, M.D., chairman of the Committee on Drugs at the American Academy of Pediatrics (AAP) and a pediatrician in Ellicott City, Md., says, "Now I can use ranitidine with as much information as doctors who use it in adults. I know the dose. I know the dosing interval."

With Neurontin (gabapentin), a drug used to control seizures, research has shown that higher doses are needed in children younger than 5 to control seizures. With Versed (midazolam), one of the most commonly used medicines to sedate children undergoing surgery, researchers found that children with congenital heart disease and pulmonary hypertension need to start therapy at a lower dose to prevent respiratory problems. Also, Versed formerly was available only by injection of the drug into a child's vein or muscle. But studies helped develop a new oral syrup, which is easier to give and less frightening to young children. (For more on label changes, see "Changing Drug Labels.")

New discoveries have revealed underdosing, overdosing, ineffectiveness, and safety problems. Gorman says, "Even though the best and brightest pediatric minds have helped us establish dosages for children, we're finding out that the dose is different than we thought in some cases. And that probably came as a surprise to most of us."

The FDA is working with the AAP to educate pediatricians about new physician labeling changes through an online continuing medical education program called PediaLink.

What's Spurring the Research?

The FDA has taken a carrot-and-stick approach to encourage pediatric studies, says William Rodriguez, M.D., the FDA's science director for pediatrics. The carrot is the voluntary pediatric exclusivity provision of the Food and Drug Administration Modernization Act of 1997 (FDAMA). And the stick has been the FDA's "pediatric rule," which required pediatric studies and was finalized in 1998. Here's an overview of each initiative:

The Pediatric Exclusivity Provision of FDAMA

The pediatric exclusivity provision has done more to spur pediatric studies than any other regulatory or legislative initiative so far. The provision extends patent protection to give companies an additional six months of marketing exclusivity if they do the studies in children requested by the FDA.

Patents protect a company's investment by giving it the sole right to sell a drug while the patent is in effect. When patents or other periods of exclusive marketing for brand-name drugs are close to expiring, other drug companies can apply to the FDA to sell generic versions, without having to repeat the original developer's clinical trials. So the trade-off is that by giving companies additional months of exclusivity, there is a delay in the availability of lower-cost generic drugs.

The FDA has interpreted the provision so that the six months of exclusivity isn't only added to the drug that was studied in the pediatric population, but also to any of the drug company's formulations, dosage forms, and indications that contain the same active part of a molecule (moiety) and have existing marketing exclusivity or patent life. So if a company markets an oral formulation and a topical cream containing the same moiety, the six months of marketing exclusivity will be added to any existing exclusivity or patent protection for both products.

The process can be initiated either by a drug company or the FDA. A drug company may submit a proposal to conduct pediatric studies to the FDA. If the FDA agrees that studying a drug may produce health benefits for children, the agency will issue a "Written Request" addressing the type of studies to be conducted, study design and goals, and the age groups to be studied. Or the agency may issue a Written Request on its own initiative when it identifies a need for pediatric data. No matter how the studies are initiated, if the FDA determines that the data submitted fairly respond to the Written Request, then the company will be granted six months of pediatric exclusivity.

The exclusivity provision also requires the FDA to publish an annual list of approved drugs for which additional pediatric information may produce health benefits.

More than 60 drugs have been granted exclusivity so far. As of Sept. 30, 2002, 601 studies had been requested and 256 Written Requests issued. The FDA estimates that about 80 percent of the studies outlined in Written Requests will be conducted.

Kauffman says the exclusivity is proof that economics plays a large role in the lack of pediatric studies. "Once the economic disincentive was removed," he says, "the dam broke completely open."

Diane Murphy, M.D., director of the FDA's Office of Pediatric Therapeutics, says "child-friendly environments"are needed when doing research on children. The office she oversees is mandated by the Best Pharmaceuticals for Children Act, signed into law in January 2002.

The exclusivity provision was renewed in January 2002 and extended through 2007 under the Best Pharmaceuticals for Children Act (BPCA). Some categories of drugs and age groups have remained inadequately studied. The incentive under FDAMA did not apply to old antibiotics and other drugs that lack marketing exclusivity or patent protection. For these products, the BPCA provides a contract mechanism through the NIH to fund pediatric studies. If a company that has a drug with existing exclusivity or patent protection chooses not to conduct the requested pediatric studies, this new mechanism through BPCA allows the Foundation for the National Institutes of Health to award grants so that third parties can conduct the needed studies.

The FDA's Pediatric Rule

In the early 1990s, the FDA implemented voluntary measures to encourage pediatric studies, but they were mostly unsuccessful. In 1997, the FDA published a proposed regulation that for the first time required manufacturers of new drug and biological products to conduct pediatric studies in some circumstances. The rule was finalized in 1998, and the first studies were required to be submitted starting December 2000.

But the rule had its critics. In December 2000, the Association of American Physicians and Surgeons, the Competitive Enterprise Institute and Consumer Alert filed a lawsuit against the pediatric rule, challenging the FDA's legal authority to require pediatric studies. And in October 2002, a federal district court overturned the pediatric rule.

HHS Secretary Tommy G. Thompson responded in mid-December 2002 by announcing that his department will push for rapid passage of legislation that would give the FDA authority to require pharmaceutical manufacturers to conduct appropriate pediatric clinical trials on drugs.

"The fastest and most decisive route for establishing clear authority in this area is to work with Congress for new legislation," Thompson said in a prepared statement. "Children need to have access to drugs that can benefit them, and these drugs need to be properly tested for pediatric use, not prescribed and sold without testing. Congress alone can speak clearly on the authority that FDA needs…"

Kauffman says turning the pediatric rule into law would be the ideal scenario. "The exclusivity provision sunsets again in 2007, with no guarantees of being renewed. We need something permanent so that we don't lose all the ground we've gained."

The pediatric rule was intended to address some of the gaps left by the pediatric exclusivity provision. Unlike the exclusivity provision, the pediatric rule was a requirement and covered both drugs and biologics—medical products derived from living sources such as vaccines, blood and blood derivatives, and new treatments for cancers.

Under the pediatric rule, the FDA could require pediatric studies of a drug submitted in a new drug application if the FDA determined the product was likely to be used in a substantial number of pediatric patients, or if the product would provide a meaningful benefit in the pediatric population over existing treatments. At the same time, the pediatric rule did not delay the availability of drugs for adults.

Changing Drug Labels

Recent pediatric drug studies have resulted in the addition of pediatric information to the labeling for more than 40 drugs. The drug labeling provides guidance for doctors and other health-care providers on how to use a drug. Here are examples of several changes that are considered significant for dosing and risk.

- **Luvox (fluvoxamine):** Treats obsessive-compulsive disorder. The dose of the drug may need to be increased up to the recommended adult dose in adolescents, but may need to be prescribed in lower than recommended doses for girls ages 8 to 11.
- **Neurontin (gabapentin):** Treats seizures. Safety and effectiveness have been established for children as young as 3. Children under 5 need higher doses than previously thought based on the studies conducted. New adverse effects not seen in adults, such as hostility and aggressive behavior, are now noted in the label.
- **Diprivan (propofol):** An anesthesia drug. A research study showed an increase in deaths when the drug was used for pediatric ICU sedation in comparison with standard sedative agents. Administration of propofol with the pain medication fentanyl may result in serious slowing of the heart rate.
- **BuSpar (buspirone):** Treats generalized anxiety disorder. Safety and effectiveness were not established in patients ages 6 to 17 at doses recommended for use in adults.
- **Versed (midazolam):** Used as a sedative. The drug was shown to have a higher risk of serious life-threatening adverse events for children with congenital heart disease and pulmonary hypertension. Research identified the need to begin therapy with doses at the lower end of the dosing range to prevent respiratory problems in this special pediatric population.
- **Lodine (etodolac):** Treats the signs and symptoms of juvenile rheumatoid arthritis. Research shows that the drug can be used in children ages 6 to 16 and that higher doses are needed in younger children.

"The exclusivity provision and the rule have worked in tandem," says the FDA's Dianne Murphy. "We have told sponsors who submit a new drug application and who are required under the rule to conduct pediatric studies that they also may qualify for pediatric exclusivity."

Gorman says the exclusivity provision is the one that has the drug industry's attention, but he has been most excited about the pediatric rule. "The exclusivity provision has been important for helping children play catch-up and that's important, but the pediatric rule puts children at the table very early in the development of drugs."

Building the Foundation

"There was no infrastructure for the research before," says Floyd R. Sallee, M.D., Ph.D., a child psychiatrist and director of the pediatric pharmacology research unit at Cincinnati Children's Hospital Medical Center. "I see the culture changing in industry and at FDA," he says. "Drug companies have hired pediatric experts and there is a larger network of expertise to draw from."

Sallee's center is part of the Pediatric Pharmacology Research Unit (PPRU) Network, a group of centers that conduct pediatric drug trials with support from the National Institute of Child Health and Human Development (NICHD). The network was established in 1994 and now includes 13 PPRUs.

Shirley Murphy, M.D., (no relation to Dianne Murphy) joined the FDA in September 2002 as director of the Division of Pediatric Drug Development. She says linkages between the FDA, NICHD, AAP, and other organizations have been important for building a foundation for pediatric research, and children are getting more and better drugs as a result.

"What it means for parents is that they can feel more secure knowing that their children are being treated appropriately," Shirley Murphy says. "FDA remains committed to keeping pediatric drug research a high priority."

Shirley Murphy cites pediatric oncology as another important area for the agency.

Several areas that will continue to receive the agency's attention include the ethics involved with studying drugs in children. The FDA's Pediatric Advisory Subcommittee has concluded that generally, pediatric studies should be conducted in subjects who may benefit from participation in the trial. Usually, this implies the subject has or is susceptible to the disease under study.

Debbie Birenbaum, M.D., an FDA pediatric team leader, says FDA experts think long and hard about the public health benefit before requesting pediatric studies. "We don't want to under study children and we don't want to over study them. It's our job to get information that will help them and protect them at the same time."

Shirley Murphy cites pediatric oncology as another important area for the agency. "The development of cancer drugs needs special consideration," she says. Differences in the biology of tumors in children and adults usually make it difficult to prescribe children drugs based on adult data. And it has been typical for new cancer drugs to reach children late—only after they have been tested in adults.

As a result of pediatric initiatives, there have been about 30 studies initiated on cancer drugs, which will help researchers gain access to potential new cancer therapies for children.

While it may be challenging to enroll children in clinical trials for some diseases, that's not the case with cancer. Most children receive their cancer therapy as part of a clinical trial. "Parents are desperate to have their children in these studies," says Patrick Reynolds, M.D., Ph.D., a pediatric oncologist with Childrens Hospital Los Angeles. "They know very well what the odds are and they want to take a chance to find life-saving treatment. They also want to help other children. They don't want to do nothing."

Reynolds is a member of the FDA's Pediatric Oncology Subcommittee, a group of outside experts who have met several times since 2000 to advise the agency on such questions as: In what phase of a drug development program should pediatric cancer studies begin? What trial designs should be used? How may data from adult studies be used in pediatric studies? How should adult and pediatric studies be coordinated when studying life-threatening diseases?

Reynolds calls both the pediatric rule and the exclusivity provision essential. "Children don't have a voice in this," he says. "Somebody has to stand up for them."

From *FDA Consumer*, January/February 2003, p. 36. © 2003 by FDA Consumer, the magazine of the U.S. Food and Drug Administration.

TOBACCO

For tobacco control advocates, the tobacco industry is public health enemy number one: It sells a commodity that will kill 500 million of the 6 billion people living today. For governments, tobacco is both a health threat and a powerful economic force that annually generates hundreds of billions of dollars in sales and billions more in tax revenues. That clash of interests fuels a debate ensnarling everything from farm subsidies and export controls to healthcare spending, taxation, law enforcement, and free speech.

By Kenneth E. Warner

"Antismoking Policies Are Hazardous to a Nation's Economic Health"

Not true, for all but a handful of countries. The tobacco industry accounts for significant economic activity in many countries through farming and product manufacture, distribution, and sales. According to a recent World Bank study, an estimated 33 million people worldwide farm tobacco either full or part time. About another 10 million workers provide materials and services to the tobacco industry (harvesting equipment, cigarette papers, insurance, shipping, etc.). China, the world's largest consumer and producer of tobacco, has an estimated 15 million tobacco farmers. Substantial tobacco sectors also exist in India, Indonesia, Thailand, Turkey, Egypt, Bangladesh, and the Philippines. Malawi and Zimbabwe are major net exporters of tobacco and depend on tobacco leaf for a far larger share of total exports (60 percent and 23 percent, respectively) than any other nation.

But typically, in the vast majority of countries, tobacco represents no more than a small fraction of gross domestic product. And in those nations with large tobacco sectors, significant economic presence does not necessarily imply significant economic dependence. If money is not spent on cigarettes, it will be reallocated to other goods and services. This alternative spending pattern, in turn, will produce essentially the same number of jobs as would spending on tobacco. The only real cost of moving from spending on tobacco to spending on other products and services is the cost of transition from one economic activity to others. But since smoking is so addictive and policies designed to reduce smoking work so gradually (over a period of many years), transition costs will be tiny. Indeed, reductions in smoking won't throw tobacco farmers out of work. Rather, fewer of their children will go into tobacco farming as a career. The transition to non-tobacco economic activity will occur through normal attrition, such as retirement and death.

Tobacco industry executives shed crocodile tears for farmers and factory workers allegedly harmed by antismoking policies, but the industry itself is frequently responsible for their economic woes. The purchase of imported tobacco cuts into domestic farming. Mechanization of cigarette production plants costs factory workers their jobs. And wholesale price hikes that enhance companies' bottom lines reduce cigarette sales, thereby threatening tobacco jobs every bit as effectively as do the tax hikes the industry so vigorously opposes.

"Smoking Causes Healthcare Costs to Skyrocket"

False. Last year, a study commissioned by tobacco giant Philip Morris made headlines worldwide when it boasted that smoking saves money for the treasury of the Czech Republic, thanks in part to the early demise of smokers, which reduces the government's obligations in healthcare, pensions, and housing costs for the elderly. The study is filled with mistakes that invalidate its finding, but it still contains a grain of truth: Smokers' shorter lives do compensate partly for their excess healthcare costs while alive.

Adult smokers experience a life expectancy reduction on the order of six years. Those smokers who die as a direct result of their habit—close to half of all smokers—are victims of a drop in their life expectancy of more than twice that amount. In the world's affluent nations, smoking is responsible for 4 to 10 percent of all healthcare spending. However, by dying earlier than their nonsmoking compatriots, smokers often avoid expensive chronic illnesses associated with old age. Consequently, a

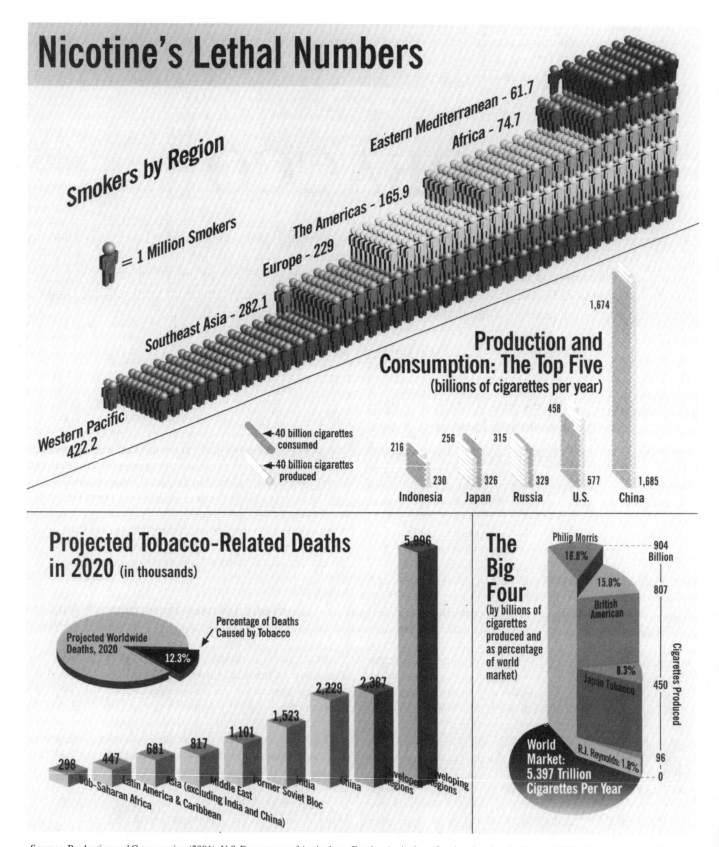

Nicotine's Lethal Numbers

Smokers by Region

= 1 Million Smokers

Eastern Mediterranean - 61.7
Africa - 74.7
The Americas - 165.9
Europe - 229
Southeast Asia - 282.1
Western Pacific 422.2

Production and Consumption: The Top Five
(billions of cigarettes per year)

← 40 billion cigarettes consumed
← 40 billion cigarettes produced

Indonesia	Japan	Russia	U.S.	China
216	256	315	458	1,674
230	326	329	577	1,685

Projected Tobacco-Related Deaths in 2020 (in thousands)

Projected Worldwide Deaths, 2020

Percentage of Deaths Caused by Tobacco
12.3%

Sub-Saharan Africa	Latin America & Caribbean	Asia (excluding India and China)	Middle East	Former Soviet Bloc	India	China	Developed Regions	Developing Regions
298	447	681	817	1,101	1,523	2,229	2,387	5,996

The Big Four
(by billions of cigarettes produced and as percentage of world market)

Philip Morris — 904 Billion
16.8%

British American 15.0% — 807

Japan Tobacco 8.3% — 450

R.J. Reynolds: 1.8% — 96

Cigarettes Produced — 0

World Market: 5.397 Trillion Cigarettes Per Year

Sources: Production and Consumption (2001): U.S. Department of Agriculture, Foreign Agriculture Service; Smokers by Region (1998); American Cancer Society and WHO; Projected Deaths: WHO and the Big Four (2000): Courtesy of The Maxwell Report

Dutch study concluded that if everyone quit smoking in the Netherlands, healthcare expenditures after 15 years would actu-ally be higher than if people kept smoking. Likewise, a study in Switzerland reported that smokers' higher costs and shorter lives amounted to almost a complete "wash" in terms of their net effects on healthcare spending.

The evidence is mixed, however. A recent analysis of all smoking-related healthcare costs in the United States (including those associated with secondhand smoke) concluded that smokers do increase U.S. healthcare costs on balance, although certainly not enough to warrant the frequently invoked label of a healthcare cost "crisis." Advocates and policymakers will have to look beyond antismoking campaigns to get a handle on healthcare costs.

"Declining Profits Have Driven Big Tobacco Into Developing Countries"

Wrong. As smoking has declined in the developed world, multinational tobacco companies have moved aggressively into middle- and low-income nations in recent years, especially in Asia and Eastern Europe. They also have established strongholds in Latin America and Africa. In all such countries, the industry employs sophisticated marketing techniques to compete with domestic brands, increase daily consumption among existing smokers, and encourage traditionally low-smoking groups (e.g., young women in many Asian societies) to "modernize" by becoming smokers. According to one study, Western marketing of cigarettes increased cigarette consumption in four Asian countries by about 10 percent.

Tobacco consumption in the West has declined at the same time that the industry has expanded into the East. But correlation is not causation. The decline in smoking in the developed world has not led to a decline in profits, since sales have fallen proportionally much slower than prices have risen. Indeed, the multinational companies' foray into new markets is a natural, inevitable outcome of conventional economic behavior. The urge to enter new markets was irresistible and independent of successes or failures in Western markets. A fortuitous set of economic circumstances created the opportunity: the bulging treasuries of multinational corporations, which permitted their overseas expansion; the general easing of trade barriers for all international commerce; and the emergence of a level of consumer income in targeted countries adequate to support consumption of Western cigarettes.

Understanding the economic causes of the industry's global expansion should allay the concerns of Western tobacco control advocates, fearful that their successes at home will create a legacy of addiction and disease abroad.

"Higher Cigarette Taxes Curb Smoking"

Absolutely. The law of demand—raise prices and quantity demanded will fall—holds for all commodities, even the most addictive. In fact, that law applies to all species. Consider laboratory rats: If forced to push a lever more times to get a dose of drug—the number of lever pushes constituting the price they face—addicted lab rats decrease the amount of drug they administer to themselves. In the case of humans and cigarettes, a

10 percent increase in price will prompt a decrease in quantity demanded by about 4 percent in rich countries and twice as much in low- and middle-income countries. Price increases are particularly effective in discouraging smoking by youth. In the handful of countries in which it has been measured, young people's price responsiveness appears to be at least twice that of their seniors.

The principal vehicle by which countries can raise tobacco prices is through taxation. Virtually all nations impose product-specific taxes on cigarettes, although these range from a small amount in many developing countries to as much as three quarters of retail price in some rich nations. Within the public health community, there is almost universal agreement that raising taxes is one of the most potent policy tools available to governments dedicated to reducing the health toll of smoking. Coincidentally, and conveniently, tax rate hikes increase tax revenues, even while smoking falls. So governments contemplating tobacco tax increases find themselves with the rare opportunity to do good while bringing home the bacon.

"Higher Cigarette Taxes Encourage Smuggling"

True, all other things being equal (but they're not). The thriving black market in cigarettes is represented by two kinds of smugglers. One group consists of individuals and gangs who bootleg cigarettes from low-tax (hence low-price) countries to nearby high-tax (high-price) countries, generally covering small distances. These so-called buttleggers are responsible for a relatively small fraction of the illicit trade in cigarettes. The other criminal element, responsible for the majority of illicit trade, worth $25 billion to $30 billion annually, consists of large-scale enterprises smuggling huge consignments of cigarettes over great distances. Buttleggers pay taxes in low-tax countries and move their product to nearby higher-priced countries. Organized smugglers avoid all taxes. Astonishingly, nearly a third of the world's legally identified cigarette exports are never registered as having been imported.

Whenever governments contemplate tobacco tax increases, the tobacco industry and its allies vigorously promote the specter of a criminal black market forged by government policy itself: Tax increases raise cigarette prices and create enticing incentives for criminal organizations to smuggle cigarettes. Proposed tax increases have been defeated by appeals to this argument and prompted Canada and Sweden to rescind previous tax hikes.

But black market trade in cigarettes has less to do with taxes than with a country's tolerance of corruption and its failure to police smuggling. Ironically, in Western Europe, smuggling problems appear to be most serious in countries with low cigarette prices. In Norway, for example, prices are high and smuggling is uncommon. In Spain, by contrast, prices are low and smuggling was pervasive until Spanish law enforcement agencies cracked down on the problem and cut smuggling from 20 to 30 percent of the market to about 2 to 3 percent.

Want to Know More?

This article is adapted from Kenneth E. Warner's **"The Economics of Tobacco: Myths and Realities"** (*Tobacco Control*, March 2000). The most recent comprehensive reviews of the economics of tobacco (including chapters on taxation and economic dependence on tobacco) can be found in Prabhat Jha and Frank J. Chaloupka's, eds., **Tobacco Control in Developing Countries** (Oxford: Oxford University Press, 2000) and in Frank J. Chaloupka and Kenneth E. Warner's "The Economics of Smoking" in the *Handbook of Health Economics* (New York: Elsevier Science Publishing, 2000), edited by Anthony J. Culyer and Joseph P. Newhouse. The former includes chapters originally developed in support of a World Bank report, **"Curbing the Epidemic: Governments and the Economics of Tobacco Control"** (Washington: World Bank, 1999).

The healthcare costs of smoking are discussed by Kenneth E. Warner, Thomas Hodgson, and Caitlin Carroll in **"Medical Costs of Smoking in the United States: Estimates, Their Validity, and Their Implications"** *(Tobacco Control*, Autumn 1999). Luk Joossens of Belgium and Martin Raw of the United Kingdom examine **"Cigarette Smuggling in Europe: Who Really Benefits?"** (*Tobacco Control*, Spring 1998) and **"How Can Cigarette Smuggling Be Reduced?"** (*British Medical Journal*, October 2000).

Evidence of the tobacco industry's direct involvement in smuggling is outlined in **"Illegal Pathways to illegal Profits: The Big Cigarette Companies and International Smuggling"** (Washington: Campaign for Tobacco-Free Kids, 2001). The Washington, D.C.-based group The Public I posted the report **"U.S. Tobacco Companies Accused of Terrorist Ties and Iraqi Sanctions-Busting"** on its Web site (February 22, 2002).

The impact of tobacco advertising and promotion evokes fevered emotions within both the public health community and the tobacco industry. J.P. Pierce, E.A. Gilpin, and W.S. Choi present a strong case on the public health side of the argument in **"Sharing the Blame: Smoking Experimentation and Future Smoking—Attributable Mortality Due to Joe Camel and Marlboro Advertising and Promotions"** (*Tobacco Control,* Spring 1999).

- For links to relevant Web sites, access to the FP Archive, and a comprehensive index of related FOREIGN POLICY articles, go to **www.foreignpolicy.com.**

And while the tobacco industry attempts to blame high taxes for smuggling, the industry itself appears to tolerate and actively encourage smuggling, as indicated by recent court cases in which tobacco company executives were found guilty of complicity in smuggling operations. In 1998, for instance, Northern Brands International, Inc. (an affiliate of R.J. Reynolds Tobacco Holdings), pled guilty to smuggling-related charges and paid $15 million in fines and forfeitures. The industry benefits from the increased sales associated with smuggling, and the multinationals benefit in particular by increased consumption of their prominent brands.

"Tobacco Subsidies Encourage Smoking"

Correct, though not always for the obvious reason. Numerous governments around the world support farmers who grow tobacco. In some countries in Africa, both governments and multinational tobacco companies assist farmers in acquiring seed and farming equipment. In many European countries, farmers receive direct governmental subsidies for their tobacco production. Export subsidies are also in effect in Europe. The result is more abundant supplies of tobacco at lower prices. However, the net effect on cigarette consumption is often remarkably small. In many developed countries, where cigarettes are highly engineered products and where taxes account for a large portion of retail price, tobacco costs constitute only a small fraction of total cigarette price, often on the order of 2 to 4 percent. The re-

maining cost comes from marketing and distribution of the final product, and of course its manufacture, which includes the expenses of cigarette paper, filters, and the hundreds of additives that end up in the tobacco.

Whether or not tobacco farm subsidies directly lower cigarette prices, the very existence of a governmental support system does inadvertently encourage smoking. In several countries, such as the United States and the United Kingdom, subsidies create a powerful political constituency that opposes both national and global efforts to restrict smoking.

"Cigarette Tax Increases Burden the Poor"

Not necessarily. In most nations, a larger proportion of the poor smoke than is the case for the rich. As a result, the poor often spend a substantially larger proportion of their income on cigarettes and bear a disproportionate share of the burden of a cigarette tax. However, while taxes hurt the poor more, tax increases may well hurt them relatively less. A British study found that a price hike of 10 percent would prompt a nearly equivalent proportional decline in smoking among the lowest social class. By contrast, among smokers in the highest social class, the price increase had virtually no impact on smoking rates. The lesson here is that the burden of a tax increase is actually experienced disproportionately by the social class most able to afford it. In addition, the poor—the group most harmed by the health consequences of smoking—benefit most from a tax increase in terms of improved health.

Meanwhile, legislators can ease the burden of an existing cigarette tax on the poor by dedicating part of the revenues from a tax increase to help low-income smokers quit. A sizable majority of low-income smokers in developed countries report that they would like to stop smoking, but they likely have limited access to professional help. The mix of greater price responsiveness among the poor and allocation of revenues toward smoking cessation can make a tax increase truly progressive, in terms of fiscal policy and public health.

"Advertising Encourages Children to Smoke"

Probably, but we don't know for sure. The targeting of children by the tobacco industry has given substantial ammunition to tobacco control activists. Stories abound of shameless marketing, whether it is Philip Morris underwriting the popular radio program "Marlboro American Music Hour" in Beijing or R.J. Reynolds sponsoring teenage tennis idols in tournaments in Hong Kong and Malaysia.

Yet the connection between cigarette advertising and increased rates of smoking remains unclear. Even when researchers do find a link, the impact of advertising tends to be modest. For instance, studies of the Joe Camel campaign in the United States demonstrate that the cartoon mascot secured a huge army of young recruits for that R.J. Reynolds brand. But nobody can prove that many of those Camel loyalists would not have started smoking—perhaps a different brand—in Joe's absence. Similarly, the emergence of aggressive Western adver-

tising of cigarettes in many Asian countries has coincided with a rapid and unprecedented growth in the number of young female smokers. (In South Korea, for example, the smoking rate among teenage girls jumped from 2 to 9 percent just one year after the government allowed U.S. cigarette imports.) Such growth might have accompanied modernization anyway, although it strains credulity to believe that such a sizable increase was not influenced by the barrage of advertising targeted at Asian girls and young women. In contrast, while public health authorities express understandable concern about the emergence of Western cigarette advertising in former Eastern bloc nations, high rates of smoking characterized all those countries well before the fall of the Berlin Wall.

Other factors—perhaps more mundane, certainly more difficult to control, and virtually immune from policy—are at least equally responsible for children smoking. Young people who smoke might be emulating parents, friends, movie and rock stars, and, on increasingly rare occasions, athletes.

A truly effective tobacco control program uses multiple policy measures (including tax increases and bans on smoking in public places) and public education initiatives (including creative, aggressive countermarketing). A ban on all tobacco advertising and promotion is essential for a truly comprehensive approach, since even a modest decrease in smoking (a 7 percent decline, according to one study on the impact of an advertising ban) is better than none at all. An advertising ban will not be a panacea, but it must be part of the solution.

Kenneth E. Warner is the Avedis Donabedian distinguished university professor of public health at the University of Michigan and director of the university's Tobacco Research Network.

Is the Drug War Over? The Declining Proportion of Drug Offenders

By Graham Farrell and David E. Carter

The explosion of the prison population, involving large increases in drug offenders as a consequence of the war on drugs, has arguably been the story of American criminal justice during the past 20 years.[1] Yet by 2000, the proportion of U.S. inmates sentenced for drug offenses had been fairly stable for a decade, with an overall decline in recent years. In 2000, the proportion of drug offenders was only 0.3 percent above its 1990 level. Is it possible that the war on drugs has not been the principal driver of prison increases for the better part of the past decade? If so, could it be that one of the more infamous eras of U.S. incarceration is coming to a close?

Blumstein and Beck's (1999) essay on trends in the prison population may well be the most recent definitive review. Blumstein is an internationally renowned expert on such issues, while Beck oversees prison-related data for the Bureau of Justice Statistics. Their 1999 review assessed trends up until 1996. It concluded that regarding the 200 percent increase in the prison population between 1980 and 1996, "the dominant factor is drug offending."

There is not necessarily any contradiction between that finding and the one suggested here, which is based on analysis of more recent data. The current study has two aims. The first is to document the fact that despite the previous long-term increases, the proportion of inmates sentenced for drug offenses was stable during most of the 1990s, and on average, declining for six years up to 2000 (for seven years to October 2001 for federal prisons, for which more recent data were available at the

time of this writing). The second aim is to outline possible explanations for the trend.

Drug Offender Trends

The analysis herein, including the data-related statement and charts, are derived from the BJS data listed in Table 1. There is little doubt why drug offenders have figured prominently in recent discourse about the prison system. From 1980 to 2000, the number of sentenced drug offenders increased more than 13 times, from 23,749 to 314,998. Between 1980 and 1990, the number of drug offenders in U.S. prisons increased annually by an average of 22.5 percent and never less than 10 percent. The increase was sharpest between 1987 and 1990, when it ranged from 27 percent to 48 percent. The war on drugs raged (see Figure 1).

The rapid rise in the number of drug offenders during the second half of the 1980s, and its continuation through the 1990s, is well-known. However, when viewed as a proportion of total inmates, the story of drug offenders is somewhat different. National trends largely reflect those of state prisons that contain the bulk of inmates, and from less than 10 percent in the early 1980s, drug offenders rose to, and stayed at a level around, one-quarter of sentenced inmates for the first half of the 1990s (see Figure 2). The fairly horizontal nature of the trend for all U.S. prisons shows that as a proportion of total sentenced inmates, the number of drug offenders changed little throughout the 1990s and declined in recent years. The proportion of the

Table 1: Total and Drug-Offense Inmates in State and Federal Prisons, 1980-2000

	State Prison Inmates		Federal Prison Inmates	
	Total	**Drug Offense**	**Total**	**Drug Offense**
1980	295,819	19,000	19,023	4,749
1981	333,251	21,700	19,765	5,076
1982	375,603	25,300	20,938	5,518
1983	394,953	26,600	26,027	7,201
1984	417,389	31,700	27,622	8,152
1985	451,812	38,900	27,623	9,491
1986	486,655	45,400	30,104	11,344
1987	520,336	57,900	33,246	13,897
1988	562,605	79,100	33,758	15,087
1989	629,995	120,100	37,758	18,852
1990	689,600	149,700	46,575	24,297
1991	728,605	155,200	52,176	29,667
1992	778,495	172,300	59,516	35,398
1993	828,566	186,000	68,183	41,393
1994	904,647	202,100	73,958	45,367
1995	989,007	224,900	76,947	46,669
1996	1,032,440	237,600	80,872	49,096
1997	1,074,809	222,100	87,294	52,059
1998	1,136,760	236,800	95,323	55,984
1999	1,189,800	251,200	104,500	60,399
2000	1,206,400	251,100	112,329	63,898

Source: Bureau of Justice Statistics

Figure 1: The Usual Suspects: Sentenced Drug-Offense Inmates, 1980-2000

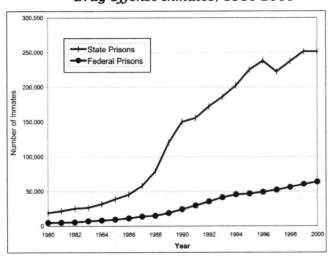

drug offenders in U.S. prisons in 2000 was the same as in 1990 (to within 0.3 percent).

Drug offenders were more prominent in the federal prison population than in the U.S. prison population as a whole. During the first half of the 1980s, approximately one-quarter of sentenced federal inmates were drug offenders. In 1990, for the first time, they surpassed the number of inmates for all other types of offenses—24,297, or 52 percent of all sentenced federal inmates, were drug offenders. That figure rose to a peak of 61.3 percent in 1994.

Distinguishing between the absolute and the relative number of drug offenders, although extraordinarily simple in analytic terms, produces two considerably different stories of the impact of the war on drugs. When absolute numbers are considered, the story of the 1990s appears similar to that of the 1980s. When relative numbers are considered, the trend across the 1990s is very different from that of the 1980s. This is because although the number of drug offenders increased in absolute terms, it did not increase relative to offenders for other crime types during the 1990s.

The trend that is the subject of this study is most apparent if the data are transformed one step further. When the annual change in the proportion of inmates is examined, an underlying trend in the makeup of the prison population is revealed. Figure 3 shows annual change grouped into five-year periods for visual clarity. The proportion of drug offenders was accelerating during the 1980s, particularly in the second half of that decade. The rate of growth slowed in the early 1990s. Since the mid-1990s, the proportion of drug offenders in U.S. prisons has decreased (see Figure 3).

The decreasing proportion of drug offenders was more marked and consistent in federal than in state prisons. In federal prisons, the proportion of drug offenders increased between 1990 and 1994, but at a declining rate. Since 1994, however, the proportion of federal drug offenders did not increase during any year. For the seven years until 2001, the proportion of federal inmates sentenced for drug offenses was either stable or decreasing. The proportion of sentenced federal inmates who were drug offenders fell 5.2 percent between 1995 and 2001. For the prison system as a whole, there was greater variation in the direction of change, but a similar tendency toward stability or a decrease in more recent years.

Skepticism: The First Response

Skepticism is a natural response to the unexpected: it is also a good research aid. The authors of this article were skeptical about the existence and significance of the trend discussed herein. The first main area of skepticism was the belief that such a trend would already be common knowledge. The second was that if it had not been widely known, perhaps that was because it was substantively insignificant?

Why Did So Few People Notice?

Several people will undoubtedly have noticed the decline in the proportion of drug offenders. Alert practitioners and analysts may have noticed it, particularly if it is more pronounced

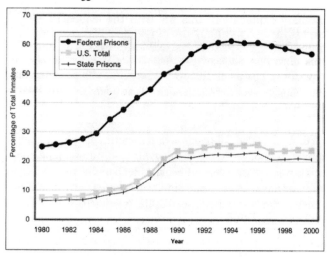

Figure 2: Prison Population: Percentage of Drug Offenders, 1980-2000

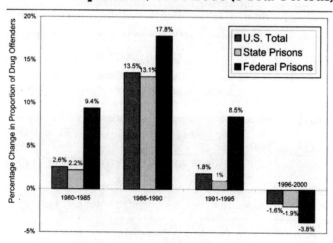

Figure 3: Percentage Change in Proportion of Drug Offenders in Sentenced Prison Population, 1980-2000 (5-Year Periods)

at the local levels (the national aggregates presented here will mask local and regional variations). However, a preliminary trawl of magazines and journals relating to prisons, combined with discussions among a small convenience sample of experts, suggest that there has been little attention paid to this underlying trend.[2] If the trend has been previously documented, then it does not appear to be a frequent subject of discussion among academic prison experts and is not prominently acknowledged in the academic or practitioner literature. Why would this be the case? Perhaps the trend is counterintuitive so that no one was looking for it, or those who noticed thought it an aberration that was too minor and brief to warrant exploration. It is more likely that it appeared trivial in light of the continuing massive increase in drug offenders.

Is It Important?

Is there any significance to the trend of a decreasing proportion of drug offenders? After all, the trend occurs in the context of continuing massive increases in the overall number of incarcerated drug offenders.

There may be much truth in the observation that the key issue is the continuing overall growth in drug offenders. However, noticing one trend does not preclude seeing another: When studying the economy, it is normal to examine overall output as well as growth, and output in different sectors and their relative growths, as well as at short- and long-term inflation and interest rates. Rates of change in economic indicators are examined to reveal underlying trends: A declining rate of increase in productivity, for example, may set off economic warning bells that go unnoticed when only output is examined. In truth, each statistical indicator provides different and complementary information. It is the same with prison statistics. Studying proportions of inmates in different categories and their relative rates of change in no way distracts from the importance of the overall trend. However, like ignoring the relative rate of annual change in the economy, ignoring the underlying dynamic of the compo-

sition of the prison population could cause certain issues to be overlooked. The issue in the current case is that the composition of the prison population has altered. More specifically, changes in the prison population have been driven less by drug offenders in recent years, and more by inmates for other offenses. Something, somewhere, has changed and it began to change quite some time ago. It may be difficult to tease out the implications that relate to the overly politicized issues of illicit drugs, the war on drugs and drug offenders. However, the fact that the trend may only be potentially significant does not detract from the need to draw the attention of a broader audience.

Rival Explanations

Why has the proportion of drug offenders been stable or declining? It is possible to speculate and develop rival explanations. Although it is unlikely to be an exhaustive list in this preliminary foray, several hypotheses are presented below. The possibility that there are multiple and overlapping explanations for the trend should also be considered. Possible explanations of a declining proportion of drug offenders include:

Reporting and/or Recording Changes. The Federal Bureau of Prisons may have changed how it categorizes inmates.

Diversion of Drug Offenders. Drug courts mushroomed in the mid-1990s, so it is possible to hypothesize that the trend is due to non-incarcerative treatment options or more lenient sentencing for drug-related offenses.

Community Re-entry. If larger numbers of drug offenders rather than other types of offenders left the prison system, then the proportion of drug offenders could decline.

Stabilization of the Global Illicit Drug Market. During the late 1980s and early 1990s, the global illicit drug market expanded significantly, particularly in relation to the illicit production of opiates, cocaine and amphetamine-type stimulants. If the expansion of the global drug market accounts for some of the increase in drug-related incarcerations, perhaps its more recent stabilization (particularly for opiates and cocaine) reduced the input of drug offenders.

Sentence Lengths. The number of prison inmates is a function of the number of new incoming inmates (the incidence rate) and outgoing inmates (the release rate), measured via sentence lengths. Perhaps drug offense sentence lengths were short compared with those of other offenses. This could produce a huge throughput of drug offenders, but little change in the total number of drug offenders when measured at any one point in time.

Presidential Terms. Although President Richard Nixon declared the war on drugs in the early 1970s, the main drug war effect coincides with the terms of Ronald Reagan and George Bush Sr. in the 1980s and early 1990s. Allowing for a lag of two or three years to reflect processing and change, perhaps the 1990s trends reflect Bill Clinton's presidency. This is speculation and probably coincidence (although the fit with presidential terms is even better when only federal inmates are considered). If it is true, then a George Bush Jr. effect might (like father, like son) produce an increase in the proportion of drug offenders around 2004 or 2005.

Change Relating to Non-Drug-Offense Inmates. Drug offenders have only declined in recent years when compared with non-drug-offense inmates. Perhaps the war on drugs has continued apace, but the war on other types of offenses has expanded. This could reflect changes either in law, law enforcement practice and priorities, prosecution, court or sentencing practices, or the overall makeup of crime (such as the possibility of increased organized crime).

Discussion

The first hypothesis—that reporting or recording practices changed—cannot be eliminated but seems unlikely to be a valid explanation since it would probably manifest itself as a sudden or one-off statistical change. The diversion, release, fewer drug crimes and reduced sentence severity hypotheses all seek explanations in terms of a decline in the number of drug offenders. Yet, since there has been no decline in the absolute number of drug offenders (see Figure 1), these hypotheses can be dismissed altogether. The presidential term hypothesis is probably spurious: It would manifest itself via more local mechanisms, such as changes in law, law enforcement and sentencing. Further, while it cannot necessarily be wholly ruled out at this stage, it also seems to be a drug offense-based explanation.

The most compelling explanation seems to be that the declining proportion of drug offenders is due to the more marked increase in non-drug-offense inmates. As a preliminary explanation, this fits with the evidence: A more explosive increase in non-drug-offense inmates began to overshadow the increase in drug offenders. The nature of this change, and how and why it occurred, however, are beyond the scope of this article. Additional research would be required to thoroughly investigate the relevant issues. Such research would require lower-level data relating to offense types, as well as, perhaps, extensive information on various aspects of the criminal justice system. Identifying a need for additional research is not unusual. Further research is still required to explore issues relating to the fact that

even when the proportion of U.S. drug offenders was at its highest in the early 1990s, it was still below the levels of several European countries (Van Horne and Farrell, 1999).

Is the drug war over? Has it been over for a decade? Almost certainly not: It may be premature to herald the end of an era. Drug offenders have stabilized, and even decreased, as a proportion of total inmates. However, the most compelling explanation is that the volume of sentenced non-drug-offense inmates has surged to the extent that they even outweigh the continuing increase in drug offenders resulting from an ongoing war on drugs. Perhaps this reflects a new war on violence and on organized and transnational crime rather than a reduction of the war on drugs. Increased attention on non-drug offenders could itself be linked to the illicit drug trade, perhaps reflecting increased sentencing for racketeering, money laundering or other linked charges, some of which may not be classified as drug offenses in prison statistics. It is worth noting that the first of the rival hypotheses, relating to classification, and the reporting and recording of inmates, could not be entirely eliminated and warrants further examination. The volume of drug offenders continues to increase so there does not seem to have been a reversal in a national trend in incarceration that has dominated prison discourse and much of criminal justice discourse for a generation.

The analysis presented herein is elementary. The intention was to document the markedly different tale of events that emerges when relative rather than absolute numbers of inmates are considered. The findings are not necessarily in contradiction with Blumstein and Beck's interpretation that drug offenders were the dominant factor in the 200 percent increase in prison inmates between 1980 and 1996. However, between 1980 and 1996, the increase in drug offenders accounted for 33 percent of the increase in the U.S. prison population.[3] Between 1980 and 2000, drug offenders accounted for 29 percent of the increase in the U.S. prison population.[4] Consequently, while the degree of "dominance" of drug offending depends on the level of disaggregation of the data, the present analysis sheds a different light on the situation. At a minimum, the decreasing proportion of drug offenders, which may well reflect the rise in non-drug-offense inmates, may warrant further examination.

ENDNOTES

[1] All federal inmate numbers are from: Federal Bureau of Prisons. 2002. *Quick facts, May 2002.* Available at www.bop.gov/fact0598.html.

State inmate numbers for 1980, 1985, 1990, 1991, 1992, 1993 and 1994 are from: Beck, A. J., and D. K. Gillard. 1995. *Prisoners in 1994.* Washington, D.C.: Bureau of Justice Statistics.

State inmate numbers for 1981, 1982, 1983, 1984, 1986, 1987, 1988 and 1989 are from: Snell, T. L. 1995. *Correctional populations in the United States, 1993.* Washington, D.C.: Bureau of Justice Statistics.

State inmate numbers for 1995, 1996 and 1997 are from: Chaiken, J. M. 2000. *Correctional populations in the United States, 1997.* Washington, D.C.: Bureau of Justice Statistics.

State inmate numbers for 1998, 1999 and 2000 are from: Harrison, P. M. and A. J. Beck, 2003. *Prisoners in 2001*. Washington, D.C.: Bureau of Justice Statistics.

[2] As our convenience sample of experts, we are grateful to professors Francis T. Cullen, John Eck, Edward J. Latessa, Patricia Van Voorhis and John Wooldredge for comments and advice on previous drafts.

[3] Between 1980 and 1996, the total prison population increased by 798,740 inmates, of whom 262,947—or 32.9 percent—were drug offenders (see Table 1).

[4] Between 1980 and 2000, the total prison population increased by 1,003,887 inmates, of whom 291,249—or 29 percent—were drug offenders (see Table 1).

REFERENCES

Blumstein, A. and A. J. Beck. 1999. Population growth in U.S. prisons, 1980–1996. In *Crime and justice: A review of research*, eds. M. Tonry and J. Petersilia, 17–62. Chicago: University of Chicago Press.

Brown, J. M., D. K. Gillard, T. L. Snell, J. J. Stephan and D. J. Wilson. 1996. *Correctional populations in the United States, 1994*. Washington, D.C.: Bureau of Justice Statistics.

Gillard, D. K. and A. J. Beck. 1996. *Prison and jail inmates, 1995*. Washington, D.C.: Bureau of Justice Statistics.

Gillard, D. K. and A. J. Beck. 1998. *Prisoners in 1997*. Washington, D.C.: Bureau of Justice Statistics.

Van Horne, S. and G. Farrell. 1999. *Drug offenders in the global criminal justice system*. HEUNI Paper series, paper 13. Helsinki, Finland: European Institute for Crime Prevention and control. Available at www.vn.fi/om/suomi/heuni/news/hp13.pdf.

Graham Farrell, Ph.D., is an associate professor in the Division of Criminal Justice at the University of Cincinnati. He was previously deputy research director at the Police Foundation in Washington, D.C., prior to which he researched international drug policy at the United Nations. David E. Carter is a doctoral candidate in the Division of Criminal Justice at the University of Cincinnati and assistant administrator for the master's degree in criminal justice with a focus in addiction studies. He holds an M.A. from East Tennessee State University.

From *Corrections Compendium*, February 2003, pp. 1-4, 28. © 2003 by the American Correctional Association, Lanham, MD 20706-4322. Reprinted by permission.

PROFESSIONAL ISSUES

Prescription drug abuse deadlier than use of illegal drugs

A surge in methadone abuse in Florida matches a national trend that also finds emergency visits for narcotic analgesics outnumbering visits for heroin overdoses.

By Andis Robeznieks
AMNews staff

The abuse of prescription drugs is sending more people to the hospital and, in Florida, more people are being sent to the morgue from prescription drug overdoses than overdoses of cocaine and heroin, according to reports from Florida medical examiners and the U.S. Dept. of Health and Human Services.

Methadone deaths rose 31% in Florida during the first six months of 2002.

Abuse of oxycodone and hydrocodone continues to rise, but a surge in methadone abuse has health and law enforcement officials particularly concerned. The Florida Dept. of Law Enforcement recently issued a public alert to raise awareness of the fact that methadone-related deaths rose 31% (from 194 to 254) in the first six months of this year compared with the last six months of 2001.

Between January and June of this year, the latest Drugs Identified in Deceased Persons report from the Florida medical examiner shows that:

- Cocaine was present in 579 deaths, and listed as the cause in 180.
- Benzodiazepine was present in 734 deaths, and listed as the cause in 150.
- Methadone was present in 254 deaths, and listed as the cause in 133.

- Heroin was present in 141 deaths, and listed as the cause in 121.
- Oxycodone was present in 267 deaths, and listed as the cause in 112.
- Hydrocodone was present in 248 deaths, and listed as the cause in 61.

Although the number of deceased persons who had oxycodone or hydrocodone in their systems increased, the number of times an overdose of those drugs was seen as the cause of death decreased 20% and 14%.

Some officials think that the decrease of deaths tied to these painkillers is linked to the increase in methadone deaths. "One theory is that doctors may be prescribing more methadone because of the bad rap oxycodone has been getting," said Vickie Marsey, a program administrator for the FDLE's medical examiner's commission.

Although there is no exact federal counterpart to Florida's medical examiner's report, the Substance Abuse and Mental Health Services Administration, an HHS agency, does compile similar statistics in its Drug Abuse Warning Network report.

In the DAWN report issued this fall, drug mentions were compiled from 458 emergency departments in 21 metropolitan areas in 2001.

"Our trends show that, in 2001, more people are showing up in emergency rooms for narcotic analgesics than for heroin," said SAMHSA spokeswoman Leah Young.

In 2001, the DAWN report estimated that 43% of the 1.1 million emergency department drug mentions were a result of abusing legal prescription or nonprescription medications. This included 135,949 mentions of anti-anxiety drugs, sedatives and hypnotics; 103,972 mentions of benzodiazepine abuse; and 61,012 mentions of improper use of antidepressants.

The number of benzodiazepine mentions increased more than 12% from 2000, and included a 16% increase in alprazolam drugs.

Florida is seeing more overdose deaths from prescription drugs than from cocaine and heroin.

National figures on methadone appear to match those of Florida. Emergency department mentions of that drug were up 37% from 2000 to 2001, and have risen some 230% since 1994.

"The trend is definitely there," Young said, but she added that the trend isn't uniform.

In the St. Louis and Philadelphia metropolitan areas, for example, she said there were more deaths from narcotic analgesics than from heroin or morphine; but in the Detroit, Seattle and Washington, D.C., areas, heroin and morphine deaths were higher.

"It seems to be all over the map," Young said. "It seems to depend on the city."

Although the news is grim, Marsey pointed to two positive items in the Florida report: Heroin-related deaths decreased 15% and methylated amphetamine-related deaths dropped 29%. In fact, of the 52 deaths in Florida related to methylated amphetamines between January and June of 2002, the drug was considered the direct cause of only eight of those deaths.

Although abuse of methylated amphetamines continues, Marsey said the drug's users are becoming aware of how dangerous they can be.

"I heard that, among the youths who use these club drugs, they now know the signs [of overdose], and don't leave their friends to die anymore," she said. "Now, they take them to the hospital."

ADDITIONAL INFORMATION

Weblink

Report, "2002 Interim Report of Drugs Identified in Deceased Persons by Florida Medical Examiners," Florida Dept. of Law Enforcement, in pdf (http://www.fdle.state.fl.us/publications/examiner_drug_report_2002.pdf)

Press release from the Substance Abuse and Mental Health Services Administration regarding release of 2001 Drug Abuse Warning Network report (http://www.samhsa.gov/news/newsreleases/020821nr_dawn2001.htm)

Laundering

American Banks and the War on Drugs

U.S. banks are the largest financial beneficiaries of the drug trade

By Stephen Bender

When discussing the war on drugs, the political class and hence the mainstream media focus their collective heft on military intervention in the South and mass incarceration in the North. The targets, almost invariably, are the poor and brown. Yet, an understanding of the drug trade's machinations is incomplete without an analysis of the crucial role transnational banks play in the laundering of drug proceeds. Indeed, Washington is proclaiming its readiness to take the "drug war" to the jungles of Colombia in an El Salvador-style intervention, while the real beneficiaries of the drug trade repose much closer to home.

That was the finding by none other than a minority report written by House Democrats on the Permanent Subcommittee on Investigations last year. "Despite increasing international attention and stronger anti-money laundering controls, some current estimates are that $500 billion to $1 trillion in criminal proceeds are laundered through banks worldwide each year, with about half of that amount moved through United States banks."

A large proportion of the conservatively estimated $250 billion in ill-gotten funds is derived from the drug trade, predominantly cocaine. That enormous sum, the Subcommittee determined, makes Uncle Sam's banks collectively the world's largest financial beneficiaries of the drug trade.

James F. Sloan, Director of the Financial Crimes Enforcement Network, (FinCEN) a subdivision of the Department of the Treasury, was also less than sanguine, when commenting on the current state of affairs. Testifying before the Congressional Subcommittee on Criminal Justice, Drug Policy and Human Resources in June of 2000, Sloan stated, "money laundering is the lifeblood of narcotics trafficking and other financial crimes.

These criminal organizations now dwarf some of the world's largest legitimate business enterprises, laundering enormous sums of money throughout the international financial system."

Raymond Baker, a career international businessperson and analyst associated with the Center for International Policy and the Brookings Institution, testified before the same Subcommittee. Noting "An absolute explosion in the volume of dirty money during this, the first decade of the globalizing world," Baker quoted U.S. Treasury Department estimates that "99.9 percent of the laundered criminal money that is presented for deposit in the United States gets comfortably into secure accounts."

So, we find testimony before Congress exploding the pious rhetoric about the drug war. If Uncle Sam is capable of interdicting only 0.1 percent of the dreaded drug kingpin's "life blood," then what exactly are we getting for our nearly $20 billion in drug war largesse?

The key institution in the enabling of money laundering is the "private bank," a subdivision of every major U.S. financial institution. Private banks exclusively seek out a wealthy clientele, the threshold often being an annual income in excess of $1 million. With the prerogatives of wealth comes a certain regulatory deference.

The General Accounting Office, (GAO), the research arm of Congress, reported in late 1999 on the difficulties surrounding the regulation of private banks. "It is difficult to measure," the report comments, "precisely how extensive private banking is in the United States, partly because the area has not been clearly defined and partly because financial institutions do not consistently capture or publicly report information on their private banking activities." As a result, estimates at the cumulative value of "private banking" assets are difficult to estimate, but the total undoubtedly reaches well into the trillions of dollars.

That U.S.-based private banks operate in a regulatory twilight zone enabling the laundering of drug profits is confirmed by the GAO. Private banks are "not subject to the Bank Secrecy Act," thus exempting banks from complying with "specific anti-money-laundering provisions… such as the one requiring that suspicious transactions be reported to U.S. authorities."

Instead of monitoring formal compliance, U.S. banking regulators "try to identify what efforts the branches are making to combat money laundering." In determining whether the offshore branches are doing an adequate job in screening for money laundering, regulators "must rely primarily on the banks' internal audit functions to verify that the procedures are actually being implemented in offshore branches where U.S. regulators may be precluded from conducting on-site examinations."

Not only is government oversight lax, but banks are willfully ignorant about their own client's account holdings, an outgrowth of the cult of secrecy surrounding private banking. The Subcommittee on Investigations report continued: "The reality right now is that private banks allow clients to have multiple accounts in multiple locations under multiple names and do not aggregate the information. This approach creates vulnerabilities to money laundering by making it difficult for banks to have a comprehensive understanding of their own client's accounts." Some banks go so far as to forbid their employees to keep information linking clients to their accounts and shell corporations. One private banker told the Subcommittee that he "had 30–40 clients, each of which had up to fifteen shell corporations and, to keep track, he and other colleagues in the private bank used to create private lists of their clients' shell companies. He said that he and his colleagues had to hide these 'cheat sheets' from bank compliance personnel who, on occasion, conducted surprise inspections to eliminate this information from bank files. When asked why the bank would destroy information he needed to do his job effectively, the former private banker simply said that it was bank policy not to keep this information in the United States."

The report then quoted the Federal Reserve's 1998 "system wide study," which analyzed the practices of seven private banks. The study concluded, "That internal controls and oversight practices over private banking activities were generally strong at banks that focused on high-end domestic clients, while similar controls and oversight practices were seriously weak at banks that focused on higher risk Latin American and Caribbean clients."

The reasons for the disparity are not complicated, the Subcommittee concluded. "Federal Reserve officials told the Subcommittee staff that private banking has become a 'profit driver' for many banks, offering returns twice as high as many other banking areas. Private banks interviewed by the Subcommittee staff have confirmed rates of return in excess of 20 percent."

In such a profitable business, competition is fierce, which leads to a whole host of other problems as outlined in a 1997 Federal Reserve report on private banking. "As the target market for private banking is growing, so is the level of competition among institutions that provide private banking services. Private banks interviewed by the Subcommittee staff confirm that the market remains highly competitive; most also reported plans to expand operations. The dual pressures of competition and expansion are disincentives for private banks to impose tough anti-money laundering controls that may discourage new business or cause existing clients to move to other institutions." In short, a rising tide of coca funds lifts all banks.

Apart from the institutional competitive forces at work, the Subcommittee found that private bankers and their clientele operate under a symbiotic relationship in which the banker identifies more closely with the client than with the duty to uphold the law.

The textbook case of this shady entente came in 1995 in a massive money laundering scandal involving the former president of Mexico's brother, Raul Salinas de Gotari, and Citibank. The case only came to light after Salinas was implicated in the assassination of Ruiz Massieu, a prominent member of Mexico's corrupt and now largely discredited Institutional Revolutionary Party (PRI). Subsequent investigations linked Salinas to the cocaine cartels that paid staggering bribes in the hundreds of millions to the political class in the early 1990s.

Citibank's private banker catering to Salinas was Amy Elliot. As the most senior private banker in New York dealing with Mexican clients, Elliot took the word of Carlos Hank Rohn (an oligarch recently linked by the Mexican press to the drug trade) in setting up the Salinas accounts. Salina's only known source of income was his annual government salary of $190,000 in addition to funds derived from his work in the "construction business" and his proximity to the president. In testimony before the Subcommittee, Elliot recounted that she estimated in June 1992 that the Salinas accounts had "[p]otential in the $15–$20M range." After multiple appeals, Salinas now sits in a Mexican prison.

In a June 29, 1993 email, shortly after the account passed the $40 million mark, Elliott wrote to a colleague in Switzerland: "This account is turning into an exciting profitable one for us all. [M]any thanks for making me look good." Salinas eventually deposited "in excess of $87 million" by way of Citibank's New York headquarters.

Although the case of Citibank and Raul Salinas generated some media interest and nudged banks to revise their internal regs, the Subcommittee found that banks had "set up systems to ensure that private banker activities are reviewed by third parties, such as supervisors, compliance personnel or auditors. The Subcommittee staff investigation has found, however, that while strong oversight procedures exist on paper, in practice private bank oversight is often absent, weak or ignored."

Another bark worse than bite facet of the drug war lies in the punishment meted out by our "zero tolerance" drug warriors to high level money laundering bankers, such as Amy Elliot and her superiors. This was a point not neglected by Kenneth Rijock, testifying before the aforementioned Government Reform Subcommittee. Rijock spoke before Congress with a background as a former "career money launderer" whose operations were based in Florida. Now a government consultant on dirty money matters, Rijock obliquely touched on the drug war's hypocrisy. "No federally chartered commercial bank has ever lost its charter for money laundering violations, no matter how serious the crime. Senior bank officers themselves are rarely indicted for money laundering; the institution simply pays a multi-million dollar fine.... Only now are we going to name and ostracize the most blatant offshore tax haven banks; we still don't indict their presidents and directors for violations of the Money Laundering Control Act." That, likely is a manifestation of the standard practice in the American justice system that "suite crime" is punished much less harshly than "street crime."

In recent years, government efforts to more effectively intercept laundered funds have been rebuffed. In 1998, the Clinton administration proposed new rules governing the reporting of banks to the government on suspicious financial transactions. The government correctly insisted that more invasive regulations were necessary to make headway against money launderers. Opponents, across the political spectrum, from the ACLU to the Cato Institute (cheered on by the banks who played a low-key role) created a firestorm of public opposition. John J. Byrne, senior council for the American Bankers Association, responded tersely to the proposed preliminary reporting to the government on suspicion of illegal activity. "We don't support the notion that we need to investigate, profile, and monitor account activity."

A subsequent attempt by the Clinton administration in January 2001 to monitor the accounts of foreign leaders laundering funds in American banks fell flat. As the *New York Times* put it: "Citigroup was among a consortium of leading New York banks that led an effort in late December to water down the new guidelines. The banks, members of the New York Clearing House, complained that the guidelines were too 'sweeping' and were based on 'unrealistic' expectations...." Although law enforcement authorities considered the proposed regulation "too weak," Justice Department officials "signed off on the voluntary guidelines." At issue was the monitoring of accounts held by foreign leaders and their families, based on the experiences of the Salinas case and others.

The point is not to apply the level of 4th Amendment protection currently enjoyed by street dealers and casual users to bankers. Rather, it is to recognize the struggle facing governments attempting to meaningfully deter drug-related money laundering. From there, consideration of decriminalization is crucial.

The problem goes deeper than one government's futile struggle. The drug trade has successfully learned to mimic the tricks of international banking and commerce, copying the methods of "legitimate" business. The favored tool in this endeavor is the use of tax havens—often used to disguise sundry forms of financial swindling. As Raymond Baker commented: "In fact, the easiest thing for criminals to do is to make their criminal money look like it is merely corrupt or preferably commercial tax-evading money, and when they do it passes readily into foreign accounts. With American and European banks and corporations aggressively competing to service gains from cor-

ruption and illegal flight capital, money laundering is almost universally successful."

The State Department admits as much when they annually categorize the world's nations based on their adherence to Washington's ground rules for drug war probity. Unsurprisingly then, Foggy Bottom finds among its "high priority" money laundering countries, the leading "free market" states: the U.S., UK, Germany, Italy, the Netherlands, Canada, and Switzerland.

While decrying the undermining of "democratic market economics" by the hemorrhaging of capital from the South, Baker conceded that the wealthy countries ultimately benefit. "The costs and benefits of the components of dirty money which we facilitate, i.e., yields from corruption and commercial tax evasion, merit clear analysis. The benefit is that it spreads several hundred billion dollars annually across North America and Europe, in bank accounts, markets and properties. The cost can be seen in the impact on both our domestic and foreign interests." Baker, the former international businessperson, then very succinctly elucidates the issue, sounding rather like a leftist. "The foreign cost of our pursuit of corrupt riches and illegal flight capital is that it erodes our strategic objectives in transitional economies and impairs economic progress in developing countries, draining hard currency reserves, heightening inflation, reducing tax collection, worsening income gaps, canceling investment, and hurting competition, all contributing to political instability."

The essential issue is neither the lack of adequate government oversight, nor the malfeasance of banks individually or collectively, although they are symptoms of the problem. Rather, the problem lies in the triumph of market forces over government and civil society.

As the late British academic Susan Strange pointed out in her 1998 book *Mad Money,* there are three distinct market forces driving the drug trade. The first is the "market for banking services" which has exploded in this era of intensified globalization of capital and integration of world markets. The second relates to the "market for hallucinatory or mood altering drugs," which has remained consistently strong for some 30 years. The final component, Stange comments, "is often overlooked in transnational organized crime... the market for [licit] tropical crops." To an impoverished peasant attempting to feed his family, it is economically irrational to grow coffee, cocoa or bananas (whose values fluctuate at meager levels) at a subsistence level when cocoa growing enables a substantially better livelihood. Moreover, it is hypocritical for the leaders of the rich countries to expect them to do so.

A further dodge lies in placing the blame on "offshore" banks. The Cayman Islands for instance, according to Ken Silverstein writing in *Mother Jones,* "with 570 banks holding $670 billion is now the 6th largest financial center in the world after London, Tokyo, New York, Berlin, and Zurich." Then again, what other options do these otherwise economically stagnant countries have? Lacking land and labor, the ability to attract capital is their "comparative advantage," and its pursuit is conducted with the otherwise much lauded "entrepreneurial spirit." It is further worth noting another facet of what *Le Monde Dip-*

lomatique last year called the "dirty money archipelago." Namely, that money launderers among others "take advantage of the existence of 250 free [trade] zones and tax havens, 95 percent of which are former British, French, Spanish, Dutch or U.S. colonies or concessions that remain dependent on the former colonial powers."

Analyzed in the broadest sense, the drug war has unleashed horrendous destruction on the very people it is supposedly designed to save. The wages of this war are eroded civil liberties, incarceration as a preferred social policy, a steady stream of violence as various gangs compete for a share in an illicit market, and the further corruption of many Latin American governments. Note however, that the powerful uniformly benefit from it. Banks reap massive profits, the military is given a further rationale for its ballast, the corporate sector obtains new investment opportunities (prisons) and markets (para-military gear

and counterinsurgency weaponry), and the state obtains a post-Cold War justification for foreign intervention. In short, a class war by other means.

The drug war, understood as a campaign to ameliorate the scourge of drug addiction, is a fraud. The greatest scandal, beyond even the connivance of the great banks in a drug trade, is that this fraud is today being deployed as a justification for war. The United States is sending $1.3 billion to Colombia to fight the "narcoterrorists," Americans are told. It was not a coincidence that Clinton accompanied 30 CEOs when he visited Cartagena to inaugurate "Plan Colombia." Unless enough Americans can see through this audacious propaganda, a lie fortified by a fraud, our government may well carry out the bloodiest pacification program since Vietnam.

Stephen Bender has written on topics of interest for the *San Francisco Bay Guardian* and Salon.com.

Survival of the druggies

Taking narcotics may be part of our evolutionary inheritance

Abbie Thomas

Sydney—IF DRUGS are so bad for us, why do so many people use them? Because they helped our ancestors survive, argue two anthropologists.

Our predilection for psychotropic substances is usually seen as a biological accident. The conventional view is that drugs fool the brain into thinking it is getting a reward when in fact it isn't.

But anthropologists Roger Sullivan of the University of Auckland and Edward Hagen of the University of California at Santa Barbara point out that our ancestors were exposed to plants containing narcotic substances for millions of years. In the April issue of *Addiction*, they argue that we are predisposed to drug-taking because we evolved to seek out plants rich in alkaloids.

Consuming such plants could have been a basic survival strategy. "Stimulant alkaloids like nicotine and cocaine could have been exploited by our human ancestors to help them endure harsh environmental conditions," Sullivan says. For example, until recently Australian Aborigines used the nicotine-rich plant *pituri* to help them endure desert travel without food. And Andeans still chew coca leaves to help them work at high altitudes.

Archaeological evidence shows that drug use was widespread in ancient cultures. Betel nut, for example, was chewed at least 13,000 years ago in Timor, to the north of Australia. Artefacts date the use of coca in Ecuador to at least 5000 years ago.

Many of these substances were potent: *pituri* contains up to 5 per cent nicotine, whereas tobacco today contains about 1.5 per cent. What's more, these drug pioneers sometimes "free-based" drugs by chewing them together with an alkali such as lime or wood ash. This releases the free form of the drug and allows it to be directly absorbed into the bloodstream.

But in Pacific cultures where chewing betel nut is still widespread, it is seen more as a source of food and energy than as a drug, Sullivan says. And some drugs do have real nutritional value. For example, 100 grams of coca leaf contains more than the US recommended daily intake of calcium, phosphorus, iron and vitamins A, B_2 and E.

And in some marginal environments, people's diets may have been so poor that they struggled to produce enough neurotransmitters of their own. Consuming plants containing substances that mimic neurotransmitters could have helped make up for the shortfall, Sullivan and Hagen speculate. They say this part of their theory could be tested by depriving animals of certain neurotransmitters and seeing if they then choose to eat food rich in substitutes.

Sullivan's adaptive model of drug use is definitely plausible, says Wayne Hall of the University of Queensland, who until recently was head of the National Drug and Alcohol Research Centre in Sydney. "There is certainly evidence that plants evolved to mimic the neurotransmitters of mammals," he says. "But the problem today is that we have much larger doses of much more purified drugs."

From *New Scientist*, March 2002, p. 30. © 2002 by the New Scientist/The New York Times Syndicate. Reprinted by permission.

UNIT 2

Understanding How Drugs Work—Use, Dependency, and Addiction

Unit Selections

Key Points to Consider

- Why are some drugs so reinforcing?

- Why do some people become dependent upon certain drugs far sooner than other people?

- Is it possible to predict one's personal threshold for becoming drug dependent or addicted? Explain

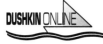 **Links: www.dushkin.com/online/**
These sites are annotated in the World Wide Web pages.

AMERSA
http://center.butler.brown.edu

Centre for Addiction and Mental Health (CAMH)
http://www.camh.net

The National Center on Addiction and Substance Abuse at Columbia University
http://www.casacolumbia.org

National Institute on Drug Abuse (NIDA)
http://www.nida.nih.gov

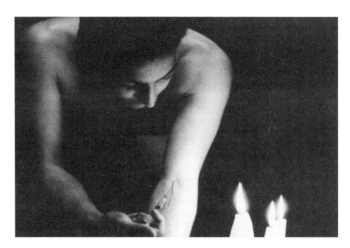

Understanding how drugs act upon the human mind and body is a critical component to the resolution of issues concerning drug use and abuse. An understanding of basic pharmacology is requisite for informed discussion on practically every drug-related issue and controversy. One does not have to look far to find misinformed debate, much of which surrounds the basic lack of knowledge of how drugs work.

Different drugs produce different bodily effects and consequences. All psychoactive drugs influence the central nervous system, which, in turn, sits at the center of how we physiologically and psychologically interpret and react to the world around us. Some drugs, such as methamphetamine and LSD, have great immediate influence on the nervous system, while others, such as tobacco and marijuana, elicit less-pronounced reactions. Almost all psychoactive drugs have their effects on the body mitigated by the dosage level of the drug taken, the manner in which it is ingested, and the physiological and emotional state of the user. Cocaine smoked in the form of crack versus that snorted as powder produces profoundly different physical and emotional effects on the user. However, even though illegal drugs often provide the most sensational perspective from which to view these relationships, the abuse of prescription drugs is being reported as an exploding new component of the addiction problem. Currently, the nonmedical use of pain-reliever drugs is occurring at rates not observed since the mid-70s. Currently, 22.1 percent of young adults, aged 18–25, report the nonmedical use of these drugs in their lifetime. The young adult rate was 6.8 percent in 1992.

Molecular properties of certain drugs allow them to imitate and artificially reproduce certain naturally occurring brain chemicals that provide the basis for the drug's influence. The continued use of certain drugs and their repeated alteration of the body's biochemical structure provide one explanation for the physiological consequences of drug use. For example, heroin use replicates the natural brain chemical endorphin, which supports the body's biochemical defense to pain and stress. The continued use of heroin is believed to deplete natural endorphins, causing the nervous system to produce a painful physical and emotional reaction when heroin is withdrawn.

A word of caution is in order, however, when proceeding through the various explanations for what drugs do and why they do it. Many people, because of an emotional and/or political relationship to the world of drugs, assert a subjective predisposition when interpreting certain drugs' effects and consequences. One person's alcoholic is another's social drinker. People often argue, rationalize, and explain the perceived nature of drugs' effects based upon an extremely superficial understanding of diverse pharmacological properties of different drugs. A detached and scientifically sophisticated awareness of drug pharmacology may help strengthen the platform from which to interpret the various consequences of drug use.

Drug dependence and addiction is usually a continuum comprising experimentation, recreational use, regular use, and abuse. The process is influenced by a plethora of physiological, psychological, and environmental factors. Although some still argue that drug dependence is largely a matter of individual behavior, something to be chosen or rejected, most experts assert that new scientific discoveries clearly define the roots of addiction to be within molecular levels of the brain. Powerful drugs, upon repeated administration, easily compromise the brain's ability to make decisions about its best interests.

Largely, drugs are described as more addictive or less addictive due to a process described as "reinforcement." Simply explained, reinforcement results from a drug's physiological and psychological influence on behavior that causes repeated introduction of the drug to the body. Cocaine and the amphetamines are known as drugs with high reinforcement potential. Persons addicted to drugs known to be strongly reinforcing typically report that they care more about getting the drug than about anything else.

Reinforcement does not, however, provide the sole basis for understanding addiction. Addiction is a cloudy term used to describe a multitude of pharmacological and environmental factors that produce a compulsive, nonnegotiable need for a drug. A thorough understanding of addiction requires an awareness of these many factors. Additionally, the recent mapping of the human genome is providing a new understanding of the genetic influence on the process of addiction. With each passing year, discoveries related to genetics influence thinking on almost all processes related to addiction.

The articles in unit 2 illustrate some of the current research and viewpoints on the ways that drugs act upon the human body. An understanding of these pharmacological processes is critical to understanding the assorted consequences of drug use and abuse. Science has taken us closer to understanding that acute drug use changes brain function profoundly and that these changes may remain with the user long after the drug has left the system. Subsequently, many new issues have emerged for drug and health-related public policy. Increasingly, drug abuse competes with other social maladies as public enemy number one. Further, the need for a combined biological, behavioral, and social response to this problem becomes more self-evident. Many health care professionals and health care educators, in addition to those from other diverse backgrounds, argue that research dollars spent on drug abuse and addiction should approach that spent on heart disease, cancer, and AIDS.

ADDICTION: LONG-TERM CHANGES

Beyond the Pleasure Principle

Sure, drugs feel good—but they're addicting because they co-opt memory and motivation systems, not just pleasure pathways.

When it comes to kicking a drug habit, going through withdrawal is the easy part. The cold-turkey alcoholic shaking with delirium tremens might not agree, but only after the body detoxifies does the real challenge begin: staying clean. Ex-addicts with the strongest resolve—and plenty of external motivation in the form of frayed relationships, probationary jobs, or incipient lung cancer—struggle to resist cravings and are susceptible to relapse even years after their last dose.

Researchers have spent decades studying the immediate effects of drugs on the brain. Drugs cause short-term surges in dopamine and other brain messengers that signal pleasure or reward. But the brain quickly adapts to this deluge; pleasure circuits overwhelmed by drugs' signals desensitize—so much so that the brain can suffer withdrawal once the binge is over.

In the past decade or so, many researchers have started to focus on a more daunting problem: the long-term consequences of drug abuse. Many drugs don't induce much pleasure after prolonged use, in part because of desensitization, or tolerance. So why do addicts keep taking their drug of choice, even when they try to abstain? To find out, researchers are seeking clues in parts of the brain that help control motivation, looking for changes that happen after weeks, months, and years of exposure to drugs.

Some of the neural changes they've found look very familiar: Addiction seems to rely on some of the same neurobiological mechanisms that underlie learning and memory, and cravings are triggered by memories and situations associated with drug use. Recent studies have revealed a "convergence between changes caused by drugs of addiction in reward circuits and changes in other brain regions mediating memory," says neuroscientist Eric Nestler of the University of Texas Southwestern Medical Center in Dallas. For instance, both learning and drug exposure resculpt synapses, initiate cascades of molecular signals that turn on genes, and change behavior in persistent ways. Understanding these processes could help addicts conquer relapse, "the core clinical problem" of addiction, says Steven Hyman, director of the National Institute of Mental Health in Bethesda, Maryland (soon to depart for Harvard University). "If we want to focus on the clinical issue that matters, we have to understand how

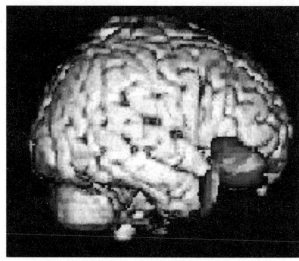

A. R. CHILDRESS *ET AL.*, *AM. J. PSYCHIATRY* **156(1)**, 11 (1999)

The face of craving. Videos containing drug-related cues stimulate the orbitofrontal cortex and temporal lobe (above) as well as deeper reward-related brain structures in addicts.

associative memories are laid down that change the emotional value of drugs and create deeply ingrained behavioral responses to those cues [that trigger relapse]."

Memories you remember

Memory researchers divide memories into those you consciously remember and those you generally don't. Consciously, people may remember a past drug-induced burst of euphoria and seek out the drug again, or they may remember that drugs stop them from feeling crummy. This type of memory is "good at explaining why people take drugs, but it doesn't explain addiction," says Terry Robinson of the University of Michigan, Ann Arbor. Plenty of people dabble in drug use for just such pleasure-related reasons, but addiction is different. Once addicted, people compulsively seek out and take drugs, even if they don't provide pleasure anymore and despite a strong will to quit—a defining feature of addiction that ties it to other compulsive behaviors.

Nonconscious memories are much more insidious, Robinson points out, and are more likely to underlie the compulsive aspect of addiction and the cravings that lead to

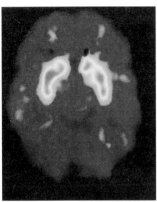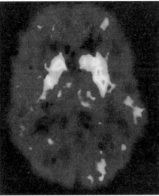

N. VOLKOW *ET AL. AM. J. PSYCHIATRY* **158(3)**, 377 (2001)

Blown out. Even 80 days after detox, a methamphetamine abuser's dopamine system (right) hasn't recovered to normal levels (left).

relapse. For instance, the paraphernalia of drug use—crack pipes, syringes, the sound of ice tinkling in a glass full of scotch—can act as cues that induce craving much like the sound of a bell caused Pavlov's dogs to salivate. Even though addicts can become conscious of the relationship between some drug-related cues and their cravings, other cues might be less obvious; for instance, they might not recognize that a certain place or smell wakens a hunger for the drug. Cues "can goad an individual to drug seeking in the absence of conscious awareness," says Robinson.

When former addicts see videos evocative of drug use, they report craving and show signs of stress, such as increased heart rate, says psychiatrist Charles O'Brien of the University of Pennsylvania in Philadelphia. Positron emission tomography (PET) shows that parts of the reward system are unusually active when people experience craving. Other researchers, particularly psychiatrist Nora Volkow of Brookhaven National Laboratory in Upton, New York, also see hyperactivation of the orbitofrontal cortex when recovered addicts see cues that induce craving for cocaine. This part of the brain is closely connected to reward pathways and is disrupted in people with obsessive-compulsive disorder. Volkow suggests that the orbitofrontal cortex is responsible for the craving and compulsion that make addicts so susceptible to relapse.

Another type of nonconscious memory, called sensitization, is less intuitive. If an animal receives a big dose of a drug—say, amphetamine, morphine, or cocaine—for several days in a row, each successive dose causes a stronger response. Behaviorally, the rat bobs its head and runs around the cage more, and inside the brain, more dopamine is released even though the drug dose is the same. The effect lasts a long time, says Robinson. His group sensitized rats to amphetamine, waited 1 year, and then gave the animals another dose. Even then, they responded more strongly than did animals without previous drug experience. Sensitization "alters neural circuitry involved in normal processes of incentive, motivation, and reward," says Robinson. This neural circuitry isn't a simple hardwired response to the drug, however: It depends on

context. If Robinson's team gives a sensitized rat another dose of the drug in a different cage from the one where it received the training doses, the animal responds normally, as if it had never experienced the drug before. Sensitization, in an environment where an animal and presumably a person has learned to expect a drug, "renders brain circuitry hypersensitive to drugs and drug-associated paraphernalia," says Robinson.

Technicolor short-circuits

Although each drug of abuse has its idiosyncratic effects, all specialize in bombarding the brain's dopamine-mediated reward circuits. Long-term abuse can wear out these pathways, reducing the number of receptors that respond to dopamine. Some of Volkow's more chilling PET scan images show the brains of former methamphetamine users: Some have been drug free for months but their dopamine systems are still not firing on all cylinders. Dopamine fuels motivation and pleasure, but it's also crucial for learning and movement. Volkow reported in the March issue of the *American Journal of Psychiatry* that the loss of dopamine transporters, a measure of how disrupted the dopamine system is, correlates with memory problems and lack of motor coordination.

Once the brain becomes less sensitive to dopamine, it "becomes less sensitive to natural reinforcers," Volkow says, such as the "pleasure of seeing a friend, watching a movie, the curiosity that drives exploration." The only stimuli still strong enough to activate the sputtering motivation circuit, she says, are drugs.

Understanding that drugs "rearrange someone's motivational priorities" can help explain some of the senseless behaviors addicts engage in, such as neglecting their families, jobs, and health, says Alan Leshner, director of the National Institute on Drug Abuse in Bethesda, Maryland. As Leshner explains, "it isn't the case that the crack-addicted mother does not love her children. She just loves drugs more."

Microscopic memories

Many recovered drug users say they fight cravings for the rest of their lives. Addiction researchers aren't sure how drugs change the brain in ways that can last a lifetime, but they aren't alone. As Nestler points out, "our field [of addiction research] and the learning and memory field have not made a lot of progress... in identifying molecular changes underlying long-term changes in memory."

They have some hunches, though, and some reasonable evidence for mechanisms that might pitch in to construct long-lasting memories or compulsions. Research on the sea snail *Aplysia* and the mouse hippocampus has uncovered a range of cellular signals that accompany learning; some of the same players are active in addiction. For example, the transcription factor CREB is necessary for learning in mice and *Drosophila*, and CREB is also boosted by drug use, suggesting that it contributes somehow to drug-mediated neural changes.

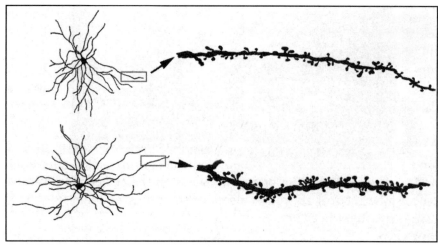

T. ROBINSON AND B. KOLB, *EUR. J. NEUROSCI.* **11,** 1598 (1999)

Memento cocaine. After drug exposure, some neurons have more dendrites and connective spines (bottom) than in untreated animals (top).

One of the best studied models of memory at the cellular level is called long-term potentiation (LTP). Memories are stored in the brain, researchers suggest, in part by changes in how neurons are interconnected. In LTP, hyperstimulation makes synapses, those points of near-contact where neurons communicate, more responsive to future stimulation—that is, it changes the connection between the two cells. In the 31 May issue of *Nature*, Mark Ungless of the University of California, San Francisco, and colleagues showed that a single dose of cocaine induced LTP in dopamine cells in a part of the brain called the ventral segmental area that is critical for addiction, suggesting that the same cellular mechanisms—albeit in different parts of the brain—are at work in memory and addiction.

Other changes in synaptic connections are more concrete: Memory researchers have found that a neuron's dendrites build more branching projections and have more synapses that connect to neurons with which the cell communicates regularly. Robinson and colleagues have found that drugs produce the same effect. When they sensitize animals to a drug, they see more dendritic branches and a greater density of neurons in the nucleus accumbens and the prefrontal cortex. Both areas are key players in processing reward signals and making decisions. These morphological changes last at least a month, Robinson says, and probably longer. Addiction researchers and memory researchers suspect that such physical changes in neurons and their connections are crucial for understanding both fields. "To me, that is the core," says Hyman. "There is no more important question in the field of addiction than understanding the mechanisms that produce and maintain altered patterns of synaptic connections."

Nestler says the basic molecular processes constructing these changes are probably the same in learning and memory and in addiction. After all, he says, "the brain is conservative" and probably has a "finite repertoire of molecular changes that it can mount in response to environmental perturbations." Nestler and his colleagues have found at least one molecule that appears to be specific for addiction, however. The protein, called Δ-FosB, builds up in the reward pathway after repeated exposure to drugs and sticks around longer than other proteins—for as long as 4 to 6 weeks after the last dose. The protein increases an animal's sensitivity to drugs and can also induce relapse if injected.

In some cases, the line between memory systems and addiction is hard to draw. For instance, Stanislav Vorel of Albert Einstein College of Medicine in New York City and colleagues reported in the 11 May issue of *Science* (p. 1175) that stimulating the hippocampus—the archetypal seat of memory in the brain—makes formerly exposed but now drug-free rats seek out cocaine. And other researchers have discovered that in some cases, dopamine in so-called pleasure circuits appears to be more important for learning—or what different labs call prediction or anticipation—than reward.

At the top of many addiction researchers' "to-do lists" is to detangle all the threads of learning and memory, motivation, and reward that make addiction addiction: Find the switch. As Leshner puts it, "we know a tremendous amount about the differences between the addicted and nonaddicted brain, both behaviorally and biologically. We know less about the transition process between the two." The processes involved in learning and memory may eventually be the key to figuring out how an often pleasurable experience—taking a drug—can change from a somewhat self-destructive hobby to a life-threatening compulsion.

–LAURA HELMUTH

IT'S A HARD HABIT TO BREAK

DISCOVER DIALOGUE WITH MOLECULAR PSYCHIATRIST ERIC NESTLER

These days it seems as if everyone is addicted—not just to heavy drugs such as cocaine but also to newly claimed obsessions such as eating, gambling, and the Internet. In his lab at the University of Texas Southwestern Medical Center, molecular psychiatrist Eric Nestler is making progress in understanding the nature of addiction and the strong similarities between different kinds of cravings. His studies show how a protein called delta-FosB modulates the brain's sensitivity to drugs, raising hopes of medical treatments that could set addicts free. Nestler discussed the science of need with *Discover* reporter Jocelyn Selim.

What are the common elements of various kinds of addictions?
Research over the past 20 years has shown that addictive drugs all produce the same net effect, which is to stimulate a "reward pathway" in a part of the brain that controls the release of dopamine. The differences come about because each drug also triggers responses elsewhere. Heroin affects the spinal column and the brain stem, slowing the respiratory rate; cocaine speeds up the heart and so can cause a heart attack.

What about people who say they're addicted to behaviors such as gambling, sex, or surfing the Internet?
There is growing evidence that these natural addictions—compulsive behaviors connected to things other than drugs—all probably have at their core the same brain reward pathways. In fact, recent brain-imaging studies show that the nucleus accumbens, the brain area associated with drug addiction, lights up both in compulsive gamblers and in people or animals shown sexual stimuli.

Do you regard tobacco, alcohol, and marijuana as "gateway" drugs?
There are people who use softer drugs who would never try the illegal ones. But because the reward mechanisms are so much the same, there is something to the gateway theory. Marijuana is obviously addictive because some people use it compulsively. Can-nabinoids, which cause the marijuana high, hang around in the body so long that withdrawal occurs imperceptibly. If you give a cannabinoid-blocking compound to a marijuana addict, all of a sudden you see severe withdrawal syndrome.

Can a drug be addictive if it produces no withdrawal symptoms?
In theory, yes. With the natural addictions—gambling, eating, etc.—you don't experience any physical withdrawal, but you do get cravings. Cocaine doesn't produce strong physical withdrawal symptoms, but it is highly addictive. Conversely, there are a lot of medications, such as the heart medication Inderal, that cause a clear physical dependence but are nonaddicting.

Ho much of addiction is genetic and how much of it is social?
Epidemiological studies tell us that about half the risk for addiction is genetic. And the degree of genetic vulnerability seems to be roughly the same for the various types of drugs—alcohol, heroin, cocaine. To put the numbers in perspective, a 50 percent genetic risk is higher than for type II diabetes or hypertension, which we often think of as genetic diseases.

Why do we have this susceptibility?
The dopamine pathway probably evolved to provide an emotional reinforcement for certain choices an animal makes about food, sex, and social interaction. Drugs of abuse came along and commandeered this pathway with a force and persistence that's not seen in the natural world.

Will there ever be a medical cure for the problem of drug addiction?
We have to be able to do better than we're doing now. Addiction and compulsive behavior are responsible for so many bad things in society: crime, loss of life, AIDS, lung cancer. I think rehab programs alone are doomed to failure until we understand the fundamental biology. Then we'll be able to develop treatments and preventive measures. Thankfully, we should have prototypes within five years.

THE BIOLOGY OF... ADDICTION

The End of Craving

A controversial new drug seems to stop addiction cold

by michael abrams

THE RATS IN STANLEY GLICK'S LAB ARE junkies. They spend their days and nights lounging around in steel cages, twiddling their claws, waiting for the next hit. Each rat has a small plastic tube protruding from the base of its skull. Once a day, for an hour, each tube is connected to an infusion pump that controls a syringe containing a common addictive substance: morphine, cocaine, nicotine, or methamphetamine. The rats are trained to pull levers for water, but for one hour each day they can use the same system to mainline as much of the drugs as they want. And they want. "Just about any drug that humans abuse, animals will self-administer," Glick says.

Glick gets the rats addicted only to get them back on the wagon later with a substance called 18-methoxycoronaridine (18-MC, for short). The new drug may be the miracle pill that addicts have always needed: A single dose of it can remarkably diminish both withdrawal symptoms and craving. By revealing its mechanism, Glick, director of the Center for Neuropharmacology and Neuroscience at Albany Medical College in New York, offers a new understanding of the brain's pleasure zones.

On the Caribbean island of St. Kitts, neuropharmacologist Deborah Mash of the University of Miami has been running clinical trials of ibogaine on addicts. Of the 272 patients she has treated, none have had major side effects, and almost all have been drug-free at least a month.

Eighteen-MC is a synthesized derivative of ibogaine, an extract of the bark of the root of the African iboga shrub. For centuries the Bwiti tribe of West Africa has used the root for initiation ceremonies and, in smaller amounts, to stay awake during long hunts. The drug's story as an anti-addictive began in 1962, when college dropout and heroin addict Howard Lotsof obtained a dose from a chemist friend. "What happened is indelibly ingrained in my mind," Lotsof says. "I was living with my parents. I felt my feet hit the ground, and I realized I had no desire to use opiates."

In 1986 Lotsof created a company called NDA International and began to supply ibogaine to a clinic for addicts in Holland. The clinic found that ibogaine works in three stages. First the addict has about four hours of waking dreams in which he seems to confront inner demons. This is followed by an eight-to 10-hour "cognitive evaluation period," during which the user analyzes the waking dream. Then comes a sleepless day or two, which Lotsof calls the "residual stimulation phase."

The clinic treated about 30 addicts and reported impressive results: After a single dose, a majority stayed off drugs for several months or more. But Lotsof was unable to find funding for follow-up studies—and they were needed: One of the patients died of unknown causes, and a study at Johns Hopkins University showed that high doses of ibogaine cause brain damage in rats. Lotsof's lack of scientific degrees, as well as his history of drug use, also raised questions.

"The personalities involved are, for lack of a better word, peculiar," says Glick. He is lanky, has a closely trimmed beard, and wears a white lab coat over black pants as if to match his Holstein-style rats. The closest he has ever gotten to drug culture is playing trumpet in a jazz band called SwingDocs. "Certainly in the beginning everybody thought that Lotsof was an absolute lunatic, and I was included. But when you hear the same things enough times from enough people who have taken ibogaine, you've got to believe that there is at least something there that is worth investigating."

> 'What happened is indelibly ingrained in my mind. I felt my feet hit the ground, and I realized I had no desire to use opiates'

In 1991 Glick and his colleagues began to look for a synthetic derivative of ibogaine without the drug's side effects. The search eventually led to Martin Kuehne, a chemist at the University of Vermont who is an expert on the anticancer drug vincristine. Vincristine is structurally similar to ibogaine, and Kuehne knew how to tinker with the compound to produce derivatives. Glick tested 15 or so of the derivatives on rats before zeroing in on 18-MC.

"Withdrawal is related to the rapidity with which the drug disappears from the nervous system," Glick says. "It really reflects the change from the drug state to the nondrug state." To test 18-MC's effect on withdrawal, Glick gave the rats a continuous supply of morphine. He then administered an opiate antagonist that removes morphine from the neurons in the brain and causes immediate withdrawal symptoms. The rats given 18-MC suffered few if any withdrawal symptoms. Unlike people who take ibogaine, who may tremble as well as hallucinate, the animals seemed normal.

Hallucinogens like ibogaine raise serotonin levels in the brain; 18-MC doesn't. At the same time, 18-MC counteracts the increase in dopamine levels that opiates create. When Glick's addicted rats received 18-MC, their dopamine levels plummeted. The next time the rats were offered their daily hour of fun, they just said no. "Here's a drug that supposedly decreases craving, that supposedly decreases self-administration, and it also appears to block a key neurochemical correlate," Glick says. "But the real question is how exactly it is doing this. And this question plagued us for several years."

Activities in the brain occur at synapses, where neurons and receptors almost touch. Neurons fire off chemicals known as neurotransmitters (of which serotonin and dopamine are two), and neurotransmitters find their way to particular receptors. By using a technique that isolates receptors, called patch-clamp electrophysiology, Glick's colleague Mark Fleck discovered that 18-MC blocks only one kind of receptor effectively (ibogaine blocks several, which accounts for its many side effects). Receptors of this kind are clustered in two very specific parts of the brain, which are connected by a channel called the habenulo-interpeduncular pathway.

Since the 1960s, scientists have known that the brain's primary reward circuit is the mesolimbic dopamine pathway. When rats are rigged with electrodes that allow them to stimulate this pathway by pressing a lever, they develop an instant and insatiable craving. "It's an amazing phenomenon," Glick says. "The rats wake up and as soon as they find the lever, they just go nuts pressing it. They'll do it to the exclusion of food and water." When Glick went back and examined similar studies done in the 1980s, he discovered that rats would behave the same way if they were allowed to stimulate another area of the brain—the medial habenula. As it happens, the medial habenula is also part of the habenulo-interpeduncular pathway. "What we believe is that we've found an alternate reward system that has been ignored for 15 years," Glick says.

The two pathways are tightly connected, and the secondary reward system seems able to modulate the activity of the primary pathway. When 18-MC binds to a receptor in the alternate circuit, it sends a signal to the main circuit that dampens its responsiveness. When the rats in a later study had 18-MC injected directly into this secondary pathway, they all but stopped administering morphine to themselves—at least for a day, and sometimes for a few weeks.

Despite the mounting evidence that 18-MC is a simple and clean way to end addiction, Glick, like Lotsof, has had trouble raising funds to test the drug on humans. The problem, he says, is guilt by association. In 1995 the National Institute on Drug Abuse hired a panel of nine academics and nine members of the pharmaceutical industry to review all the existing ibogaine research. After hearing presentations from Lotsof and others, 16 of the panel members reportedly voted to end trials of ibogaine in humans. Unfortunately, Glick says, 18-MC was tarred by the same brush. "I keep fighting the same battles over and over again," he says. "People lump 18-MC with ibogaine, and I'm constantly making the same point—that we've got something that is a hell of a lot better."

In the meantime, Glick gets about three calls a month from addicts and their families. "They're desperate for anything that will help," he says. "They've tried everything. They always want to know when can I give them 18-MC, and it's really hopeless. I'm just not in the position to do that yet."

From *Discover* magazine, May 2003, pp. 24-25. © 2003 by Michael Abrams. Reprinted by permission.

Hungry for the Next Fix

Behind the relentless, misguided search for a medical cure for addiction.

Stanton Peele

AS DIRECTOR OF the National Institute on Drug Abuse (NIDA), Alan Leshner toured the country with a PowerPoint presentation featuring brain scans. The show was a slightly more sophisticated version of the Partnership for a Drug-Free America's famous ad showing an egg frying in a pan. As he flashed magnetic resonance images (MRI's) on a screen, Leshner would say, in effect, "This is your brain on drugs."

Leshner's message was threefold: First, certain drugs are inherently addictive. Second, scientists have discovered the neurochemical processes through which these drugs cause addiction. Third, that understanding will make it possible to develop drugs that cure or prevent addiction. Leshner's traveling PowerPoint show epitomized NIDA's reductionist approach to drug abuse: Take a brain, add a chemical, and voilà, you've got substance dependence.

Leshner left NIDA at the end of November. Coincidentally, Enoch Gordis, head of the National Institute on Alcohol Abuse and Alcoholism (NIAAA) since 1986, retired around the same time. Like Leshner, Gordis sees addiction as a biological problem with a pharmaceutical solution. He believes scientists have "the ability based on new knowledge from neuroscience research to develop pharmacologic treatments that act on brain mechanisms involved in alcohol dependence."

The view of addiction espoused by Leshner and Gordis is at odds with what we know about the actual behavior of drug users and drinkers—including evidence from government-sponsored research. These studies indicate that treatment is neither necessary nor sufficient for overcoming addiction. The main factor in successful resolution of a drug or alcohol problem is the ability to find rewards in ordinary existence and to form caring relationships with people who are not addicts. By looking instead for a magical elixir just over the horizon, NIDA and the NIAAA give short shrift to the individual circumstances that are crucial to understanding why some people abuse drugs.

'A Medical Illness'

NIDA's official mission is, in its own words, "to lead the Nation in bringing the power of science to bear on drug abuse and addiction." Leshner, who has a Ph.D. in physiological psychology, took the agency's helm in 1994. During his tenure NIDA's budget doubled to $781 million, money devoted mainly to biological research that approaches addiction as a disease.

Although drug use "begins with a voluntary behavior," Leshner said in a 2001 interview with *The Journal of the American Medical Association*, it ceases to be voluntary after it repeatedly affects the "pathway deep within the brain" common to all drug addiction. "There's no question it's a medical illness," he said, "and once you have it, it mandates treatment. It's a myth that millions of people get better by themselves."

> Addicts act very much like other human beings: They pursue pleasure or relief, and most will change their behavior when it causes them serious harm, so long as they have reasonable alternatives.

Leshner's model of addiction emphasizes the special power of drugs. After all, he did not travel around the country with MRI images showing how shopping, gambling, or eating potato chips affects the brain. Thus it was startling to see him concede that drug abuse may be fundamentally similar to excessive involvements with other activities that give pleasure or relieve stress. "Over the past 6 months," he said in the November 2 issue of *Science*, "more and more people have been thinking that, contrary to earlier views, there is a commonality between substance addictions and other compulsions." Some of us have been making this point for years, and it does not fit very well with the idea that drugs create addicts by transforming their brains.

As evidence for this view, Leshner would point to MRI scans of experienced drug users, which he claimed differed in characteristic ways from images of ordinary brains. He also cited studies of drug-induced brain changes in animals. He liked to display a map—reminiscent of a phrenology chart—showing which areas of the brain are involved in drug use and addiction.

But Leshner's seemingly scientific claims have never jibed with reality. Consider what the sociologist Lee Robins and the psychiatrist John Helzer found when they headed a team that interviewed veterans who had been addicted to heroin in Vietnam. Only one in eight became readdicted at any time during the three years after they came home. This was not because the rest were abstinent: Six in 10 used a narcotic after returning to the U.S., and a quarter of the previously addicted men used heroin regularly. Yet only one in five of those who used a narcotic after they got home, including only half of those who used heroin regularly, became readdicted.

At the National Institute on Drug Abuse, studies of human behavior have taken a back seat to research involving brain scans, special breeds of rats, and monkeys tethered to drug-dispensing catheters.

The Vietnam situation, of course, was unique. Young men were torn from their homes, sent to a strange and dangerous environment, and offered easy access to heroin. Then they returned to normal life. Still, the results surprised Robins and her associates, who commented: "It is uncomfortable presenting results that differ so much from clinical experience with addicts in treatment. But one should not too readily assume that differences are due to our special sample. After all, when veterans used heroin in the United States… only one in six came to treatment." In other words, looking only at addicts who are treated provides a skewed view of addiction. Indeed, the vets who were treated after they got home actually were more likely to pick up the habit again.

Rats vs. People

Any doubts about the relevance of the Vietnam veterans study are allayed by findings from long-term studies of drug users in

the United States. Long-term cocaine users, for example, generally do not become addicts. And when they do go through periods of abuse, they typically cut back or quit on their own. They may not do so as rapidly as others (and they themselves) wish they would. But addicts act very much like other human beings: They pursue pleasure or relief, and most will change their behavior when it causes them serious harm, so long as they have reasonable alternatives.

According to the National Household Survey on Drug Abuse (overseen by the Substance Abuse and Mental Health Services Administration), about 3 million Americans have used heroin. Of these, one in 10 report using the drug in the last year, and one in 20 say they've used it in the last month. The percentages for cocaine are similar. In both cases, daily use is so rare that the government does not provide figures for it. These findings indicate that the vast majority of heroin and cocaine users either never become addicted or, if they do, soon manage to moderate their use or abstain.

This pattern has been confirmed again and again by government-sponsored research. At NIDA, however, studies of human behavior have taken a back seat to research involving brain scans, special breeds of rats, and monkeys tethered to drug-dispensing catheters.

Given NIDA's biological orientation, it may seem odd that the main form of treatment the agency advocates (pending development of a wonder drug for addiction) involves adopting a new set of quasi-religious beliefs and meeting regularly with like-minded individuals. But NIDA's take on addiction has much in common with the view promoted by Alcoholics Anonymous and its imitators. Both see addiction as a disease involving loss of control that can be overcome only through abstinence.

NIDA's support for drug treatment based on A.A.-like principles, the dominant approach in the United States, flies in the face of its avowed commitment to rigorous science—a conflict illustrated in the last issue of NIDA's newsletter published under Leshner. A front-page article announced the disastrous long-term consequences of heroin use, based on a study that followed a group of addicts for more than 30 years. "The death rate among the members of the group is 50 to 100 times the rate among the general population of men in the same age range," the article said. "Even among surviving members of the group," the lead researcher added, "severe consequences such as high levels of health problems, criminal behavior and incarceration, and public assistance were associated with long-term heroin use."

Yet the subjects of this study were criminal offenders in California who were forced to attend abstinence-oriented, A.A.-style group sessions between 1962 and 1964. In other words, they benefited from just the sort of treatment NIDA advocates. Undaunted, Leshner began his column in the same issue of the newsletter with the cheery news that "NIDA's quarter century of research has produced a basic unequivocal message—drug addiction is a treatable brain disease." Yet today's preferred treatment is indistinguishable from the programs those California convicts attended in the 1960s.

Sugar: The Miracle Cure

If Leshner and Gordis are right, A.A.-style therapy will ultimately be replaced, or at least supplemented, by drugs that block addiction. The leading candidate so far is naltrexone, which is reputed to curb the urge for both heroin and alcohol. Naltrexone has been approved for treatment of alcohol dependence, and Gordis, an M.D., promoted the drug as the first in the pharmacopoeia he envisioned for alcoholism.

A study published in December made that prospect seem unlikely. The researchers divided 600 alcoholics into three groups: One received naltrexone for a year, another was given naltrexone for three months followed by nine months of sugar pills, and the third group took just the placebo. The subjects began the study drinking, on average, on two out of every three days, 13 drinks on each occasion. One year after their treatment began, these men were drinking one-quarter as frequently and consuming somewhat less when they did drink. But the reduction was about the same for the men who took the fake pills as it was for those who were given naltrexone.

Announced in *The New England Journal of Medicine*, these findings were incomprehensible to anyone who accepts the view of alcoholism promoted by the NIAAA. Aside from the evidence against naltrexone's effectiveness, it was stunning that sugar pills enabled severe alcoholics to reduce their drinking without abstaining completely, which alcoholism experts in the United States teach is impossible. Yet every major study of alcoholism carried out during Gordis' tenure at the NIAAA yielded the same sort of results. It's just that Gordis spent much of his energy denying what his own agency had found.

In 1992 the NIAAA surveyed more than 42,000 randomly selected Americans in the National Longitudinal Alcohol Epidemiologic Survey. Census Bureau interviewers questioned each respondent about his or her lifetime drug and alcohol use. Of special interest were 4,585 respondents who at some time in their lives were "alcohol dependent" (what most people call alcoholic). Of this group, only about a quarter were ever treated for alcoholism (including A.A. as treatment). But the treated group was no more likely to have improved, as measured by either abstinence or drinking without abuse. In fact, more treated (33 percent) than untreated alcoholics (28 percent) were continuing to abuse alcohol.

One reason untreated alcoholics did better was that many more of them reduced their drinking without abstaining. Among people who at some point in their lives had qualified as alcohol dependent but were never treated, nearly "6 in 10" or "more than half" (58 percent) in the untreated group were drinking without a diagnosable problem. Including all the treated and untreated alcoholics in this random sample of Americans, half were drinking without abusing alcohol.

Driven Not to Drink

The NIAAA sponsored another ambitious study—the largest trial of psychotherapy ever conducted. Completed in 1996, the study was known as Project MATCH because it was aimed at determining whether different treatments could be "matched" to specific types of alcoholics to produce optimum results. One of the therapies, based on A.A.'s 12 steps, was called "12-step facilitation." A second was dubbed "coping skills therapy." The third was "motivational enhancement therapy." Nearly half of the 1,700 or so subjects underwent hospital treatment first; the rest entered the MATCH treatments directly.

All the therapies performed equally well, but one was considerably simpler than the others: Motivational enhancement involved four sessions with each alcoholic, compared to 12 for the two other types of therapy (although, on average, subjects attended only two-thirds of the sessions scheduled for any of the therapies). Motivational enhancement brings into focus and strengthens the individual's own drive for sobriety, but it leaves the mechanics of sobriety to the alcoholics themselves.

Although the Project MATCH subjects had few counseling sessions (especially in motivational enhancement therapy), their drinking was periodically assessed following treatment. These interactions with the project, intended solely for research purposes, seem to have had the effect of keeping alcoholics focused on controlling their drinking.

Whatever treatment alcoholics received in Project MATCH, few abstained for even a year. Gordis and his colleagues instead emphasized dramatic reductions in drinking by the subjects. Whereas they averaged 25 days of drinking a month prior to treatment, after a year they were drinking only six days out of the month. Moreover, the average number of drinks they consumed each time they drank dropped from 15 to three.

In all three of these prominent studies—the naltrexone trial, the NIAAA's national survey, and Project MATCH—the results were essentially the same. Even with clinical alcoholics, minimal treatments were as successful as more elaborate ones, and the best indicator of success was the alcoholics' ability to cut back their drinking rather than quit altogether. But how can sugar pills or a few sessions of motivational enhancement help alcoholics control their drinking? The basic ingredients for successful treatment are 1) identifying a problem with the agreement of the addict, 2) believing change is possible, 3) placing primary responsibility on the addict for carrying out the change, 4) accepting reductions in use as well as abstinence, and 5) following up to let addicts know someone cares and wants to make sure they stay on course.

Beyond Abstinence

In the face of studies that cast doubt on traditional notions about alcoholism, Gordis seemed to consider it his duty to explain why they actually confirmed the conventional wisdom. Project MATCH in particular presented a serious P.R. problem for the NIAAA: It spent more than $30 million without fulfilling its purpose of identifying principles for matching alcoholics to treatments. This is how Gordis spun the results: "The good news is that treatment works. All three treatments… produced excellent overall outcomes."

Although Gordis relied on reduced drinking as a measure of success to put the best gloss on Project MATCH, he has always quashed any revision of the abstinence-oriented goals that characterize virtually all American alcoholism treatment. Responding to a 1997 *U.S. News and World Report* story on Moderation Management, a program for reducing alcohol consumption among problem drinkers, Gordis sternly warned that "current evidence supports abstinence as the appropriate goal for persons with the medical disorder 'alcohol dependence' (alcoholism)."

While abstinence may be a desirable goal for these individuals, not many accomplish it. Project MATCH engaged the top clinical practitioners and researchers in the United States in designing and supervising treatment for alcoholics. As a result of this attentive, sophisticated care, which is unlikely to be matched by any program an alcoholic could find in the real world, about a quarter of the subjects abstained for as long as a year.

Gordis' attitude seems to be: "Most alcoholics won't abstain after treatment, but they should! And we are not going to accept anything less than this worthy, if unreachable, goal." His attitude is especially disturbing since Project MATCH found that reductions in drinking were beneficial. The subjects' liver functioning typically improved, and they displayed fewer problems associated with drinking. Surely, better health and less destructive behavior are worthy goals.

Since Gordis spoke for the U.S. alcohol treatment establishment, his rigidity condemned American alcoholics to limp along, most continuing to drink, with little chance of finding assistance in limiting their drinking or reducing its negative consequences. We will never eliminate drinking and drug use. But we might be able to reduce the harm they sometimes cause if we could eliminate the pseudoscientific moralism dispensed by the likes of Leshner and Gordis.

Stanton Peele (www.peele.net), a psychologist and attorney, is the author of several books on addiction.

A new treatment for addiction

The FDA recently approved buprenorphine for the treatment of opiate addiction. Psychologists helped develop the drug and will provide key services to patients treated with it.

BY ETIENNE BENSON
Monitor **staff**

Approximately one million Americans are dependent on heroin, prescription painkillers and other opioids, but the vast majority of them—as many as 800,000—aren't receiving any treatment.

Opiate substitutes that prevent withdrawal are among the most effective treatments for such addictions, when combined with psychological counseling, researchers say. But until recently, only two such drugs—methadone and levo-alpha-acetyl methadol (LAAM)—were available, and only licensed treatment clinics were authorized to dispense them. Many addicts avoid opiate treatment programs (OTPs) because of their inconvenience or perceived stigma, and even those who would like to enroll sometimes can't because of limited treatment slots.

The approval of a new medication by the Food and Drug Administration (FDA) last fall, however, could reshape the landscape of opiate addiction treatment in the United States, making pharmacotherapy available and attractive to patients who previously shunned it, say researchers.

Psychologists have played a key role in developing the medication—buprenorphine—by conducting the basic and clinical research that defined its unusual pharmacology. They are continuing to shape its use by influencing training programs for physicians. And they are developing the behavioral and psychosocial treatments that are a critical part of any effective substance abuse treatment program.

And as the network of physicians who are certified to prescribe buprenorphine grows, it should also provide new opportunities for psychologists to get involved in pharmacotherapy-based substance abuse treatment by making such treatments available in a wide variety of settings and increasing the number of patients who use pharmacotherapies—and who therefore need the counseling and behavioral treatments that psychologists can provide.

"It's a very, very exciting time to be involved with buprenorphine work," says psychologist Leslie Amass, PhD, of the Friends Research Institute in Santa Monica, Calif., who has been studying the use of buprenorphine as a treatment for opiate addiction since the early 1990s.

"For those of us who have been involved with the medication from very early on, it's rewarding to see it get to this point and be offered to patients."

Unique pharmacology

Buprenorphine has been under development for several decades, during which time psychologists have discovered a great deal about its unusual pharmacology, says Amass.

Their discoveries have been made possible, in large part, by support from the National Institute on Drug Abuse (NIDA) and other government agencies concerned with substance abuse. NIDA's Division of Treatment Research and Development, headed by Frank Vocci, PhD, has played an especially important leadership role, says Geoff Mumford, PhD, APA's science policy director.

Like heroin, methadone and many prescription painkillers, buprenorphine acts on the brain's mu-opioid receptors to cause analgesia, euphoria and other effects. But unlike them, it is a partial agonist—a drug that has mechanisms of action that are similar to pure agonists, such as heroin, but with less potency. Even when it occupies almost all of the brain's mu-opioid receptors, buprenorphine has only about 40 percent of heroin's effect, says psychologist Mark Greenwald, PhD, of Wayne State University's Addiction Research Institute in Detroit.

Another pharmacological factor that makes buprenorphine well-suited to addiction treatment is its high affinity for the mu-opioid receptor, says psychologist James Woods, PhD, of the University of Michigan, who has studied buprenorphine's pharmacology in animals.

"It has an absolutely fascinating course of action," says Woods. Even after it's been removed from the blood by elimination and metabolism, he says, buprenorphine stays firmly attached to the brain's receptors, blocking the effect of other drugs with lower affinities. That means that opiate-dependent individuals who take buprenorphine won't get any additional kick from using other opiates, such as heroin.

Buprenorphine's stickiness has another advantage, says Greenwald. Because it clings to the receptor long after it has been administered, it can make the detoxification process gentler—more like sliding down a hill than falling off a cliff. "You get a softer landing, if you will, as you detoxify someone from buprenorphine," he says. It also means that buprenorphine doesn't have to be administered every day to be effective.

But while buprenorphine's stickiness and partial-agonist effects make it ideal for many addiction treatment applications, they also limit its effectiveness with the most heavily dependent individuals, researchers say. In such individuals, buprenorphine's insistent weakness—its ability to monopolize mu-opioid receptors while providing only a fraction of the effect of drugs such as heroin—can actually trigger withdrawal symptoms.

Although buprenorphine has been tested extensively in humans and nonhuman animals, there is still much to learn, researchers say. "There are very elemental things about the way it interacts with the receptor that we don't understand yet," notes Woods.

In ongoing efforts to resolve those uncertainties, psychologists' scientific training has been and will be critical, says Greenwald. "Their ability to design controlled studies—using valid and sensitive models that are relevant to drug dependence—gives them a unique opportunity to contribute," he notes.

Translation to practice

Psychologists have also played a key role in determining how buprenorphine can best be used clinically. The consensus is that, as with other medications used to treat addiction, buprenorphine will be most effective when paired with psychological treatments.

"No one feels that buprenorphine alone is going to be that successful in the treatment of a complex disorder such as addiction without appropriate counseling, psychotherapy, etc.," says psychologist Charles Schuster, PhD, of Wayne State University, who has been involved in both the research and regulatory aspects of buprenorphine's development.

"Now that the medication has been approved, psychologists trained in substance abuse treatment will be essential partners in this important new treatment paradigm," agrees H. Westley Clark, MD, JD, director of the Center for Substance Abuse Treatment (CSAT) at the Substance Abuse and Mental Health Services Administration (SAMHSA).

Clark notes that the legislation that authorized office-based prescription of buprenorphine—the Drug Abuse Treatment Act of 2000 (DATA)—explicitly acknowledges the importance of behavioral treatments. The law requires certified physicians to have the capacity to refer patients to qualified behavioral health treatment providers.

One of the psychologists who has studied buprenorphine the longest is Warren Bickel, PhD, of the University of Vermont. Bickel and his colleagues have shown that buprenorphine can still be effective when given on alternate days or even every third, fourth or fifth day. That, Bickel notes, could make a huge difference in states such as Vermont, where patients sometimes have to drive for hours to get to the nearest certified doctor or OTP.

The availability of buprenorphine in physicians' offices offers great opportunities, but it also raises new challenges, says Bickel. For instance, OTPs provide integrated pharmacotherapy and psychotherapy in a single setting—something that many patients who go to their physicians for buprenorphine won't find, he says.

"It's imperative that these patients not only receive medication, but also receive the additional services that they really need to do well," he says. "But getting that to happen, I think, is the challenge that faces us in this new era."

As buprenorphine use spreads, there is also the risk that the drug might be diverted from patients to abusers. Rickitt Benckiser Pharmaceuticals offers two formulations of the drug: Subutex, which contains just buprenorphine, and Suboxone, which contains a combination of buprenorphine and naloxone, an opiate antagonist. Neither formulation appears to have a large potential for abuse relative to other opioids. (Suboxone, which is expected to be the standard formulation, is an effective opiate substitute when taken under the tongue, but can trigger withdrawal if injected.)

But the FDA isn't taking any chances. Wayne State psychologist Schuster has been picked to lead a large-scale surveillance effort that includes ethnographic reports, surveys of physicians, monitoring of chat rooms, news groups and other Internet resources, and interviews with patients—all in the hopes of catching signs of buprenorphine abuse before it spreads.

The surveillance effort is slated to run for five years, with Schuster's research team providing quarterly reports to an advisory group. "If a problem is emerging, we want to catch it early," he says.

Building a network

Buprenorphine's transition from a promising experimental drug to a prescription medication was made possible by two events: the enactment of DATA and the FDA's approval, both of which were the culmination of many years of research and lobbying. But turning it into an effective treatment will require building a network of certified physicians and psychologists prepared to offer the kinds of therapy that are essential to the medication's success.

> **"Buprenorphine offers yet another opportunity to demonstrate the important contribution that psychologists can make in partnership with our physician colleagues."**
>
> *Norman B. Anderson*
> *APA CEO*

To aid patients and treatment providers in finding local physicians who can prescribe buprenorphine, CSAT offers on online Buprenorphine Physician Locator at http://buprenorphine.samhsa.gov/bwns_locator. Meanwhile, progress in training physicians—using curricula that have been shaped by psychologists—has been rapid.

For its part, APA has been trying to help build the buprenorphine network by encouraging appropriately trained psychologists to make themselves available to referral resources. In a recent letter to state psychological associations, APA CEO Norman B. Anderson, PhD, emphasized the importance of collaboration in realizing buprenorphine's potential. "Buprenorphine offers yet another opportunity to demonstrate the important contribution that psycholo-gists can make in partnership with our physician colleagues," he wrote.

ON THE WEB

- **Substance Abuse and Mental Health Services Administrations:** http://buprenorphine.samhsa.gov
- **Food and Drug Administration:** www.fda.gov/cder/drug/infopage/subutex_suboxone
- **American Society for Addiction Medicine:** www.asam.org/conf/Buprenorphineconferences.htm
- **Reckitt Benckiser Pharmaceuticals:** www.suboxone.com

FINDING THE FUTURE ALCOHOLIC

Scientists may soon be able to identify children who are likely to become alcoholics. But will society be able to prevent their addiction?

By Steven Stocker

Many alcoholics tell the same story: Before they took their first drink they felt constantly anxious, irritable, or depressed. Afterwards, they felt normal for the first time in their lives.

The first time Judy drank alcohol, she knew it was for her. "It was a sort of 'Eureka!' experience. It wasn't so much that I felt good, it was just that I suddenly felt right," she says.

Judy had been a shy, depressed teenager in high school, but in college she blossomed, largely under the influence of alcohol. Drinking helped her socialize, dance, and even write. But eventually alcohol began to show its downside, contributing to the breakup of her first marriage and causing problems at work. After 13 years of heavy drinking, Judy quit and is now in her twentieth year of recovery.

Researchers speculate that people who abuse alcohol are trying to self-medicate some type of brain abnormality. Alcohol temporarily quells the symptoms of this abnormality, but when its effects wear off the symptoms return, worse than ever. To keep them under control, people continue to drink—greater amounts and more frequently—until they become dependent on alcohol.

People from families of alcoholics respond differently on certain blood and electroencephalogram (EEG) tests, raising the possibility that either these tests, or perhaps tests for genes associated with these abnormal responses, might be able to identify children who are more likely to become alcoholics. Once identified, they could be treated with medications and/or behavioral therapies to prevent them from becoming dependent on alcohol.

The Personality of the Alcoholic

C. Robert Cloninger, a psychiatrist at Washington University in St. Louis, has proposed that there are two fundamental personality types among alcoholics. The first, like Judy, is anxious, inhibited, eager to please others, and rigid. The second resembles an action hero: confident, impulsive, socially detached, and constantly seeking new experiences. The second type is also aggressive, getting into bar fights when drunk and often crossing the line into criminal behavior.

Research suggests that the anxious, inhibited type of alcholic may have a brain that is hypersensitive to stress.

The two personality types were first identified in studies of adopted men and women in Sweden, where careful records are kept on alcoholics. Because the alcohol-related behaviors of these people were more similar to their biological parents than to their adopted parents, researchers suspected that distinct genes were contributing to the development of the two alcoholism personality types.

More recent studies indicate that the two types of alcoholic personalities—inhibited and impulsive—respond differently on biological tests, supporting the notion that their differences are associated with distinct genes. For example, research at the Johns Hopkins University School of Medicine suggests that the anxious, inhibited type of alcoholic may have a brain that is hypersensitive to stress. This hypersensitivity can be detected by measuring the blood level of the hormone cortisol that is secreted in response to a chemical stressor.

Hypersensitivity to stress might be caused by a deficiency in the brain of *endogenous opioids*, compounds similar to morphine and heroin that occur naturally in the brain and the body and slow the release of stress hormones such as cortisol, according to neuroendocrinologist Gary Wand, who is conducting the Johns Hopkins research.

These natural opioids provide people with a sense of well-being. When the effects of the opioids are blocked, people feel depressed, tense, tired, and confused, and they have a hard time concentrating, performing poorly on reasoning and memory tasks.

Theoretically, people with opioid deficiency would feel tense all the time, as if they were in the middle of final exams week every second of their lives.

Wand believes that the high cortisol producers may be using alcohol to self-medicate their underlying opioid deficiency. Alcohol releases opioids in the brain, which would bring the opioid levels up to where they should be, at least temporarily.

Monkeys reared without adults, with only same-aged peers, show prolonged immaturity, including fearfulness and emotional instability. Such experiences have long-term effects on the brain and behavior, increasing risk for alcohol abuse during adolescence and impaired neurotransmission in some systems of the adult brain.

Another reason that high cortisol producers would like alcohol better than normal cortisol producers is that high cortisol levels produced by chronic stress make the brain's reward system more responsive to potentially addictive substances such as alcohol. As a result, high cortisol producers get more "bang for the buck" from an alcoholic drink.

Although Wand thinks that opioid deficiency is genetic, he leaves open the possibility that it is acquired during childhood. "Households with alcoholics are generally dysfunctional, where there's a lot more stress, so we may be looking at the adverse effects of chronic stress on the development of brain opioid activity," he says.

Anxiety and Alcoholism In Monkeys

In a recent study conducted by psychologist James Dee Higley and others at the National Institutes of Health Animal Center in Poolesville, Maryland, researchers induced stress in six-month-old rhesus monkeys by separating them from other monkeys to which they were emotionally attached. The monkeys' blood cortisol levels were measured during the separation. When the monkeys were four years old, the scientists gave them access to alcohol and found that the monkeys who drank the most alcohol were also the ones who had produced the highest levels of cortisol when stressed as infants. The monkeys

continued to produce high levels of cortisol throughout their life span.

The researchers call these high cortisol-producing animals their "uptight" monkeys. They cower in their cages, hugging themselves and sucking their thumbs. They seldom approach other monkeys or rise to a high social rank. Higley notes that when uptight monkeys drink alcohol they seem to be self-medicating, because alcohol causes them to stop exhibiting anxious behaviors and to interact better with the other monkeys.

Let's assume that high cortisol levels in response to stress during development can help to produce uptight humans who self-medicate their chronic anxiety with alcohol, just like the uptight monkeys. Theoretically, if we could identify these at-risk children, perhaps using a genetic test, we could find ways to prevent them from becoming alcoholics.

Substance abusers may turn to drink and drugs because their brains are hyperactive and they are trying to calm themselves down.

One possibility, Wand speculates, is to treat them with antidepressants, such as Prozac or Zoloft, that have been shown to be effective in treating anxiety disorders. Another possibility is to treat them with a new class of medications being developed that blocks the action of CRH, the hormone that triggers the release of stress hormones. CRH also acts as a neurotransmitter in the brain, where it mediates that tense, aversive feeling you get when you're unpleasantly stressed. Higley and his colleagues will be administering one of these new CRH blockers on a long-term basis to a group of their uptight monkeys starting in infancy to see if it can prevent them from developing their passion for alcohol.

Understanding the Hyperexcitable Brain

Unlike the shy and depressed Judy, Eric represents the impulsive, antisocial type of substance abuser who generally starts drinking and taking drugs earlier than the anxious type. Eric smoked his first joint at age 10, started drinking alcohol at 14, and began using cocaine at 17.

Even if we don't force every child to take alcoholism vulnerability tests, controversy is still inevitable when we start medicating those who score positive on the tests.

"I was always hyper. I lived for excitement—fighting, chasing girls," says Eric. "I was always seeking attention. I felt that, if I didn't get enough attention, I was going to do something to get it." He remembers that when he was five or six years old he broke a fish tank in his elementary school because he felt that his teacher wasn't paying enough attention to him.

Substance abusers such as Eric may turn to drink and drugs because their brains are hyperactive and they are trying to calm themselves down. This theory, proposed by neuroscientists Henri Begleiter and Bernice Porjesz at the State University of New York Health Science Center in Brooklyn, is derived from EEG studies of alcoholics and their offspring. They found similar brain-wave responses to stimuli between alcoholics and their sons.

EEGs will probably never be used to screen all children for potential alcoholism because it is too time-consuming and cumbersome, according to Begleiter. Studying brain-wave responses in children at risk for alcoholism is principally a step toward identifying genes that confer a vulnerability to alcoholism, since genes that contribute to a reduced brainwave response to stimuli should also contribute to this vulnerability. Once the genes are identified, tests for these genes could be conducted using blood samples taken from children, and medications could be given to the children who test positive for the genes. The medications would reduce the overexcitation in their brains, thereby theoretically reducing their inclination to drink alcohol when they get older.

Preempting Alcoholism: A Scenario

Let's assume that scientists eventually develop genetic or other tests that reliably identify children at risk for alcoholism. And let's say further that we start giving these tests to every 10-year-old in the country. One day, a child will refuse to take the genetic test. How should society react?

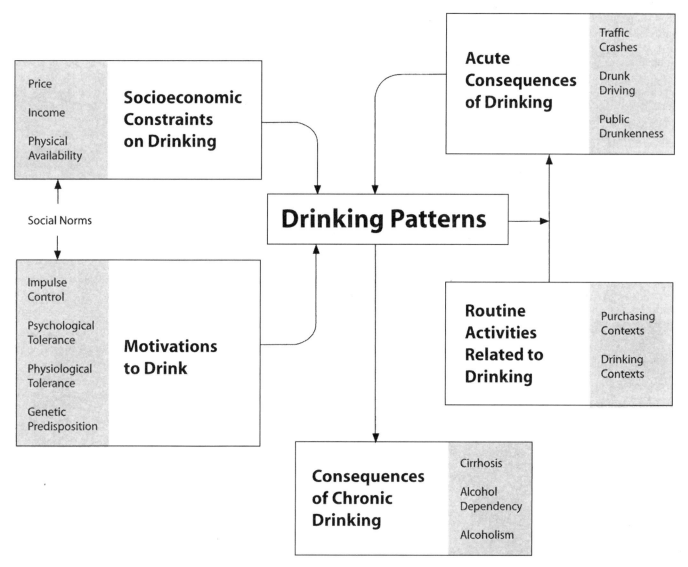

Alcoholism is not just about genetics. This schematic illustration shows the interlinked components of drinking behavior: the motivations to drink, socioeconomic constraints on drinking, health and other consequences of drinking, and routine activities.
Source: *Alcohol Health and Research World*/NIAAA

"Society has yet to compel anyone to take a genetic test or even a test for an infectious disease such as AIDS no matter how damaging their future behavior may be," notes Gary Wand. He points to court cases in which rape victims wanted to know the HIV status of their perpetrators, but the courts ruled that rapists could not be forced to take HIV tests.

Even if we don't force every child to take alcoholism vulnerability tests, controversy is still inevitable when we start medicating those who score positive on the tests. Given that the biological forces

contributing to alcoholism are probably complex, it will be a long time before clinicians agree on which medications are best. And inevitably, many parents will not want to give their children psychoactive medications.

James Dee Higley of the National Institutes of Health sees a situation developing that is similar to what we have now with Ritalin and attention deficit disorder (ADD). Ritalin and other mild stimulants have been shown to help children with ADD pay attention, but many parents are reluctant to give these drugs to their children.

However, giving medications to children is probably not the only way to prevent alcoholism. "I suspect that we could prevent much of the alcoholism that occurs simply by altering rearing conditions and teaching good parenting skills," says Higley. This is because environmental factors—such as interactions in the family, school, or neighborhood—contribute as much to the development of alcoholism as bad genes do.

Higley argues that he can produce a monkey that consumes vast quantities of alcohol no matter what its genetic makeup is simply by taking it away from its mother at birth and raising it in a cage with three other monkeys of the same age. "Monkey mothers do two things extraordinarily well," he explains. "First, they reduce arousal in their infants by comforting them so that, in time, the infants learn how to reduce their own arousal. And second, they react negatively when the infants behave inappropriately."

In the absence of its mother, the infant monkey develops into an anxious adult, because it has never learned how to reduce its own arousal, and also into an impulsive adult, because it has never learned how to limit its behavior. It drinks alcohol when given the opportunity because it constantly feels bad—a sort of monkey form of existential nausea—and has learned that alcohol can make it feel better. In other words, the motherless monkey is like a hybrid of the two types of human alcoholics: the anxious type and the impulsive type.

In the future, both medications and behavioral treatments will have roles to play in preventing these two types of alcoholism. In some instances, medications will be useful, like Ritalin in the more severe cases of ADD. In other cases, we must teach parents how to be better parents.

About the Author

Steven Stocker is a science writer who has published articles in *The Washington Post* and *Baltimore City Paper*. He has also written for magazines published by the National Institute on Drug Abuse and the National Center for Research Resources, both of which are components of the National Institutes of Health. His address is 18712 Curry Powder Lane, Germantown, Maryland 20874. Telephone 1-301-216-2071; e-mail sstockerl@earthlink.net.

Originally published in the May/June 2002 issue of *The Futurist.*, pp. 41-46. Used with permission from the World Future Society, 7910 Woodmont Avenue, Suite 450, Bethesda, MD 20814. Telephone: 301/656-8274; Fax: 301/951-0394; http://www.wfs.org. © 2002.

Drug abuse in the balance

Researchers, regulators and drug developers met recently to assess the state-of-the-art in drug-abuse liability assessment.

BY ETIENNE BENSON
Monitor staff

In the 1880s, Sigmund Freud noted that cocaine had a number of pleasing effects—euphoria, tiredness, heightened mental acuity— and thought it might even help one of his friends, Ernst von Fleischl-Marxow, recover from a devastating morphine addiction. Needless to say, he was wrong. Fleischl's cocaine addiction proved to be much worse than his morphine addiction had been, and eventually—but too late for Fleischl—Freud realized his mistake and retracted his support for the drug.

Preventing that kind of disaster from recurring is one of the reasons that researchers since have tried to develop rigorous, reliable methods of determining whether new medications have any potential for abuse, and why U.S. lawmakers have developed strict regulations for the medical use of drugs with high abuse potential.

But with new drugs constantly being developed—some of which have pharmacologies fundamentally different from those of cocaine, her-oin and other conventionally abused drugs—that challenge continues to grow. At a recent conference in Bethesda, Md., researchers, drug developers and federal regulators met to assess the state-of-the-art in drug-abuse liability assessment (ALA) and to draw up a list of recommendations and research priorities for the field. The conference was sponsored by the College on Problems of Drug Dependence (CPDD), APA and a number of other professional and scientific societies.

Identifying key questions

The central question in ALA, according to Wayne State psychologist Charles Schuster, PhD, one of the meeting's organizers and a former director of the National Institute on Drug Abuse, is about how to balance the needs of patients who might benefit from new medications with the need to reduce the incidence of drug abuse.

"A variety of new medications are being developed that have interest-ing therapeutic usefulness for the treatment of a variety of psychiatric disorders, but that also have the potential for misuse and abuse," he says. "How can we properly evaluate them so that we can prevent drugs with high abuse potential from being marketed without any warning to physicians, and without regulation? And also, on the other hand, ensure that regulators in the federal government don't overly regulate drugs and thereby prevent access to drugs with great medical potential?"

Another key question, says Virginia Commonwealth University psychologist Robert Balster, PhD, who presented one of the meeting's background papers, is whether the techniques that have served researchers well in assessing the abuse liability of older drugs will succeed when applied to the new kinds of drugs moving through the pipeline.

"We know best how to perform scientific research on drugs that are similar to heroin, cocaine, alcohol and barbiturates," he says. "We don't know so much about drugs with other kinds of pharmacologies, such as ketamine-like drugs [e.g., PCP] or cannabinoids."

Determining the best way to track the abuse of a drug after it has been released into the market is also a high priority, says meeting organizer Chris-Ellyn Johanson, PhD, of Wayne State University.

That question has gained more importance recently, she says, because the Food and Drug Administration (FDA) has increased its emphasis on risk management. Instead of asking pharmaceutical companies only to demonstrate that a drug has low abuse potential in studies that take place before the drug is marketed, she says, the agency is now also asking them to answer the question, "If you have evidence that a drug is being abused, how are you going to handle it?

"It's now realized that regardless of how much you study a drug [before marketing it], we don't have perfect models, so things can slip through," says Johanson. "The problem is that the survey systems that are in place don't really get you that evidence until several years down the pike." With the rise of the Internet, it has become easier than ever for drug abusers to share information about the abuse potential of new medications through e-mail, chat rooms and Web sites. Now researchers are trying to find similarly effective ways of tracking patterns of drug abuse. One solution may lie in post-marketing surveillance, the subject of a conference presentation by Theodore Cicero, PhD, of Washington University.

The goal of post-marketing surveillance is to detect a drug-abuse "signal"—an early warning that a new medication is being abused by patients or the drug abusing population. In some cases, post-marketing surveillance might show that the

FDA's restrictions on new drugs are tougher than they need to be, says Johanson; in other cases, unexpected abuse of a drug after marketing could lead to tightened restrictions.

Drawing conclusions

The conference's final conclusions and recommendations will not be published until this spring, when they are expected to appear in a special issue of the journal *Drug and Alcohol Dependence*, but a preliminary outline was presented at the end of the meeting. According to APA Science Policy Director Geoff Mumford, PhD, who helped organize the meeting, the outline largely affirmed that existing animal and human laboratory methods provide valid assessments of abuse potential, but it also pointed out avenues for improvement.

"There was general agreement that the science base for drug-abuse liability assessment is strong," he says, "but the discussions also highlighted some new opportunities."

For example, it would be easy to collect data relevant to drug abuse from patients as part of most clinical trials, he says, but that rarely happens. The panel also made the following recommendations:

- The drug-abuse liability assessment field should identify a set of measures and methods that are essential to valid drug-abuse liability assessment.
- Although an effective scientific framework for assessing the abuse liability of new drugs is in place—one that relies heavily on laboratory-based behavioral tests in animals—researchers should continue to update and refine that framework to incorporate new findings and to address questions raised by new drug classes.

- Current methods of post-marketing surveillance are limited in their usefulness; new techniques should be developed to monitor drug abuse in various communities.

The results of the meeting will help fill a temporary gap left by the dissolution of the Drug Abuse Advisory Committee, which was commissioned by the FDA in 1978 to provide expert advice on drug-abuse liability assessment, says Mumford. The committee was dissolved in 2000 and then reconstituted as a standing subcommittee of the Drug Safety and Risk Management Advisory Committee in 2002.

The meeting also accomplished another important result: lowering the barriers to communication that separate the diverse professional groups that participate in ALA. According to Drug Enforcement Administration psychologist Christine Sannerud, PhD, for instance, such meetings provide valuable opportunities for federal regulators to explain how the results of scientific research enter into the scheduling process.

Meeting organizer Johanson agrees. "It's unusual to have all the stakeholders—academic, government and industry—together in a single meeting," she says, "but it is very important that all of these people talk to each other."

Psychologists whose background papers were presented at the meeting included Robert Balster, PhD, of Virginia Commonwealth University, and Nancy Ator, PhD, Roland Griffiths, PhD, and George Bigelow, PhD, of Johns Hopkins University. A number of other psychologists also played ciritical roles in the meeting as organizers, expert panel members and representatives of professional, government and industry organizations.

From *Monitor on Psychology*, January 2003, pp. 38-39. © 2003 by the American Psychological Association.

OPIOIDS For people with chronic suffering, these powerful pills are a godsend. For others, they're a prescription for abuse and misery.

IN THE GRIP OF A DEEPER PAIN

BY JERRY ADLER

THEY WERE INVENTED TO STOP PAIN, THE KIND THAT TRAVELS up the spinal cord, and they're remarkably effective at it: the synthetic opioids developed since the 1970s can mute the agony of slipped disks, deteriorating joints, tooth decay and even terminal cancer. If that was all they did, then it wouldn't be much of a problem; most people acquire the drugs innocently enough by prescription and take them only as long as they need to, and even the risk of dependence may be worth running, if the alternative is lifelong pain. The problem with painkillers is they also work on existential pain, the kind that originates in the mind—such as might be experienced by a right-wing radio host who doesn't have Bill Clinton to torture anymore. Cindy McCain, the wife of the Arizona senator, took Vicodin, a common opioid, for back pain, but she found it also helped her get through the "Keating Five" investigation involving her husband. "The newspaper articles didn't hurt as much, and I didn't hurt as much," she wrote in NEWSWEEK in 2001. "I've had clients describe Vicodin as 'a four-hour vacation'" from daily stress, says Robert Weathers, clinical director at Passages, a Malibu, Calif., super-deluxe rehab facility catering to clients who can afford monthly charges north of $30,000.

And more and more people are making that unfortunate discovery, it seems. Illegitimate use of OxyContin (a trade name for oxycodone), one of the drugs to which Rush Limbaugh was allegedly linked, has skyrocketed in recent years. At least 1.9 million Americans have admitted taking it illegitimately at least once, the Drug Enforcement Administration recently reported. "Right now it's one of the most abused prescription drugs," says one DEA official. "It's certainly the most dangerous."

Limbaugh's other narcotic of choice, according to news reports, was hydrocodone, the generic name for a family of drugs including Vicodin, Lorcet and Lortab. These drugs also have a high potential for abuse—although the DEA lists them on Schedule III, a lower level of control than OxyContin, a Schedule II drug—and they accounted for slightly more emergency-room visits than oxycodone last year. Both classes of drugs work the same way, by locking on to a chemical receptor called *mu*, which blocks the transmission of pain in the spinal cord. Taken quickly and in large doses, the drugs also stimulate the production of dopamine in the brain, which can produce effects that mimic street narcotics. Long-term use of Vicodin has been linked, in very rare cases, to hearing loss; there's no published data yet on OxyContin. There's one other big difference, which helps explain why OxyContin has such a high profile in the DEA's view. Its great virtue is that it can be formulated in time-release tablets, packing as much as 12 hours worth of medication in one dose; hydrocodone pills, by contrast, usually last only about four hours. But that also opens the door to abuse; if you can defeat OxyContin's time-release function by pulverizing the pills and then swallowing, snorting or dissolving and injecting the powder, you can get seriously high. People can and do become addicted to hydrocodone, which is more widely prescribed than OxyContin. But Vicodin and its relatives also contain acetaminophen (Tylenol), creating a built-in disincentive to overdose: winding up in the hospital with liver failure.

HOW PAINKILLERS WORK

Millions rely on them for legitimate medical relief. But the illegal use of these drugs has jumped in recent years, as have related visits to the emergency room. Here's how opioids function in the body, and how they can lead to addiction.

1 TARGET SITES: Opioids travel through the bloodstream to the brain, where they interrupt incoming pain signals.

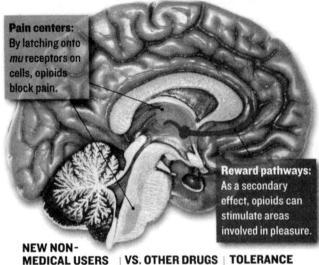

Pain centers: By latching onto *mu* receptors on cells, opioids block pain.

Reward pathways: As a secondary effect, opioids can stimulate areas involved in pleasure.

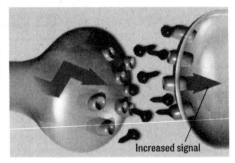

2 NORMAL BRAIN: The chemical dopamine jumps between brain cells in the reward pathway, producing pleasurable feelings.

3 BRAIN ON OPIOIDS: Painkillers can stimulate the release of extra dopamine, strengthening reward signals and pleasurable sensations.

NEW NON-MEDICAL USERS

2 million		
1		
1965		2001

VS. OTHER DRUGS

Millions of users in 2002, 12 yrs old+

Marijuana	25.7
Painkillers	11.0
Cocaine	5.9
Ecstasy	3.2
Heroin	0.4

TOLERANCE When users take these drugs excessively, their brains become accustomed to an overstimulated reward pathway.

SOURCES: NATIONAL INSTITUTE OF DRUG ABUSE, SUBSTANCE ABUSE AND MENTAL HEALTH SERVICES ADMINISTRATION. WRITTEN BY JOSH ULICK. GRAPHIC BY KARL GUDE AND TONIA COWAN–NEWSWEEK

Purdue Pharma, acutely aware of the negative publicity around OxyContin, is working furiously to protect its $1.5 billion brand. It has committed $150 million to measures including public-service ads and the distribution of fraud-resistant prescription pads to physicians (try to photocopy it, and the word "void" miraculously appears). The company is also researching ways to make OxyContin less addictive, by adding a compound such as naltrexone that binds to the same receptors in the brain and blocks the action of oxycodone. The trick is to formulate the naltrexone so that it gets into the bloodstream in large amounts *only when the pill is crushed in order to get high*. Purdue's goal—probably five or so years off—"is to make it less desirable enough that abusers won't be interested in it," says Dr. Paul D. Goldenheim, the company's chief scientist.

The company obviously can't talk about individual patients, even famous ones. Goldenheim says, though, that it's extremely rare for a person with no history of substance abuse to become addicted to OxyContin after us-

ing it correctly. Outside authorities agree with that assessment. Goldenheim is drawing an important distinction between "dependence" and "addiction." Most people who take a powerful drug like OxyContin long enough will become physically dependent on it and suffer withdrawal symptoms (including pain, restlessness and nausea) if it's taken away; doctors deal with this by tapering down the dosage to zero and then, if all goes well, it's over. Or, if the pain is chronic, the patient stays on the drug indefinitely. In principle there's no more shame or harm in being dependent on painkillers than on, say, beta blockers for high blood pressure.

BY CONTRAST, A DRUG ADDICT has a psychological craving as well, which returns even when the physical dependence is overcome. That is what makes addiction so notoriously hard to treat; Limbaugh, who headed straight for rehab after signing off last week, has admitted attempting to kick his habit at least twice before. The state of the art, for people who can afford it, is a monthlong stay in a residential facility that offers both medically supervised withdrawal and psychological and spiritual counseling, usually based on the 12-step program. The best-known treatment center is Hazelden, based in Minnesota but with centers in four other states as well. For all forms of addiction, Hazelden claims that 53 percent of its patients stay clean for a year—in other words, after spending four weeks and $19,000, almost half its clients relapse within months. Nationwide, 12-step programs do poorly in treating painkiller abuse: relapse rates after a year approach 80 percent.

The other route to getting clean is a protocol developed in the past decade sometimes known as "rapid detox." It involves delivering a large intravenous dose of naltrex-

one to a patient under anesthesia—a dose so large it would be intolerable if the patient were conscious. The Waismann Institute in Beverly Hills, which pioneered the technique, says its program—which takes three to four days and costs around $10,000—has a 65 percent one-year success rate. "Our patients don't want to go to a 30-day program and 'talk about it' with a bunch of drug addicts," Dr. Cliff Bernstein says dismissively. "They just want to be off the drugs." Either way, it's not an easy thing to do. As long as there is pain, people will try to escape it—and sometimes wind up with something worse.

With CLAUDIA KALB, DEBRA ROSENBERG, MARY CARMICHAEL and ANNE UNDERWOOD

UNIT 3

The Major Drugs of Use and Abuse

Unit Selections

Key Points to Consider

- How is it that specific drugs evolve, develop use patterns, and lose or gain popularity over time?

- How does the manner in which a drug is ingested help define its respective user population?

- How does the manner in which a drug is used influence the severity of consequences related to that drug? Or does it?

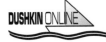 **Links: www.dushkin.com/online/**
These sites are annotated in the World Wide Web pages.

Drugs, Solvents and Intoxicants
http://www.termisoc.org/~harl/

QuitNet
http://www.quitnet.org

The following articles discuss those drugs that have evolved to become the most popular drugs of choice. Although pharmacological modifications emerge periodically to enhance or alter the effects produced by certain drugs or the manner in which various drugs are used, basic pharmacological properties of the drugs remain unchanged. Crack is still cocaine, ice is still methamphetamine, and black tar is still heroin. In addition, tobacco products all supply the drug nicotine, coffee and a plethora of energy drinks provide caffeine, and alcoholic beverages provide the drug ethyl alcohol. These drugs all influence how we act, think, and feel about ourselves and the world around us. They also produce markedly different effects within the body and within the mind.

To understand why certain drugs remain popular over time and why new drugs become popular, one must be knowledgeable about the effects produced by individual drugs. Why people use drugs is a bigger question than why people use tobacco. However, understanding why certain people use tobacco, or cocaine, or marijuana, or alcohol is one way to construct a framework from which to tackle the larger question of why people use drugs in general. One of the most complex relationships is the one between Americans and their use of alcohol. More than 76 million Americans have experienced alcoholism in their families.

The most recent surveys of alcohol use estimate that 120 million Americans currently use alcohol. About 54 million are estimated to have engaged in binge drinking (five or more drinks on one occasion), and currently there are 10.7 million drinkers between the ages of 12 and 20. Alcohol prevails as the most popular recreational drug of choice, and its use is commonly associated with the use of most illicit drugs. Of the current 11.2 million heavy drinkers, 30 percent (3.3 million people) are illicit drug users. There is also a long-standing and significant relationship between the use of alcohol and the use of tobacco. An estimated 66.5 million Americans report current cigarette use. The majority of Americans, however, believe that alcohol is used responsibly by most people who use it, even though 10 percent of the American population is believed to be suffering from various stages of alcoholism. The use of alcohol is a powerful force within our national consciousness about drugs.

Understanding why people turn initially to the nonmedical use of drugs is a huge question that is debated and discussed in a voluminous body of literature. One important reason why the major drugs of use and abuse, such as alcohol, nicotine, cocaine, heroin, marijuana, amphetamines, and a variety of prescription, designer, over-the-counter, and herbal drugs, retain their popularity is because they produce certain physical and psychological effects that humans crave. They temporarily restrain our inhibitions; reduce our fears; alleviate mental and physical suffering; produce energy, confidence, and exhilaration; and allow us to relax. Tired, take a pill; have a headache, take a pill; need to lose weight, take a pill. There is a drug for everything. Some drugs even, albeit artificially, suggest a greater capacity to transcend, redefine, and seek out new levels of consciousness. And they do it upon demand. People initially use a specific drug, or class of drugs, to obtain the desirable effects historically associated with the use of that drug. Heroin and opiate-related drugs such as Oxycontin and Vicodin produce, in most people, a euphoric, dreamy state of well-being. The abuse of these prescription painkillers is one of the fastest growing, and alarming, drug trends. Cocaine and related stimulant drugs produce euphoria, energy, confidence, and exhilaration. Alcohol produces a loss of inhibitions and a state of well-being. Nicotine and marijuana typically serve as relaxants. Ecstasy and other "club drugs" produce stimulant as well as relaxant effects. Various over-the-counter and herbal drugs all attempt to replicate the effects of more potent and often prohibited or prescribed drugs. Although effects and side effects may vary from user to user, a general pattern of effects is predictable from most major drugs of use and their analogs. Varying the dosage and altering the manner of ingestion is one way to alter the drug's effects. Some drugs, such as LSD, and some types of designer drugs produce effects on the user that are less predictable and more sensitive to variations in dosage level and to the user's physical and psychological makeup.

Although all major drugs of use and abuse have specific reinforcing properties perpetuating their continued use, they also produce undesirable side effects that regular drug users attempt to mitigate. Most often, users attempt to mitigate these effects with the use of other drugs. Cocaine, methamphetamine, heroin, and alcohol have long been used to mitigate each other's side effects. A good example is the classic "speedball" of heroin and cocaine. When they are combined, cocaine accelerates and intensifies the euphoric state of the heroin, while the heroin softens the comedown from cocaine. One currently popular trend is to mix energy drinks with alcoholic beverages to mitigate the drowsiness associated with drinking alcohol. Some alcoholic beverage companies are producing recipes to capitalize on this trend. Other related drug trends, availability, price, and the public's perception of the drug's safety often influence the degree to which some drugs remain popular.

Drug abuse in America spans the spectrum of legality. To associate only illegal drugs with abuse and criminality is shortsighted. In terms of drug-related social impacts, any discussion of major drugs could begin and end with the topics of alcohol and nicotine. The pursuit of drugs and the effects they produce may be influenced by, but not bound by, legal status. For the student of drug-related phenomena, an attachment to the concepts of legality or illegality for purposes of comprehensively rationalizing drug-related reality is inappropriate. For example, annual alcohol-related deaths far outnumber deaths from all illegal drugs combined.

IS POT GOOD FOR YOU?

Well, no. But the latest research suggests the health risk from occasional use is mild, and it might ease certain ills

By JOHN CLOUD
SAN FRANCISCO

I never smoked pot in junior high because I was convinced it would shrivel my incipient manhood. This was the 1980s, and those stark this-is-your-brain-on-drugs ads already had me vaguely worried about memory loss and psychosis. But when other boys said pot might affect our southern regions, I was truly terrified. I didn't smoke a joint for the first time until I was 21.

SMOKE IT In a California clinic, James Ruiz participates in a study evaluating whether marijuana eases intractable nerve pain

By 12th grade, about half of young Americans have tried marijuana, which put me in the geeky other half. I used to think this was a good thing, since I never developed a taste for pot and avoided becoming dependent. But as the medical-marijuana movement flowered and weed's p.r. improved, I often wondered if I shouldn't have relished it as a kid, before I had a personal trainer to tsk-tsk my every vice. Shrinking testicles? Mushy brains? I came to see these as grotesqueries invented by antidrug propagandists.

GROW IT Under Proposition 215 in California, police may not seize or destroy [a] pot plant

It turns out that the study of marijuana's health effects is at once more complex and less advanced than you might imagine. "Interpretations [of marijuana research] may tell more about [one's] own biases than the data," writes Mitch Earleywine in *Understanding Marijuana: A New Look at the Scientific Evidence*, published in August by Oxford. For example: "Prohibitionists might mention that THC [delta-9 tetrahydrocannabinol, the smile-producing chemical in pot] often appears in the blood of people in auto accidents. Yet they might omit the fact that most of these people also drank alcohol. Antiprohibitionists might cite a large study that showed no sign of memory problems in chronic marijuana smokers. Yet they might not mention that the tests were so easy that even a demented person could perform them."

INHALE IT A pharmaceutical company in Britain is testing this whole-marijuana extract delivered in a spray

The science of marijuana—especially its potential medical uses—is malleable because it's so young and so contradictory. Although preliminary data are promising, scientists haven't definitively shown that the drug can safely treat nausea or pain or anything, really. Some experts claim the U.S. government has sabotaged medical-marijuana research, and there is evidence to support them.

Even so, in the past few years scientists have made rapid advances in their basic understanding of how *Cannabis sativa* works. By 1993, researchers had found the body's two known receptors for cannabinoids, the psychoactive chemicals in the plant (THC is the main one, but there are at least 65 others). Since then, there has been important new work in several fields that users, potential users and former users should know about—and that voters should take into account before deciding whether to legalize pot.

So much new research has appeared that in November the *Journal of Clinical Pharmacology* and the National Institute on Drug Abuse will publish a 100-page supplement devoted entirely to marijuana. The *Journal* gave Time an advance look; it's a comprehensive review that will annoy both sides in the drug war. You won't find clear evidence that pot is good or evil, but the research sheds light on some of the most important questions surrounding the drug:

Can it kill you?

NO ONE HAS EVER DIED OF THC POISONing, mostly because a 160-lb. person would have to smoke roughly 900 joints in a sitting to reach a lethal dose. (No doubt some have tried.) But that doesn't mean pot can't contribute to serious health problems and even death—both indirectly (driving while stoned, for instance) and directly (by affecting circulation, for example). A paper published last year in the journal *Angiology* found 10 odd cases in France of heavy *herbe* smokers who developed ischemia (an insufficient blood supply) in their limbs, leading in four cases to amputations. It's not clear that marijuana caused the decreased blood flow, but the vascular problems did worsen during periods of heavy use. Another 2001 paper, in *Circulation*, found a nearly fivefold increase in the risk for heart attack in the first hour after smoking marijuana—though statistically that means smoking pot is about as dangerous for a fit person as exercise.

Does it make you sick?

MARIJUANA MAY DIRECTLY AFFECT THE immune system, since one of the body's two known receptors for cannabinoids is

located in immune cells. But the nature of the effect is unclear. A recent study showed that THC inhibits production of immune-stimulating substances. But cigarette smokers may do greater harm to their immunity than pot users, who tend to smoke less. A study published earlier this year found that tobacco smokers but not marijuana smokers had high levels of a type of enzyme believed to inflame the lungs. Dr. Donald Abrams, professor of clinical medicine at the University of California, San Francisco, found that short-term cannabis use doesn't substantially raise viral loads of HIV patients. (People with HIV sometimes smoke marijuana to stimulate appetite.) In fact, his study participants who smoked pot enjoyed significantly higher increases in their lymphocytes (cells that help fight disease) than those who took a placebo.

Can it give you cancer?

DATA ON CANCER ALSO GENERATE mixed conclusions. A 1999 study of 173 patients with head and neck cancers found that pot smoking elevated the risk of such cancers. (Smokers of anything should also worry about lung cancer.) But it's not clear that THC is carcinogenic. The latest research suggests that THC may have a dual effect, promoting tumors by increasing free radicals and simultaneously protecting against tumors by playing a beneficial role in a process known as programmed cell death.

Is it addictive?

THOSE WHO BELIEVE YOU CAN'T BEcome physically or psychologically dependent on marijuana are wrong. At least three recent studies have demonstrated that heavy pot smokers who quit can experience such withdrawal symptoms as anxiety, difficulty sleeping and stomach pain. On the other hand, the risk of becoming dependent on marijuana is comparatively low. Just 9% of those who have used the drug develop dependence. By comparison, 15% of drinkers become dependent on alcohol, 23% of heroin users get hooked, and a third of tobacco smokers become slaves to cigarettes.

Does it make you stupid?

POTHEADS ARE DUMBER THAN NONUSERS, but only a little. Earlier this year, the *Journal of the American Medical Association* published a study of 102 near-daily marijuana users who wanted to quit. The authors found that the longer subjects had toked up, the worse their memories and attention spans. But they were hardly like Gobi, the *Saturday Night Live* wastoid who is so ruined he can barely talk. Participants who had used cannabis regularly for an average of 10 years fared significantly worse on only two of 40 indices of cognitive functioning (they had particular trouble estimating how much time had passed during a test). Those stout folks who had been smoking pot for an average of 24 years did significantly worse on 14 of the tests. But scientists can't say that marijuana causes such problems. "These long-term users may have been worse off in the first place, before they ever smoked marijuana," says Dr. Harrison Pope, a Harvard psychiatrist who wrote an editorial accompanying the study arguing that "we must live with uncertainty" on whether pot causes long-term cognitive impairments.

What about sex?

THE LATEST STUDIES SUGGEST I NEEDN'T have fretted so much about pot's gonadal consequences. "Marijuana might interfere with [kids'] ability to go through puberty," says Dr. Adrian Dobs, co-author of a paper on the endocrine effects of the drug in the upcoming *Journal of Clinical Pharmacology*. "But the abnormalities seen are not really clinically significant." Despite tales of male potheads growing breasts, the long-term effects on adult glands are uncertain.

Do the sick really benefit?

SO IF MARIJUANA CAN BE HARMFUL to healthy people—but usually isn't—could it actually be good for the sick? This is where the science gets scraggier—and in the absence of data, politics takes over. What we know is that healers have accumulated copious anecdotes on weed's powers over the past 4,700 years. *Understanding Marijuana* author Earleywine credits a (possibly mythical) Chinese emperor with introducing the

What Marijuana Does to Your Body

Negative effects	Positive effects
BRAIN Causes changes in brain chemistry. Marijuana hinders the neurotransmitter acetylcholine, a chemical that triggers various types of signals throughout the nervous system.	**PAIN** Increases sense of euphoria. May help minimize pain from migraine headaches and from the spread of cancer
MOOD AND BEHAVIOR Leads to difficulty in concentration, attention to detail and learning new, complex information. Also impairs time perception as well as certain aspects of memory—at least in the short term	**EYES** Reduces intraocular pressure; helping those afflicted with glaucoma
HEART Increases the work of the heart. The changes in heart rate and blood pressure are the same as those found in a person under high stress	**SPASTICITY** Believed to help calm spasms from spinalcord injury, MS and possibly epilepsy. In the early 1900s, cannabis tinctures were marketed as antispasmodics
LUNGS Is more irritating to (50% more tar than tobacco) and has a greater effect on the upper airways (sinuses and larynx) than tobacco. May cause lung, head and neck cancer	**STOMACH** Helps restore appetite in people who have lost weight from cancer or AIDS
SEXUAL PERFORMANCE May reduce the number and quality of sperm and damage their mobility, possibly affecting fertility	**NAUSEA** Combats nausea from chemotherapy and helps minimize vomiting
BLOOD FLOW Decreases blood flow to the limbs, which in extreme cases may require amputation	

plant as a treatment for gout around 2700 B.C. But the emperor also thought his pot potion would help memory, making him the first of many fans to aggrandize the drug's medical potential. The ancient Greek doc Galen even used the drug to treat flatulence.

The A.M.A. issued a report last year summarizing the body of knowledge about medical marijuana. It's shockingly slim. Dr. Abrams in San Francisco has produced some of the clearest evidence to date of pot's therapeutic value. Even though his clinical trial was designed merely to investigate whether marijuana is safe for HIV patients, he also turned up data that anyone who ever had the munchies already knew: pot makes you hungry. Test subjects who smoked marijuana gained an average of 6.6 lbs. during the trial, compared with 2.4 lbs. for the group taking the placebo. Some other findings from the A.M.A. report:

NAUSEA Patients who are HIV-positive or undergoing chemotherapy can have trouble keeping food down, so anything that helps them eat is significant—though not necessarily for the reasons marijuana boosters think. Pot's ability to enhance appetite may have more to do with its high and less to do with any direct effects on nausea. Only 20% to 25% of patients in two 1980s trials could completely control vomiting with marijuana; other drugs work better for emesis. Still, the A.M.A. recommended more studies on marijuana for those who don't respond to the other drugs, and it notes that for those feeling sick, inhaling a substance may be more palatable than swallowing a pill.

GLAUCOMA Marijuana does reduce pressure on the eyeball, about 25%, but the drug isn't always practical as a glaucoma treatment. Many who have the disease are elderly and can't tolerate pot's tendency to raise heart rates.

SPASTICITY Marijuana can help people with spasticity (extreme muscle tension) and tremor due to multiple sclerosis and trauma. But the drug hasn't been rigorously compared with the standard antispastic treatments.

PAIN In patients with postoperative pain, THC is more effective than a placebo, and some reports suggest smoking pot may reduce the need for highly addictive opioids. But the A.M.A. says better-designed studies are needed to properly evaluate pot as a painkiller. Several are under way. In California, five teams of researchers are conducting studies of marijuana as an analgesic, particularly for cancer and nerve pain.

The A.M.A. concludes that the lack of "high-quality clinical research… continues to hamper development of rational public policy" on medical marijuana. Which raises the question, Why, after five millenniums, doesn't such research exist? Two possible answers: First, the government may have rejected cannabis studies to avoid any challenge to its view that pot is dangerous and medically useless. Second, pot may just be dangerous and medically useless.

The drug wasn't always so controversial in the scientific establishment. The *U.S. Pharmacopeia*, a doctors' listing of remedies begun in 1820, first included cannabis in 1870. The *Pharmacopeia* didn't drop pot until its 1942 edition, the first published after cannabis was outlawed in 1937. Eventually most physicians began to view the drug as little more than a crude intoxicant. They tended to favor new-fashioned drugs that were refined by pharmaceutical firms into pure chemicals. Raw marijuana contains some 400 compounds.

STUDY IT Dr. Donald Abrams of San Francisco has investigated whether smoking pot can be safe for patients

It wasn't until the '70s that modern methods were applied to test the medicinal effects of cannabis. As Earleywine recounts, a UCLA study designed to confirm police reports that pot dilates pupils found instead a slight constriction. That's how doctors discovered the drug could help glaucoma sufferers by reducing intraocular pressure. In the years after that discovery, 26 states opened therapeutic research programs.

But the Federal Government, which by then controlled the only legal supply of marijuana, had just passed the Controlled Substances Act of 1970. That law placed marijuana in Schedule I, the designation for drugs without valid medical use. State health officials found it difficult to persuade their federal counterparts to give them cannabis for research, as doing so would undermine the law, at least in spirit, by suggesting there were medical uses. (Only seven states got pot. One was Tennessee, which is why Al Gore's sister was able to try the drug before losing her battle with lung cancer in 1984.)

Then, in 1985, the Food and Drug Administration (FDA) approved dronabinol, an oral form of synthetic THC, to treat chemotherapy-induced nausea. Many doctors believed dronabinol, marketed as Marinol, could provide the benefits of the plant without the impurities. By the mid-'80s, the availability of Marinol and the escalating drug war had killed the state research programs. But Marinol turned out to have shortcomings. Because it enters the blood through the stomach, it doesn't work as fast as smoked marijuana. Because it is essentially pure THC, its users can get too high. "Marinol does tend to knock people out," says Abrams, the San Francisco doctor who has conducted trials with both Marinol and pot. "Our patients [taking Marinol] spent a lot of time in bed, and that wasn't the case with those smoking marijuana."

Such problems appeared in only "a small portion of the patients in our clinical trials," says Dr. Hjalmar Lagast, a vice president for Solvay Pharmaceuticals, which makes Marinol. He notes that the drug comes in three strengths, allowing doctors to pick the right dose. By the early '90s, at the height of the U.S. aids epidemic, many patients so preferred marijuana to Marinol that they would use the street drug regardless of legality or safety. Abrams and a few others began pushing the government to permit new studies of marijuana to find out what these patients were doing to themselves.

Officials again resisted, and some researchers became convinced the government would never allow evidence of pot's possible benefits to emerge. In 1999, Paul Consroe, a professor of pharmacology at the University of Arizona, failed to win FDA approval for a clinical trial of marijuana for aids and cancer wasting. He believes the FDA turned him down because of political pressure. "If you want to study its harmful effects, you can get all the money you want," says Consroe. "But for this one, I would have spun my wheels forever." (An FDA spokeswoman declined to comment.)

It took Abrams five years, but he finally pushed his study through. A stubborn and irreverent oncologist who had watched hundreds of aids patients suffer brutal nausea, he won government approval in 1997 for the first clinical trial of marijuana in more than a decade. Marijuana proposals at the time required the approval of three agencies—the FDA, the Drug Enforcement Administration and the National Institute on Drug Abuse—and the DEA and NIDA had resisted. A DEA official worried in a letter about the political fallout if Abrams found positive results. "The government is saying there are no studies proving the medical benefits," Abrams fumed in 1996. "But they're also not letting studies be conducted."

"The government says it wants more studies, but they make it harder to get marijuana for research than any other drug."
—RICK DOBLIN

Not true, says Steven Gust, special assistant to the director of NIDA, who has worked at the agency 15 years. "Ever since I've been here, there's been no prejudice against studying the medical applications of marijuana. Frankly, good proposals weren't coming in. The people you've talked to had a bad experience getting approval, and that's going to color their perception."

Whatever the case, Abrams and Gust agree that the government and medical-marijuana researchers are now working together. Abrams has two approved studies under way, and the State of California has founded a new, grander version of its old therapeutic research program. The Center for Medicinal Cannabis Research, which opened at the University of California two years ago with a yearly budget of $3 million, currently supports 11 studies that have received federal approval.

To be sure, many scientists—especially in the government—still squirm at the very idea of medical-marijuana research. Despite encouraging anecdotal reports, the National Institutes of Health hasn't initiated a study of cannabis therapeutics in two decades, leaving California's young center as the only U.S. research institution doing the basic science. Marijuana remains the only drug that researchers must acquire directly from the feds. If the FDA and DEA approve, scientists can get even ecstasy from outside labs, but NIDA is the sole source for cannabis, requiring a third bureaucratic layer. "In an era of privatization, it's shocking that the government insists on a monopoly so that it can choose not to provide marijuana to projects it doesn't like," says Rick Doblin, founder of the Multidisciplinary Association for Psychedelic Studies, a nonprofit pharmaceutical firm. (For 18 months, Doblin's association and the University of Massachusetts Amherst have unsuccessfully sought a license to grow research-grade cannabis at the university.)

Not every country is as pot-phobic as the U.S. Scientists in Britain, which has effectively decriminalized personal use of small amounts of pot, have moved well beyond the preliminary work being done in the U.S. Britain's GW Pharmaceuticals plans to publish results of a large study of its new marijuana product, a whole-cannabis extract rendered into a mouth spray. That way, patients avoid the lung damage of smoking. The British government is likely to make the spray available for prescription if published results are as good as the company promises.

In this country, new drug products like GW's spray rarely appear without cordial cooperation among pharmaceutical companies, research institutions and government officials. Such partnership could take years to develop. But the politics has leaped well ahead of the science, meaning voters will decide long before physicians whether medical marijuana is an oxymoron.

The Dangers of Diet Pills

Just because they're sold in health-food shops and drugstores doesn't mean they're safe. Not only are some weight-loss supplements ineffective, some are outright harmful—even lethal.

BY JENNIFER PIRTLE

Anyone who has tried to lose weight fantasizes about a magic bullet, a little pill that can painlessly melt away the pounds. That's exactly what marketers play to when they churn out all manner of powders and potions that promise to fight hunger, rev up metabolism and make fat evaporate. Every year, Americans spend $30 billion on weight-loss products and programs, hoping that the claims on the package will actually work. And women turn to these pills twice as often as men do.

"Hope springs eternal," says Ruth Kava, Ph.D., director of nutrition at the American Council on Science and Health, in New York City. "Everyone wants an easy way to weight loss." But the worst-case scenario the hopeful envision is that the product is a bust and they'll have wasted their money. Most don't expect that they might be gambling with their health—or their very lives.

DYING TO BE THIN

The ingredients in over-the-counter (OTC) weight-loss products capturing consumer attention lately is ephedra, or ma huang, an herb that has chemical properties similar to amphetamines and that acts on the appetite-control center of the brain. It's available in more than 200 dietary supplements, including well-known brands such as Metabolife and Xenadrine. (A synthetic version of the stimu-

lant is also used in some decongestants and asthma drugs.)

Ephedra was in the news last fall, when the military reported more than 30 deaths linked to the substance. It came roaring back into the news in February, when Steven Bechler, the 23-year-old pitcher for the Baltimore Orioles, collapsed and died of heatstroke. He had been taking Xenadrine RFA-1, which contains ephedra, and the medical examiner said that the substance likely contributed to his death.

Coincidentally, just days after Bechler's death, a study commissioned by the National Institutes of Health was released, which analyzed more than 1,500 "adverse event reports" related to herbal ephedra and reviewed 52 clinical trials of ephedra for weight loss or athletic performance. This report, conducted by the nonprofit RAND public policy research organization, showed some evidence that ephedra did promote modest short-term weight loss: Users lost a couple of pounds more a month than those taking a placebo. But it also found that there were side effects, including nausea, vomiting, jitteriness and palpitations. Additionally, the study showed a possible link between ephedra use and heart attack, stroke, seizures, serious psychiatric symptoms and even death, but concluded that further study is needed in order to prove a direct relationship.

BUYER BEWARE: A GUIDE TO WEIGHT-LOSS SUPPLEMENTS

CATEGORY/PRODUCTS	TYPICAL PROMOTIONAL CLAIM	HOW THEY SUPPOSEDLY WORK	WHAT'S IN THEM	WHAT EXPERTS SAY
Ephedra-free appetite suppressants: Dexatrim Results, Eat Less Blend, Xenadrine EFX, Zantrex-3 **Ephedra-free appetite suppressants:** Metab-olife 356. Metab-O-LITE, Stacker 2, TrimSpa, Xenadrine RFA-1	To curb and control appetite so you eat less, create a feeling of fullness, increase your metabolism and boost energy	The ones containing stimulants stimulate the nervous system to affect the hunger center in the brain to make you feel full.	Despite recent headlines about the potentially deadly dangers of ephedra, many products still contain the ingredient (also known as ma huang); others contain fiber that expands in your stomach to fill you up. Still others may contain vitamins, minerals, different forms of caffeine, herbs such as ginseng, licorice root, fenugreek seed, yerba mate or bitter orange peel extract.	The FDA advises against taking products containing ephedra, which has been linked to strokes and heart attacks. Some appetite suppressants can create psychological dependence because their chemical structure is similar to amphetamines. Others can cause insomnia, drowsiness, irritability or depression. Herbs are untested and may have harmful side effects.
Fat burners: Supplements labeled conjugated linoleic acid (CLA) or chromium picolinate (many brands); Hydroxycut, Nutrilite Trim Advantage Weight Management Support Pack, Estrolean	To encourage the breakdown of fat; boost energy; suppress appetite	Increase glucose metabolism in muscle cells, thus increasing fat breakdown and sustaining energy	CLA, chromium picolinate, hydroxyl citric acid (HCA), also may contain caffeine and herbs	Some of these products may affect blood sugar and insulin levels—potentially bad news for diabetics. At best, there's little convincing evidence they work for weight loss. Some herbs that are untested could have harmful side effects.
Fat blockers: Chitosan (many brands), Chitosol, FatAbsorb, Fat Cutter Plus	To grab and hold on to the fat from your food and carry it out of your body	Inhibit the intestinal enzyme that works on fat, so fat passes undigested through the large intestine. Instructions are to take product just before consuming fatty foods.	Chitosan, an ingredient derived from shellfish (a problem for those who are allergic); some (such as Fat Cutter Plus) may contain ephedra, caffeine and herbs	Side effects can include cramping, diarrhea and intestinal discomfort—common problems when a lot of fat passes through the bowel. May also increase the risk of fat-soluble vitamin deficiency (A, D, E and K). If you block fat, you block these vitamins.
Carb blockers: Carb Cutter, Carb Block, Carb Trapper Plus, Sugar Blocker	To prevent body from absorbing sugar	By blocking starch-converting enzymes in saliva and/or in the intestines so that carbohydrates pass through the digestive tract instead of going to the blood	Often contain trademarked "proprietary blends" with ingredients such as gymnema sylvestre leaf and fenugreek seed extract; also may contain chromium picolinate, vitamins and herbs	Claims are unproven. But even if these ingredients did work, there's no proven correlation between carbohydrates and obesity and no guarantee that blocking them would cause weight loss.
Other "natural" weight loss supplements: Acutrim Natural, Cider Vinegar Tablets (many brands), Dexatrim Natural Green Tea, PatentLEAN, Puralin	To be an all natural, safe, effective way to lose weight, reduce toxins, boost energy	Same as above categories, depending upon particular product. Labeling claims play on the widespread assumption by many consumers that anything natural is safer and more effective.	Herbal blends may contain green tea extract, caffeine, ginseng; PatentLean contains 3-Acetyl-7-Oxo-Dehydroepiandrosterone, "produced in our adrenal glands"; Puralin contains Calcareacarbonica, carbo vegetabilis, and other ingredients. Cider vinegar contains just that.	Natural origins do not guarantee effectiveness or safety. As with any diet supplement, natural ingredients may cause reactions with other drugs. Ask your doctor.

How to Read a Diet Label

If you've ever stood in the supplements aisle of the drugstore or health-food shop, searching for something to help you battle the bulge, you know how confusing the display of products can be. If the sheer number of choices isn't enough to make your head spin, the alphabet soup on the labels certainly will.

Though the Federal Trade Commission polices claims made in print advertisements and on radio, label claims fall under the jurisdiction of the FDA, which imposes less stringent requirements. Under FDA guidelines, manufacturers may describe the supplement's effects on the body, but they must also include a disclaimer on the label that reads: "The statements have not been evaluated by the FDA. This product is not intended to diagnose, treat, cure or prevent any disease." While this may be within the letter of the law, it provides little protection to the consumer.

Another concern, completely separate from whether an ingredient is safe or harmful, is how much of it is actually contained in the product. Dosages are not standardized, and supplements often contain dozens of ingredients. "We don't know if what is supposed to be there will be there or not—or at what strength," says Ruth Kava, Ph.D., director of nutrition at the American Council on Science and Health. "We also don't know if it will react with other prescription and over-the-counter products a person may be taking."

A recent study by Consumerlab.com, an independent evaluator of health and nutrition aids, looked at levels of chromium, conjugated linoleic acid, and pyruvate (three ingredients used in weight-loss supplements and that some experts believe to be safe) to confirm their identity and amounts. Several products did not indicate the correct amount of the ingredient that was actually contained in the product. One supplement, for example, contained less than 5 percent of the amount of the chromium claimed on the label, another product met its claimed amount of chromium, but it was a different form: chromium (VI)—the type implicated as causing cancers in the case portrayed in the movie *Erin Brockovich*. "This review is a microcosm of the problems we've found with other supplements," said Tod Cooperman, M.D., Consumerlab's president, in the study. "If consumers are going to use a supplement, they should be able to get what they expect—nothing less and nothing more."

You Tried *What* to Lose Weight?

The unglamorous truth is that the best way to lose weight in the long run is to change your eating habits and exercise more. Yet millions of us continue to search for the quick fix. Some of the calorie cure-alls range from the scary to the silly. Three of the more offbeat ones you may have heard of include:

- **Appetite-suppressing eyeglasses:** These eyeglasses with colored lenses claim to project an image to the retina that dampens the desire to eat. The FDA says there is absolutely no evidence that they work.
- **Slimming soap:** An "amazing seaweed soap" promised users they would lose weight by lathering up—and even quoted a *Wall Street Journal* article purportedly supporting its powers. However, they conveniently failed to include a paragraph from the original article that quoted a medical anthropologist, who said she had

heard of no links between seaweed and weight loss, and a mocking quote from an herbalist saying that "eating the soap may be a more effective slimming plan than bathing with it."
- **Weight-loss slippers:** Reported to be all the rage in parts of Asia, they are now available for $44.95 on the Internet. The slippers are deliberately made too short, so that the heel of each foot hangs over the back edge. The slippers offer a cross between reflexology and magnet therapy. A bulging center applies pressure to the feet's arches, while magnets located inside the slippers supposedly stimulate the nerve endings in the soles. Promotional materials promise that the slippers will "increase your metabolism naturally. The side effect is you lose weight." There is no evidence that the slippers work.

In late February, the FDA proposed new labeling requirements on products containing ephedra to warn consumers that it could have life-threatening consequences. But, as of press time, the government has stopped short of proposing an outright ban, pending further study, and the drug remains widely available. Some supplement manufacturers have already voluntarily removed ephedra from their products, but other untested stimulant substances may well be ready to step in and fill the void, says Sidney Wolfe, M.D., director of Public Citizen's Health Research Group in Washington, D.C. "We've seen this movie before."

To wit, in 2000 the FDA requested the phenylpropanolamine, or PPA, an ingredient used in hundreds of OTC weight-loss aids, be removed from products when it was discovered that it increased the risk of stroke. Although the process took a while, that ingredient now seems to have disappeared from store shelves and Internet sites. Dexatrim and other products were reformulated and later reintroduced without PPA.

"But even before the FDA action against PPA," says Dr. Wolfe, "companies were already hawking products with ephedra, which was even worse." Despite the call for more study, Dr. Wolfe says the FDA has enough evidence to ban ephedra, which he thinks will happen soon. If it is banned, what will be the next possibly dangerous ingredient? "We already know," says Dr. Wolfe. "It's bitter orange, or syneprhine (also known as citrus aurantium). Companies are already marketing this largely untested stimulant."

How is it possible that products with such potentially serious health risks are allowed to come to a drugstore near you in the first place? Part of the problem can be attributed to the passage by Congress of the Dietary Supplement Health and Education Act (DSHEA) in 1994. Before then, the FDA regulated what are now called dietary supplements (including vitamins, herbs and OTC diet pills) as a special category of food to ensure that they were safe and wholesome and that their labeling was truthful. But under DSHEA, the rules were relaxed and supplements were no longer subject to the pre-market safety evaluations required of new food ingredients.

The result is that manufacturers are left to police themselves and take responsibility for diet pills being safe and label information being truthful and clear. The FDA is responsible for taking action against a dietary supplement proven to be unsafe *after* it has reached the market. That means that the FDA can remove a product from the shelves if claims made by a manufacturer are not met, or if there is compelling evidence that the product is harmful. Short of that, your health is in the hands of the companies selling you these pills.

Where does all this leave consumers? "While some over-the-counter diet pills may be based on solid nutrition science," says Julie O'Sullivan Maillet, Ph.D., president of the ADA, "others are gimmicks with little or no research to show that they are effective or safe, especially in the long run." And, unless you're a chemist who can decipher the complicated labels, it's almost impossible to tell the difference.

"Weight loss supplements are quick fixes that, for the most part, don't deliver on their promises," says Neal Barnard, M.D., president of the Physicians Committee for Responsible Medicine. "Just using supplements won't work in the long run, and won't make you healthy, either."

In fact, says Dr. Wolfe, "They are an extraordinary waste—of whomever might die next."

Why Rx may spell danger:

'Do you know the difference between use and abuse of prescription medicines?

Kathiann M. Kowalski

"Morphine Helped Cause Death of Delaware Teen," read the Columbus Dispatch headline. According to the coroner's report, a mixture of morphine and over-the-counter allergy medicine killed 15-year-old Samantha. Less than two weeks earlier, the same combination had killed a high school senior in Licking County, Ohio.

In Los Angeles, more than a dozen students at two high schools got sick after taking the stimulant Ritalin. Police later arrested five teens. They had sold or given away the pills to other students.

While prescription medicines are used legally for certain purposes, they are not safe for everyone. Abuse can kill.

By Prescription Only

Prescription drugs are medicines that have been approved by the Food and Drug Administration for specific purposes. They can be used legally only under the direction of a physician. The doctor can tell if a patient has a certain condition and can prescribe the proper dosage, based on the person's age and weight. Also, the doctor can advise the patient about possible side effects or interactions with other medicines.

Thanks to prescription medicines, doctors can effectively treat a wide range of medical conditions. Have you ever had to see the doctor for a severe headache or muscle strain? If over-the-counter pain relievers did not work, your doctor might have prescribed a stronger analgesic to reduce pain.

Opioids and opiates are another kind of pain killer. They work by attaching to certain receptors in the brain and spinal cord and blocking pain messages from going to the brain. A hospital may give morphine intravenously after surgery, for example. Or, a doctor may prescribe pills, such as Percocet, Percodan, or Darvon. (Heroin and opium are also opiates, but they have no legitimate medical use.)

Central nervous system depressants include barbiturates, such as Mebaral or Nembutal. Doctors may prescribe them for severe insomnia, or sedation while performing surgical procedures. Tranquilizers such as Xanax, Valium, and Librium are also central nervous system depressants. They help patients who suffer from severe anxiety disorders, panic attacks, or severe stress.

Stimulants are drugs that enhance brain activity and increase the body's heart and breathing rates. Stimulants can help some patients with narcolepsy (a sleeping disorder) and depression.

… 10 percent of 12th graders said they had used prescription narcotics other than under a doctor's orders.

Stimulants can also treat ADHD (attention deficit hyperactivity disorder). Ritalin and Adderall are examples. They help young people with this condition function normally. "If the diagnosis has been made carefully, and the treatment is taken as it's prescribed, there's a very low risk of user addiction," notes Richard Brown, M.D., at the University of Wisconsin Medical School.

Prescription drugs do a lot of good when they are prescribed and used properly. Sometimes, though, people abuse them.

How Abuse Occurs

A small percentage of drug abusers start out by taking medicines that were prescribed for them. More often, however, teens who abuse these drugs take medicine that is not prescribed for them. Sometimes a "friend" gives it to them at school. Other times, they steal a couple of pills at a time from friends or family members. Or, they may buy from dealers at school, work, or elsewhere. In one recent case, Boston police arrested a teen for robbing a pharmacy at gunpoint.

Unfortunately, the number of teens who abuse prescription medicines is substantial. In the 2002 Monitoring the Future survey, 10 percent of 12th graders said they had used prescription narcotics other than under a doctor's orders. The category included medicines such as Vicodin, OxyContin, Percocet, and Dilaudid.

Similarly, 10 percent of the 12th graders surveyed had used barbiturates. Eleven percent had used tranquilizers. Within the 30 days before the survey, 4 percent had used Ritalin without a doctor's supervision.

When doctors prescribe medicines, they consider a patient's medical history, including age and weight, allergies, other medicines that the patient uses, and so forth. While the patient may still need to beware of side effects or interactions, someone who has a legitimate prescription knows it is meant for him or her and can feel confident that the medicine is what it is supposed to be.

Teens who take drugs that were not prescribed for them cannot be sure what they are. If a 120-pound teen steals a pill meant for a 220-pound man, that teen risks a serious overdose. That's why it's dangerous to use someone else's medicine.

"People should be especially cautious if they have some kind of ongoing medical problem," notes Dr. Brown. "They may not be aware that a certain medication may be dangerous for them."

Drug Interactions and Reactions

Some medicines interact with other drugs. Some trigger serious allergic reactions.

… when someone who doesn't have a legitimate medical problem takes them [prescription drugs], they feel the effects much more, and that leads to more use

Different drugs present specific health risks. Tranquilizers, barbiturates, and narcotics all slow the central nervous system. Potential health consequences include confusion, memory problems, loss of coordination, and impaired judgment. Depres-

sants can also cause dangerously slow breathing, coma, and even death.

Stimulants speed up the central nervous system. Undesirable side effects can include sleep disorders, irritability, aggression, and hyperactivity. More serious health consequences can include irregular heartbeat, elevated body temperature, and fatal seizures or heart attacks.

Mixing prescription drugs with each other, with alcohol, or with other drugs multiplies their risks. Doctors call this a synergistic effect. Even though the allergy pills that Samantha took were over-the-counter medicine, the depressant in them magnified the potent effects of the morphine.

With their judgment impaired, teens are also more likely to engage in risky behavior. That includes impaired driving, sexual activity, and criminal behavior. Accidents, injuries, HIV and other sexually transmitted diseases, pregnancies, and arrests all become more likely.

Addiction: A Downward Spiral

Beyond their immediate health risks, many prescription medicines are also addictive. "Usually when people with legitimate medical conditions take these medicines, they don't feel euphoria. They feel relief of symptoms," says Dr. Brown. "But when someone who doesn't have a legitimate medical problem takes them, they feel the effects much more, and that leads to more use. Eventually, when kids take enough of the medicine and if they have a genetic predisposition, they can end up addicted." No one can know beforehand whether or not he or she has a genetic predisposition to become addicted to any drug.

"Prolonged use of these drugs eventually changes the brain in fundamental and long-lasting ways, which explains why people cannot just quit on their own, and why treatment is essential," Glen Hanson of the National Institute on Drug Abuse explained to a Senate committee last year. "In effect, drugs of abuse take over the brain's normal pleasure and motivational systems, moving drug use to the highest priority, thereby overriding all other motivations and drives. These brain changes are responsible for the compulsion to seek and use drugs that we have come to define as addiction."

As people become addicted, their lives spiral downward, out of control. They steal or incur debts to maintain their habit. Performance in school and work drops. Personal relationships deteriorate.

"No adolescent ever starts drinking or using drugs thinking he or she is going to become addicted," notes Dr. Brown. "That's the real trap of it all. Adolescents feel invincible. They feel they'll be able to control it. But before they know it, they're addicted. It's very difficult to break an addiction."

Medicine is supposed to help you function better, not worse. If one medicine is not right for you, another one may work better.

Complications arise when some teens who start out with valid medical problems become addicted. The addiction needs to be dealt with, but the underlying medical problem may still need attention. "Often we can find other medicines that are less addictive, tighten up supervision under which they're administered, and provide mainstream addiction treatment along with some more specialized treatment for the legitimate medical diagnosis," notes Dr. Brown.

Face to Face with Your Doctor

You know prescription medicines can help a lot of health problems. But you also know now that some medicines can cause addiction. What should you do when you see the doctor?

First of all, be completely honest. If you have any history of using alcohol or other drugs, say so. Don't assume that the doctor can figure it out or doesn't need to know. If a teen complaining about severe anxiety uses alcohol, for example, the doctor may decide not to prescribe certain tranquilizers. Also tell your physician about any addiction issues in the family.

Ideally, you'll be able to see your doctor one-on-one, so you can speak more freely. Most doctors will respect a teen's confidentiality. If you have any concerns, ask upfront. Doctors aren't in the business of judging patients, but helping them.

Also tell the doctor about all medicines you take—both by prescription and over-the-counter. Even vitamins or herbal supplements can interact dangerously with medications.

Be honest about your symptoms. No one else can tell you how much pain you should or shouldn't feel. Pain is a subjective experience. Too often, teens with chronic diseases such as sickle cell anemia or arthritis may suffer more than necessary.

Ask a lot of questions too. Exactly what is the medicine, and how is it supposed to work? What is the dosage? What if you forget a dose? Should you take the medicine with food? What side effects might you expect, and how should you deal with them? Should you take all of the medicine until it's gone, as doctors recommend for antibiotics? Or, should you use the medicine only as needed? Often it helps to take notes.

If a particular medicine gives you a really good feeling, tell your doctor. Feeling euphoria (as opposed to just relief of symptoms) is a potential danger sign for addiction.

On the other hand, a medicine may make you groggy or have other bad side effects. It may not be the right medicine for you. Sixteen-year-old Chris got morphine at the hospital after his arm surgery. When that made him sick, the doctor gave him Percocet instead.

"It took the pain away within minutes and lasted several hours," recalls Chris. "The only thing that I did not like was that all I wanted to do was sleep." The doctor then put him on Vicodin. Once he got home, however, Chris did not need the strong medicine. He was able to manage by taking ibuprofen and icing his shoulder instead.

Medicine is supposed to help you function better, not worse. If one medicine is not right for you, another one may work better. Your doctor might also recommend non-drug treatments, such as using ice or heat.

Be responsible with your medicines. Never share them with anyone. Even if a medicine is right for you, it could harm someone else. At home, store your medicines out of sight.

Last but not least, take any medicines exactly as prescribed. After all, that's just what the doctor ordered.

The Dangers of OXYCONTIN

When OxyContin went on the market in 1995, the drugmaker promoted it to doctors as a relatively safe narcotic. The round pills had a time-release mechanism for their synthetic version of morphine, oxycodone. Instead of giving patients a euphoric high, the drug could provide strong and sustained pain relief for chronic conditions like cancer and arthritis.

Soon, however, abusers looking for a quick high began chewing tablets or snorting crushed pills. Others dissolved them in water and injected the mixture. These methods quickly put dangerously high levels of oxycodone into the bloodstream.

OxyContin is known by the street names "oxy," "oxycotton," and "hillbilly heroin." In some rural areas, large numbers of people became addicted.

Abuse spread from rural areas to suburbs and cities. OxyContin became the subject of serious fraud, theft, and drug trafficking problems. Meanwhile, some patients who really needed the medicine had trouble getting it.

OxyContin abuse has killed many people, including teenagers. The Drug Enforcement Agency estimated that OxyContin played a part in more than 460 deaths during a two-year period.

The drug's maker has been working on a newer version. An added ingredient would block the drug's effect if someone chewed or crushed the pill. But the new version is not available yet. Meanwhile, the company has been named in more than a dozen lawsuits.

The bottom line? Experimenting with drug abuse is always dangerous.

over-the-counter drugs can pose risks too

You don't need a prescription to buy over-the-counter (OTC) medicines. Yet they can still present risks.

Some cough and cold medicines contain alcohol or other depressants. Other medicines have decongestants that speed up the heart rate. Still other medicines may contain both kinds of drugs.

Abusing these medicines to get a high or spaced-out feeling can be dangerous. Mixing them with alcohol, prescription medicines, or other drugs is even more risky.

for more information

National Institute on Drug Abuse. "Information on Drugs of Abuse—Prescription Drugs." http://www.drugabuse.gov/drugpages/prescription.html

reality check

do you know the rules at school?

Your school has rules about whether, when, and how students may take any medicines at school. The goal is to protect the safety of all students.

Review your school's policy on prescription and over-the-counter medicines at school. Then decide how you should act in each of these cases. Be ready to discuss each in class.

1. You are supposed to take a prescription medicine every four hours. What do you need to do to take it at school?
2. You have a terrible headache. What is the proper way for you to get an over-the-counter medicine to relieve the pain?
3. A friend says she's having terrible cramps with her period. She asks if you have anything she can take. What should you do?
4. Your friend starts having an asthma attack. He left his inhaler at home. What can you do?
5. You feel nervous before a big exam. A friend offers a pill to help you calm down. What do you do?

From *Current Health 2*, April/May 2003, p. 6. © 2003 by Current Health 2.

Addicted to anti-depressants?

The controversy over a pill millions of us are taking

Scores of patients call Paxil, a top-selling antidepressant, their emotional lifesaver.
But some say that getting off the drug has been physically torturous.
Now they're asking, Why weren't we warned?

By Stephen Fried

It wasn't until she felt the zaps— sharp, electrifying jolts causing sizzles of pain behind her green eyes—that Adrienne Bransky knew she was in trouble. "It was the worst pain I'd ever had in my life," she says.

She'd felt flu-ish all day during the conference she was attending, but her Chicago firm had flown the 29-year-old strategic management consultant to New York to troll for new contacts in the world of corporate mergers, so she tried to tough it out. The dizziness, nausea and vertigo got so bad, though, that she finally retreated to her hotel room.

She changed from her tailored suit into her old, comfy sweatpants and lay down on the king-size bed. Nothing helped—she couldn't stop the world from spinning. And then she felt that first zap. "Oh, my God," she said aloud as she burst into tears. "What was that?"

"If I moved my head," she recalls now, "it was like I was seeing in slow motion and the rest of my brain had to catch up. And when it caught up, I got the jolts, which just killed!"

Lying in the darkness, she wished she could talk to her husband, Aaron, a medical student, but he was unreachable at the hospital. Eventually, she contacted her personal physician and reported the symptoms, but the internist was baffled.

Then Bransky mentioned that her psychiatrist was weaning her off her antidepressant. She had been taking Paxil (paroxetine), among the most popular of the selective serotonin reuptake inhibitors (SSRIs), the class of psychiatric medicines that also includes Prozac and Zoloft. Bransky had been on Paxil ever since suffering what she refers to as a "breakdown" in her midtwenties, when she says she was "severely depressed and obsessed with running away from my life or killing myself." Paxil helped her in a matter of weeks, and she had been taking it successfully for four years, maintaining a moderate dosage of 30 mg per day. She'd asked her doctor to help wean her off the drug because she wanted to try to get pregnant.

Mysteriously—and violently—ill

Virtually all drugs may trigger side effects, and Bransky knew firsthand that Paxil can make your weight go up and your libido go down, something the drug's manufacturer, GlaxoSmithKline (GSK), acknowledges. But no one had ever told her that *quitting* the drug could cause problems. So she hadn't anticipated any.

Bransky's internist had a gut feeling that the Paxil was somehow to blame for her symptoms and told her to page the psychiatrist who'd prescribed the drug. The psychiatrist, however, assured her that as long as she had gradually reduced her dosage as instructed, Paxil could not be the culprit, Bransky says.

Mystified and violently ill, Bransky booked a flight home for the following morning. Then she curled up in a fetal position and cried herself to sleep.

> *"I thought that if I ever had to go through that hell again, I would kill myself."*

At the emergency room back in Chicago, doctors ran tests for everything from vertigo to serious neurological conditions; all were inconclusive. Bransky's internist continued to suspect Paxil, but she rarely prescribed the drug and didn't know its safety profile well. So she checked with the psychiatrist and ultimately deferred to her expert opinion that Bransky's discontinuation of her antidepressant wasn't to blame. Bransky was eventually sent home, where she lay in bed with no answers, still waiting for the shocks and the dizziness to stop.

"It was like I was drunk on an out-of-control cruise ship," she remembers.

Finally, about three weeks after the symptoms first appeared, they began to dissipate. At the one-month mark, she still felt drunk, but at least the cruise ship had docked in calm harbor. Eventually, Bransky was able to return to the office.

Don't take any drug until you read this!

Adverse drug reactions, commonly known as side effects, can occur when you start or stop taking a new medication, or at any time in between. You can minimize your risks by following these simple steps, developed in consultation with Brian L. Strom, M.D., director of the Center for Clinical Epidemiology and Biostatistics at the University of Pennsylvania School of Medicine.

Before you take a new medication, tell your doctor about all your old ones—prescription, over-the-counter and naturopathic. Also mention any drugs that have caused you problems in the past.

Ask your doctor if the drug she is prescribing is new to the market. If it's been available for less than a year, its potential side effects can't possibly be well-known yet. If you're being switched to a new drug for a condition your doctor has treated successfully in the past with something else, be especially curious. Doctors sometimes suggest swapping your old drug for another simply because your health insurer made a deal to buy the new one for less.

Never stop taking a prescribed medication—even for just a few days—without approval from your doctor.

Still, the memory of her world spinning out of control remained vivid.

"I thought that if I ever had to go through that hell again, I would kill myself," she says.

An army of angry patients

That episode occurred in 1998, and it would take more than a year for Bransky to feel sure that Paxil had, in fact, triggered her medical crisis. Yet even today—after experiencing a second episode of what she refers to as "Paxil withdrawal" and switching to another drug—she admits that Paxil "worked amazingly well. It saved me." The drug gets similarly ecstatic reviews from legions of other patients—most of them female, since the majority of those taking Paxil, and all antidepressants, are women. But an estimated one in 10 patients will experience problems if the drug is abruptly discontinued, and one in 20 may develop

more serious symptoms, similar to Bransky's, according to a leading expert on SSRI discontinuation, Jerrold F. Rosenbaum, M.D., chair of psychiatry at Massachusetts General Hospital in Boston. With approximately 25 million prescriptions written for Paxil last year, it's likely that hundreds of thousands of patients are affected.

A growing number of these patients assert that they they weren't adequately warned about how hard it can be to stop taking Paxil. Some have joined a major lawsuit in California that charges GSK with deliberately withholding information about "withdrawal." (Similar suits have been filed in at least 14 other states.) The firm handling that suit has heard from more than 6,000 prospective clients, and of the 35 named plaintiffs in the suit—those with the most typical symptoms and strongest cases—two thirds are women. Bransky is one them. "I'm not looking to get anything out of this financially," she says, "but these pharmaceutical companies are not educating doctors and patients!"

There is no question that Paxil and the other SSRI medications have revolutionized the treatment of depression. They have relieved symptoms for millions of patients worldwide, becoming one of the pharmaceutical industry's blockbuster categories in the process. For the past several years, Paxil has been the top-selling drug for GSK, with some $2.67 billion in global sales last year (second only to Zoloft among the SSRIs).

But ever since the first SSRI, Prozac, came on the market in 1987, there have been questions about the potential for significant side effects. For years, the SSRI manufacturers and the Food and Drug Administration only glancingly acknowledged the fact that the drugs can cause sexual problems—everything from dampening of libido to complete inability to have an orgasm—affecting perhaps as many as half of all patients; they can also cause weight gain. Such problems are among the reasons that many patients have a love-hate relationship with their psychiatric drugs and often look forward to a day when they can manage without them.

Given this yearning to stop taking antidepressants, it is bitterly ironic that

some of the worst side effects can hit when patients least expect them: The moment they try to get *off* the drugs. Many patients suffer nothing more than flulike symptoms. But the more extreme cases, frequently involving Paxil, include symptoms like severe nausea, dizziness, disorientation and "zaps"—the feeling of a lightning jolt in the brain. Studies report that these patients often miss days or weeks of work and still don't feel *right* even after they return to their normal routines. Many find that the only thing that makes them feel better is going back on their medication. Talk to them and you find that most knew nothing about the risk of withdrawal when they were put on antidepressants: They received no warnings from their doctors and read no prominent advisories in GSK's package insert; FDA regulation did not protect them. The message to the rest of us? When your doctor starts you on a prescription drug, particularly one that's relatively new to the market, you may not get the whole story on its side effects. And the whole story, argue women like Bransky, is exactly what you need to stay safe.

Drug company denials

While these side effects can occur with all SSRIs, they occur more frequently with Paxil, according to sources such as *The Journal of Clinical Psychiatry*. This is especially troubling because Paxil is FDA-approved to treat more symptoms than any other SSRI, including anxiety, panic disorder, social phobia (clinical shyness) and, most recently, post-traumatic stress disorder. Physicians also favor Paxil because it's thought to be the fastest-acting SSRI.

The Paxil discontinuation syndrome and the reasons for it were explored anecdotally in reports throughout the mid-nineties. Then in 1997, papers by Dr. Rosenbaum and others cited studies that proved the symptoms existed and could be serious. Why might Paxil cause more problems when halted than other SSRIs? Dr. Rosenbaum and his colleagues explained that the drug stops working as quickly as it starts, exiting the body in four days. (Prozac, by contrast, can linger up to four weeks.) Apparently, this abruptness causes a sudden chemical imbalance and in some cases makes patients physically ill.

Those who have had the most difficult experiences getting off Paxil, along with some vocal physicians and health care advocates, claim that patients are becoming "addicted" to their antidepressants and are experiencing true withdrawal. They are harshly critical of GSK's actions—and inaction—over the years. "What shocks me, to be quite honest, is not the existence of this very nasty side effect but the way [GSK has] denied it," says British pharmaceutical safety activist Charles Medawar, whose lobbying helped persuade his government to change the drug's label warnings in the United Kingdom. "There is clear evidence of withdrawal, and a risk of dependence exists for a minority of users."

GSK refutes such charges and says the symptoms critics call "withdrawal" are, in most cases, little more than a rapid relapse of the psychiatric illness the drug was prescribed for. "Many of these discontinuation symptoms overlap with the symptoms of anxiety and depression," says Alan Metz, M.D., GSK's vice president, psychiatry, clinical research and medical affairs. "It may be difficult to distinguish discontinuation symptoms from a relapse of the underlying illness." According to prescribing materials for Paxil, these symptoms are usually "mild" and "may have no causal relationship to the drug," "did not require medical intervention" and, in any case, "have been reported for other selective serotonin reuptake inhibitors." In other words, the symptoms are minor and common to all SSRIs. Dr. Metz strongly denies the harshest accusation, that Paxil is addictive, pointing out: "With addictive medications, it's very clear that the longer you take them, the more likely you are to become dependent. If this were to occur with Paxil, it should get worse when the patient takes the drug for long periods. But we found that the symptoms were less frequent in the longer-term studies."

Dr. Metz does admit, however, that the company discovered long ago that tapering the dose, rather than stopping the drug cold turkey, appeared to prevent many patients from suffering discontinuation symptoms. (Tapering doesn't help everyone, though, as Bransky's case illus-

trates.) In fact, all GSK clinical trials with Paxil since 1994 have included a tapered regimen. But it took the company nearly eight more years, until December 2001, to directly acknowledge the problems of discontinuation symptoms and suggest tapering to patients and physicians in Paxil's FDA-approved prescribing information. Because of that delay, advocates say, hundreds of thousands of patients may have needlessly suffered when they stopped taking the drug suddenly.

"We all hope that we won't have to take these pills forever. That's why drug companies need to be more responsible."

Martha Folmsbee, a 40-year-old microbiology graduate student at the University of Oklahoma, says she is one of those patients. Her Paxil "withdrawal" experience began when her fanny pack, which had her medication, was stolen while she was at a scientific conference in Los Angeles. Folmsbee had been on Paxil for a year, and while it effectively controlled her depression, she was uncomfortable with the idea of taking the drug indefinitely. She decided to use the pilfering of her pills to see how she felt without Paxil. Several days later, she had her answer: She was in agony. "I was vomiting and had horrible diarrhea, constant nausea, migraines and extreme weakness," she recalls. Her doctors, like Bransky's, could determine nothing from numerous tests. But when she started taking Paxil again and all the symptoms miraculously disappeared, she felt certain that she had experienced Paxil "withdrawal."

"I was told by a doctor that I had just relapsed, but these weren't symptoms of my depression, which I know well," Folmsbee says. "When Paxil was abruptly withdrawn, I was *physically* sick, with awful vomiting, diarrhea, disorientation and confusion." She tried to wean herself off the drug, but the "withdrawal" symptoms returned whenever she got down to 5 mg. It took a year of lowering her dose by minute increments to finally wean herself completely. "The hardest part is that you don't have an organized support network like the ones people rely on to

get over many other addictions," she says. "My family helped pull me through. Even so, it took all my determination."

The question of addiction

So what truly goes on in patients' bodies when they try to go off Paxil? Many experts believe they are experiencing neither relapse of psychiatric symptoms nor true withdrawal. "It's a classic rebound effect," says John Urquhart, M.D., professor of pharmaco-epidemiology at Maastricht University in the Netherlands. Rebound effects occur when a body system that has been artificially regulated by medication is suddenly left to its own devices again—and temporarily over-regulates before finding a new happy medium. The harsh post-Paxil symptoms might just be the serotonin system sputtering as it readjusts. Other commonly used drugs can cause rebound effects when stopped—for example, getting off some beta blocker medication can cause anything from severe anxiety to a full-blown heart attack. Many patients don't know about rebound effects, says Dr. Urquhart, because "what happens to patients when they stop taking drugs turns out to be a major blind spot in drug development. Companies invariably invest major efforts in studying the onset of drug action but hardly ever study the 'offset' of drug action."

The big difference between beta blockers and Paxil, however, is that the rebound effects of heart drugs are well-known by physicians and pharmacists, and the warnings on their labels are far more prominent than those on Paxil's. In a 1997 study, 70 percent of general practitioners surveyed and 28 percent of psychiatrists didn't know that SSRIs could cause discontinuation symptoms; only 17 percent of general practitioners and only 20 percent of psychiatrists were consistently cautioning their patients about how to slowly taper off the drugs. And for years, the FDA allowed GSK to describe Paxil as "non-habit-forming" in its print and TV ads, even though critics say this scientific claim is false.

In a California federal court hearing last August, U.S. district judge Mariana Pfaelzer banned, in the name of "public interest in health and safety," all ads making the claim that Paxil wasn't habit-forming. The court order was quickly reversed, but last October GSK voluntarily dropped the troublesome language. And new ads running this winter included a warning that patients should consult their doctors before discontinuing the drug.

For Monica Keller, a 40-year-old accountant for Ticketmaster who is a member of the California suit, those concessions are too little, too late. "For years, they claimed it wasn't habit-forming. That was the biggest lie!" she fumes. Keller originally took Paxil for panic attacks and was incapacitated for more than a month with "withdrawal" symptoms; they vanished the day after she resumed taking the drug. It took her more than two years of repeated attempts before she finally quit Paxil for good. "It *is* habit-forming," she says. "And I was a drug addict."

An online underground

For quite a while, Adrienne Bransky didn't believe her physical breakdown at the conference had anything to do with her antidepressant. When the episode ended, she was happy not to think about it. She got pregnant in 1999, several weeks after her worst symptoms abated, and her mood remained fairly stable during her first and second trimesters. In the middle of the third trimester, however, she became depressed and even entertained what her husband describes as suicidal thoughts—"although I don't think she would have done anything to herself," he says. Finally, her condition seemed too dangerous to leave untreated. Her doctors decided she had to go back

on Paxil. Once again, her depression quickly lifted. If anything, she experienced postpartum elation after giving birth to her son.

Life went on. Soon Bransky was back at work, the baby was doing fine and Paxil was, once again, her wonder drug. Then about a year later, she began having "breakthrough symptoms," signs of depression indicating that her current dosage of medication was no longer adequate to control her illness. Bransky had switched psychiatrists when she and Aaron moved to Milwaukee for his residency; her new doctor suggested an increase in her dosage of Paxil. That seemed logical, but Bransky wanted to do some research on the Internet first. There she discovered the growing controversy over "Paxil withdrawal."

She quickly tapped into a cluster of Web sites that constitute the "Paxil withdrawal" underground—a community of advocates and patients trying to inform the public about the syndrome and help one another break free of the drug. That's when Bransky told her doctor she "just wanted off Paxil," no matter how bad quitting might make her feel. After reading countless discontinuation accounts that sounded strikingly similar to her own, she simply couldn't bring herself to give one more penny of her money to GSK. So she endured a second wave of flulike symptoms and disorientation. This time, however, she was better prepared: At the suggestion of her new psychiatrist, Bransky added Prozac to her pharmacological cocktail during the weaning process. With the longest half-life of all the SSRIs, Prozac keeps

regulating serotonin long after Paxil has left the building. The combo technique is now recommended by sources like *Prescriber's Letter* and *Harvard Mental Health Letter*.

Eventually, Bransky got pregnant again, and in her second trimester the depression returned, full force. She and her doctor decided to try a lesser-known antidepressant called Celexa, marketed by Forest Laboratories, in the hopes that it would cause fewer side effects and discontinuation problems. So far, so good: Bransky says she has had "no issues" with the drug, and her depression is currently in check.

She remains a member of the California suit, however, and follows the case closely. While she was relived when GSK dropped the "non-habit-forming" lines and added a warning to its new ads, she continues to worry that patients will start taking the drug without any knowledge of the complications they could encounter while getting off it. "Most people don't want to rely on antidepressants all their lives," she says. "We all hold out the hope that we don't have to take these pills forever. That's why pharmaceutical companies need to be more forthright and responsible and need to put more money into educating doctors about the risks of withdrawal. Maybe then you'll have fewer patients going through the hell I went through."

Stephen Fried is the author of Bitter Pills: Inside the Hazardous World of Legal Drugs. *His latest book is* The New Rabbi: A Congregation Searches for Its Leader.

From *Glamour*, April 2003, pp. 178-180, 262. © 2003 by Glamour.

WHEN DRINKING HELPS

Sorting out for whom a nip might prove therapeutic

BY JANET RALOFF

Downing a cocktail or other alcoholic drink at least three to four times a week appears to substantially cut a man's risk of heart attack, Boston-area researchers reported in early January. Less than a week later, a U.S.-Canadian team of epidemiologists focusing on African Americans announced it had found no clear benefit to people drinking the same amount of alcohol per week. These reports joined other seemingly conflicting studies on the health impacts of alcohol that have emerged in the past few years.

Some research found that regular, moderate drinking not only helps preserve mental clarity in both young and elderly people but also increases blood-sugar control in people with diabetes. Other studies linked low but regular consumption of alcohol with an increased risk of certain cancers and a stunting of children exposed to alcohol in the womb. These subtle detrimental effects, of course, add onto the potentially catastrophic acute events caused by alcohol-impaired judgment.

With dozens of conflicting reports spilling out each year, is it any wonder that the public is confused about alcohol and health?

Yet, in probing the scores of published papers on alcohol's impacts, researchers have begun to discern a few trends. Chief among them: Alcoholic beverages can offer large pharmacological benefits, especially to people at elevated risk of heart disease. Various studies have begun unveiling why (*SN: 1/5/02, p. 8*).

In fact, argues Jurgen Rehm of the Centre for Addiction and Mental Health in Toronto, because alcohol's benefits appear primarily from slowing the progression of chronic diseases that usually emerge in or after middle age, there seems to be little health justification for drinking alcohol before age 40.

Among older adults, however, benefits of moderate drinking "appear to be huge," notes Tim Stockwell, director of the National Centre for Research into the Prevention of Drug Abuse at Curtin University of Technology in Perth, Australia. Data in his country indicate that among people who regularly down a few

drinks a day, "there are approximately 6,500 lives saved each year by alcohol's protective effects on cardiovascular disease." Even factoring in alcohol-associated deaths from breast cancer and other malignancies, he says, "the net benefit for [moderate] drinking here appears to be about 5,000 lives a year."

"Although I think alcohol can be part of a healthy lifestyle, it's not a necessity," says Eric B. Rimm of the Harvard School of Public Health in Boston. Moreover, he adds, one wouldn't want to push abstainers to start drinking if they have cultural, religious, or other prohibitions against it—or an inability to hold their drinking to a few glasses per day. And drinking should never, he says, be portrayed as a substitute for exercise, eating a healthy diet, or giving up cigarettes as the best ways to stave off heart disease.

"There are probably many cases where some people should be told to drink a little more."

—ERIC B. RIMM

But among people who now drink occasionally, Rimm says, the accumulating evidence of alcohol's potential benefits is "so overwhelming that there are probably many cases where some people should be told to drink a little more."

RISKS IN ABSTAINING Alcohol is without question a poison. People die from binging, and many children enter the world with a retardation that traces to prenatal alcohol exposure. In fact, Rehm says, more than 60 diseases have been linked to excessive consumption of alcohol.

Although one might expect those risks to increase linearly with consumption, they don't. Stockwell points to hundreds of studies showing that a little daily drinking is more healthful than either abstaining or drinking to excess.

Epidemiologists refer to this as alcohol's "J-shape curve, for the contour that the risk data take when plotted on a graph. That provocative contour emerged strongly in a new review of 35 studies on stroke performed by researchers at Tulane University in New Orleans. In the Feb. 5 *Journal of the American Medical Association*, Kristi Reynolds and her colleagues confirm "a J-shaped association between alcohol consumption and the relative risk of… ischemic stroke," a disorder that traces to blockages in the brain's blood vessels.

Two years ago, Rehm and his colleagues reported a J-shape curve for alcohol consumption and premature deaths from all causes in their 11-year study of 5,200 U.S. men and women.

Economists at Duke University in Durham, N.C., published data 2 years ago showing a J contour in alcohol's impacts on disability claims. For 6 years, Jan Ostermann and Frank A. Sloan followed 12,650 people initially in their 50s or 60s. People drinking one or two drinks a day were least likely to report a disabling event, such as stroke or arthritis, "whereas abstainers generally were most likely to be disabled."

No matter how many possibly confounding factors they investigated, Sloan says, "we could not make the effect go away."

Rimm's team also observed a disadvantage for abstainers in a new 12-year study of heart-disease risks in 38,000 male health professionals. Overall, the researchers report in the Jan. 9 *New England Journal of Medicine*, disease risk fell as the volume of regularly consumed alcohol rose.

SWEET NEWS A J-shape curve has emerged in alcohol's effects on diabetes and also on cognition. Last spring, federal scientists at the Beltsville (Md.) Agricultural Research Center linked alcohol consumption directly to blood sugar and insulin benefits in a trial with 63 healthy postmenopausal women.

In one 8-week phase, the women drank orange juice laced with 15 grams of alcohol each night before bed; in another, they drank juice containing 30 grams a night, the equivalent of two drinks. To keep other aspects of the diet from affecting the parameters being measured, the scientists administered carefully controlled meals to every woman throughout the trial. Such costly, controlled-feeding trials represent the gold standard of nutritional studies.

In the May 15, 2002 *Journal of the American Medical Association*, David J. Baer and his colleagues report that the women's insulin values, blood sugar, and cholesterol were healthiest during the two-drink-per-day regimen.

Although this trial used straight ethanol in juice, other studies have shown that certain pigmented compounds, called phenolics, that show up in beer and red wine can have their own healthful effects on people's hearts and blood sugar.

Pierre-Louis Teissedre and his colleagues at the University of Montpellier, France, gave diabetic rats phenolics-enriched white wine for 6 weeks in amounts equivalent to a person's intake of a half-liter per day. Afterward, the rats' blood quashed oxidative reactions—a major cause of diabetes complications—as well as the blood of healthy rats did. The treated animals also showed slightly improved control of blood-sugar concentra-

tions. The findings appear in the Jan. 1 *Journal of Agricultural and Food Chemistry*.

The researchers then further enriched the wine with phenolics to achieve what Teissedre describes as pharmacological doses. In just-completed tests, this doctored wine "corrected the diabetes" by bringing control of the animals' blood sugar into a normal range, Teissedre reports.

One interesting observation: The antidiabetes effect diminished when the animals received phenolics without alcohol.

A clear J-shape curve is also showing up in studies of alcohol's effects on cognition. For instance, a year ago, Dutch researchers found that moderate drinkers have a lower risk of Alzheimer's disease and dementias than do abstainers or heavy drinkers (*SN: 2/2/02, p. 67*).

While that study was in the works, Constantine G. Lyketsos and his colleagues at Johns Hopkins University in Baltimore investigated effects of long-term drinking on reasoning, memory, decision making, and psychomotor speed in nearly 1,500 people. Scores on the test used in the study typically drop about 1 point per decade during early adulthood and 2 to 3 points per decade for people in their 60s. But in the new 13-year study, both young and old adults who regularly drank outperformed abstainers of the same age.

The finding was particularly robust for women, the Johns Hopkins team reported in the Oct. 15, 2002 *American Journal of Epidemiology*. Nondrinking women declined a point more on the test during the study than did moderate, habitual drinkers. For perspective, Lyketsos notes, "people with Alzheimer's disease tend to decline an average of 3 to 4 points on this scale every year, so a 1-point drop is not negligible." In fact, he concludes, because even heavy drinkers outperformed teetotalers, "the findings suggest that maybe the worst thing you can do is not drink."

TROUBLING TESTIMONY Such statements trouble Nancy L. Day of the Western Psychiatric Institute and Clinic in Pittsburgh. Many women don't know they're carrying a child until well into their pregnancy, she notes, and her data indicate that "no amount of alcohol is healthy during pregnancy"—at least for the child.

Over the past couple decades, she and her colleagues have been measuring the growth and development since birth of 565 children from low-income, inner-city families. In the October 2002 *Alcoholism: Experimental and Clinical Research*, Day's group reported that 14-year-old children who had been exposed in the womb to alcohol were—as they had been at birth—shorter and leaner than the offspring of women who eschewed alcohol during pregnancy. The finding was true even for the women who downed just one or two drinks per month during their first trimester—a finding that "blew us away," Day told *Science News*.

By age 14, children of the lightest drinkers averaged 3 pounds less than nondrinkers' children; offspring of the heaviest drinkers, 16 pounds less. Though smoking during pregnancy also yields smaller babies, those kids "usually catch up within the first year or so," Day notes.

What concerns her most is that teenage children of drinkers had a smaller average head circumference—"a very crude measure of brain size"—than nondrinkers' teens had. Indeed, her latest findings show that fetal-alcohol exposure correlated with subtle changes in information processing that could impair learning.

For adults, drinking alcohol has also been tied to cancer. Many analyses show a steadily increasing risk of breast cancer as the average daily consumption of alcohol increases. For example, one 1998 study found that alcohol equivalent to one drink a day increases the risk of breast cancer by about 9 percent.

Characteristics of drinking can have an effect, too. People who down a significant share of their alcohol outside of meals, for instance, face at least a 50 percent higher risk of cancer in the oral cavity, pharynx and esophagus than do people who drink only at meals (*http://www.sciencenews.org/20030215/food.asp*).

BINGEING BACKFIRES A growing number of studies are finding new risks from binge drinking, which is usually defined as downing five or more servings of alcohol in one day. Lyketsos and his colleagues found in their study that people who typically binged had more cognitive decline than did heavy, frequent drinkers consuming comparable volumes of alcohol.

Indeed, Rehm and Christopher T. Sempos of the University of Buffalo's Department of Social and Preventive Medicine suspect that bingeing may account for the results of their team's analysis of drinking and health in 2,000 African Americans.

They analyzed 19 years' of dietary data for blacks in the National Health and Nutrition Examination Survey (NHANES). The epidemiologists compared alcohol consumption per week with death from any cause. In the January *Alcoholism: Experimental and Clinical Research*, they report that the data for the African-Americans didn't follow the J curve, but risk of death "increased with increasing average consumption."

FORTIFIED WHITE—Domaine Virginie of Bezier, France, has begun marketing Paradoxe Blanc as "the first white wine offering the same health benefits as red wine." The chardonnay, developed at the University of Montpellier, is enriched with phenolics that are good for the heart.

Rehm and Sempos note that the survey asked only how many servings of alcohol people typically down in a week. If the answer was 10 to 14, for example, but that amount was consumed only over the weekend, that's bingeing, Sempos says.

In fact, the researchers cite three studies since 1995 indicating that the African-American community has a higher proportion of abstainers and bingers than the white population does. Moreover, says Thomas K. Greenfield of the Alcohol Research Group in Berkeley, Calif., some studies have reported "that because of larger containers and higher-alcohol-content products marketed to African-Americans, surveys [like NHANES] may even underestimate the heavy quantities consumed by ethnic minorities."

Fuzzy reporting of consumption patterns compromises data from most alcohol surveys, Rehm observes. That's why many researchers would prefer data from experiments in which people drink alcohol only under researchers' supervision.

Shela Gorinstein of the Hebrew University-Hadassah Medical School in Jerusalem says her team expects to begin just such a clinical trial soon. Some lucky recruits will get free beer for 10 years.

Binge drinking holds steady:

College students continue to drink despite programs

By Alvin Powell
Gazette Staff

College students have continued binge drinking at about the same rate over the past 10 years, despite increases in alcohol education programs and substance-free on-campus housing, and a decrease in high school binge drinking, according to a Harvard School of Public Health study.

The positive trends have been offset by an increase in heavy drinking by students who do drink, with an increase in the percentage of frequent binge drinkers to 22.8 percent from 19.7 percent in 1993.

"This to us indicates very strong forces are continuing to support drinking on campus," said Henry Wechsler, director of College Alcohol Studies and a lecturer on social psychology at the Harvard School of Public Health. "The drinking style on campus is still one of excess."

About 44 percent of college undergraduates reported binge drinking at least once in the two weeks prior to being surveyed, according to findings in the 2001 College Alcohol Study, whose results were released March 25. The study, which was also conducted in 1993, 1997, and 1999, also indicated that, of students who drink, 70 percent engage in bingeing. The study defines binge drinking as having five or more drinks on one occasion for men and four or more drinks on one occasion for women. Frequent binge drinkers binged on at least three occasions in the previous two weeks.

The survey includes responses from more than 10,000 full-time students at 119 four-year colleges located in 38 states. Wechsler declined to identify individual schools, saying it's a problem of all colleges, not just those involved in the survey. He did say that selective schools such as those in the Ivy League had results similar to other institutions. Results were published in two articles in the Journal of American College Health's March issue.

The surprising thing in this year's study was the steady 44 percent rate despite other positive changes, Wechsler said. That indicates not that those changes were failures, Wechsler said, but that they alone can't fix the problem.

"I think what colleges need to do is go beyond the kinds of programs in place at most schools aimed at educating students to a restructuring of the whole environment, both campus and the community," Wechsler said.

Counterbalancing the positive changes are entrenched forces that promote drinking, Wechsler said. Fraternities and sororities continue to be centers of campus drinking, he said, with 75 percent of those living in frat or sorority houses reporting binge drinking in the survey. While that number is actually down from 83 percent in 1993, it's still indicative of a problem, Wechsler said.

Another problem area is college athletics, Wechsler said, with drinking commonly being associated with athletic events and, outside those events, athletes often involved in heavy drinking.

Economics are also working against a downward trend in heavy drinking, Wechsler said. Typical college campuses are ringed by bars and liquor stores that market heavily on campus, offering low prices and easy access.

While the overall bingeing rate held steady, the overall picture of college drinking hasn't been completely static, Wechsler said. There has been a trend of polarization, with more students abstaining and heavier drinking by those who drink. More students are living in substance-free housing on campus, rising from 17 percent in 1993 to 28 percent in 2001. Rates of bingeing at all-women colleges have risen, from 24 percent in 1993 to 32 percent in 2001. Despite that increase, bingeing rates at all-women colleges are still lower than for women at coed institutions.

While fewer high school students are bingeing, underage drinking at college campuses continues to be a problem. Underage students accounted for about half—48 percent—of the drinking on campus.

Student housing was a major factor in the level of drinking, Wechsler said, with 75 percent of those living in frat or sorority houses reporting bingeing, 51 percent living in dormitories, 50 percent in off-campus housing without their parents, 36 percent living in substance-free housing, and 25 percent living at home with their parents.

The study did provide cause for hope. Wechsler said that states with tough underage drinking laws reported lower rates of underage drinking, showing that those laws are working.

Colleges and universities need help from the surrounding communities to tackle this problem, Wechsler said, with tougher laws, limits on on-campus alcohol marketing, and higher prices for alcohol. Colleges, for their part, he said, should look into the connection between drinking and athletics and fulfill their longstanding promises to crack down on fraternity- and sorority-related drinking.

Finally, Wechsler said, parents should take an active role, talking to their children about alcohol use and—at a minimum—refrain from bringing alcohol to their underage children in the dormitories, as some students reported.

"I think parents should take the problem of drinking alcohol seriously for their underage students," Wechsler said. "I think the one thing we need to do is get real about this. It's a serious problem and people are groping for quick and easy solutions. And there aren't any."

---

alvin_powell@harvard.edu

MORE THAN A KICK

On its own, nicotine might promote tumors and wrinkles

BY KENDALL MORGAN

Nicotine shifts the body into high gear. Whether from a puff on a cigarette or a patch stuck to the skin, the drug enters the bloodstream and bathes the internal organs. But scientists generally attribute nicotine's power solely to the activity it sparks in the brain. That stimulation makes smokers feel good, even euphoric. It's also what makes them crave more. Physicians, however, generally finger tobacco's thousands of other chemical constituents, including known carcinogens—not nicotine—for cigarettes' nastiest side effects. Each year, tobacco accounts for 400,000 deaths among 48 million smokers in the United States alone.

TROUBLE MAKER— Nicotine, cigarettes' chemical lure, might also be an accomplice in many of the ailments spawned of tobacco.

Beyond its addictive appeal, nicotine itself might have devastating consequences throughout the body, some scientists now say. Acetylcholine—the natural nerve-signal carrier that nicotine mimics—is a jack-of-all-trades. The chemical acts on many cells, including those in the lungs and skin. Therefore, nicotine may goad many tissues into hyperactivity—a possibility that raises scientists' suspicions about its role in disease.

"It's an eye opener. Nicotine isn't just a drug that stimulates neurons. It does the exact same thing to cells outside of the nervous system," says dermatologist Sergei A. Grando of the University of California, Davis, who studies nicotine's effects on skin.

A handful of recent studies has suggested a link between nicotine and ailments ranging from sudden infant death syndrome (*SN: 9/14/02, p. 163*) to cancer. Scientists have found that the stimulant spurs the formation of blood vessels that could feed tumors and promote plaque buildup in arteries (*SN: 7/7/01, p. 6*). The body may also convert nicotine into the chemical precursors of the carcinogen that scientists call NNK (*SN: 10/28/00, p. 278*).

The latest experimental work strengthens the connection between nicotine and disease and highlights additional ways that the chemical might promote tumors, age skin, and stall wound healing. Researchers say the drug may also literally cook proteins in the blood.

DEATH CAN BE GOOD Nicotine probably doesn't cause cancer, but new research suggests it might keep cancer cells alive. And it apparently does so in two different ways.

First, the drug prevents a cellular form of suicide, called apoptosis, that normally eliminates nascent cancer and other damaged cells, says clinical oncologist Phillip A. Dennis of the National Cancer Institute in Bethesda, Md.

In many cancers—including those of the breast, ovaries, prostate, and brain—a protein that normally keeps apoptosis under control gets stuck in its active form and thus shuts down the suicide sequence. More recently, Dennis' team discovered that the same molecule, called either Akt or protein kinase B, jams in the on-position in most lung cancer cells. The finding led the team to wonder whether constituents of tobacco activate Akt in the lung.

To find out, they tested the effect of nicotine and its derivative NNK on normal lung cells in lab dishes. Nicotine activated Akt at concentrations comparable to those that have been measured in smokers' blood, and the cell-suicide rate fell by 60 percent, the team reports in the January *Journal of Clinical Investigation*. It took more stress—ultraviolet radiation exposure, for example—to kill nicotine-activated cells than normal cells required, Dennis says.

Nicotine-treated cells acted abnormal in other ways, too. In lab dishes, lung cells usually stop growing when they become crowded, Dennis explains. "When treated with nicotine, lung

Not all bad

A once-good-for-nothing drug improves its reputation

The properties that make nicotine a health hazard might also make it a useful therapy for more than smoking cessation. "Nicotine is a drug—not a poison or carcinogen—but a drug," says Sergei A. Grando of the University of California, Davis. "Nicotine is often a bad guy," he adds, "but it can also be a good guy."

For one, nicotine can help alleviate the mind-numbing symptoms of Alzheimer's disease. Alzheimer's patients lack the normal number of one type of receptor that binds acetylcholine in the brain, making them less responsive to that nerve signal. The deficit leads to learning and memory problems, says neurobiologist Alfred Maelicke at Johannes-Gutenberg University in Mainz, Germany.

A similar shortfall plagues people with schizophrenia and epilepsy, among other disorders, he adds. In such cases, intermittent nicotine boosts to the brain can help, Maelicke says. Nicotine patches may also fight depression (*SN: 5/11/02, p. 302*). And there's more good news. Although regular nicotine use can delay wound healing, a new study finds that the stimulant speeds healing in mice with diabetes—a disease that normally impairs wound healing.

Prompted by his earlier discovery that nicotine spurs blood vessel growth, John P. Cooke of Stanford University wondered whether the drug might help close wounds. His team injured diabetic and nondiabetic mice and then applied a solution containing nicotine to some of the animals in each group.

After 5 days, diabetic mice receiving the nicotine treatment had healed substantially more than diabetic mice not getting the drug had, the team reported in the July 2002 *American Journal of Pathology*. Nondiabetic mice didn't benefit from the treatment with nicotine.

That result makes sense to Grando. "Like any drug, the dose is important," he explains. "At low doses, nicotine can favor faster wound healing, while in larger doses it has the opposite effect."

The challenge in all nicotine's possible uses is to identify people for whom the drug's benefits outweigh its risks and to develop targeted delivery methods, says Phillip A. Dennis of the National Cancer Institute in Bethesda, Md.—K.M.

cells kept growing to the point of coming right out of the plastic," he says.

NNK also enhanced cell survival by stimulating Akt. Therefore, NNK might exacerbate nicotine's cancer-promoting ability, Dennis suggests.

Nicotine's boost to cell survival could be important to other cancers associated with tobacco, including those of the head, neck, kidney, and bladder, he says.

Nicotine has a second talent for enhancing tumor growth, two lines of research suggest. The drug makes tumor-nurturing blood vessels sprout. Tumors can only grow to a certain point before they must be fed, says John P. Cooke of Stanford University. "They don't continue to grow and become malignant unless they can call blood vessels into themselves," he says.

Cooke's team has found that nicotine increases the speed at which human blood vessel cells grow in lab dishes. What's more, lung-tumor cells in mice given nicotine-laced water expanded faster than those in mice not given the drug (*SN: 7/7/01, p. 6*).

Nicotine may encourage blood vessel formation by stimulating the production of vascular endothelial growth factor, or VEGF, a second team of researchers has found. Vascular-system researcher Brian S. Conklin, now at Baylor College of Medicine in Houston, and his colleagues knew that VEGF shows up in the majority of cancerous tumors. It's also a player in plaque formation along blood vessel walls. Because vascular disease and cancer are both linked to smoking, Conklin and his colleagues wondered whether nicotine might ramp up blood concentrations of the growth factor.

The team tested the effects of nicotine and cotinine—the primary product of nicotine breakdown in the liver—on blood concentrations of VEGF in a pig artery. Both compounds hiked concentrations of the growth factor, the researchers reported in the February 2002 *American Journal of Pathology*.

FULL SPEED AHEAD Just as nicotine sparks activity in nerve and tumor cells, it speeds up normal cellular activity in the skin. For example, some cells exposed to nicotine might go through the same life stages in 10 days that would normally take 10 weeks, says dermatologist Grando.

Such hyperactivity occurs in cells called dermal fibroblasts that control the skin's texture by regulating the production of support proteins including collagen and elastin. When skin gets wounded, these fibroblasts send out proteins that clean the site. The cleanup crew acts like "biological scissors," Grando says, clearing the way for healing to begin.

In the February *Laboratory Investigation*, the team reports that nicotine sends fibroblasts into inappropriate activity. In the laboratory, the researchers exposed human fibroblast cells to the drug. Enzymes normally unleashed to clean wound sites were deployed in the absence of injury. Those proteins then chewed up the scaffolding that keeps skin flexible and strong. That effect would leave skin sagging and wrinkled, Grando explains.

On the other hand, in regular users of tobacco, another mechanism of skin healing slows down as a result of nicotine's ability to speed cells up. Normally at a cut, skin cells called keratinocytes crawl out from the edge of a wound and cover the broken surface. Acetylcholine sets those cellular healers in motion. That led Grando and his colleagues to ask whether nicotine interferes with keratinocyte migration.

The researchers grew human skin cells in lab dishes and treated some cells with growth factors and others with growth factors in combination with nicotine. Nicotine-treated cells started to move as if on a healing mission but stopped short of the distance that cells not given nicotine traveled, the team reported 2 years ago. The span traveled by keratinocytes declined further as more nicotine was added to the lab dishes.

The fast-paced lifestyle that nicotine induces in cells might explain why, Grando says. Nicotine cuts skin cells' active life

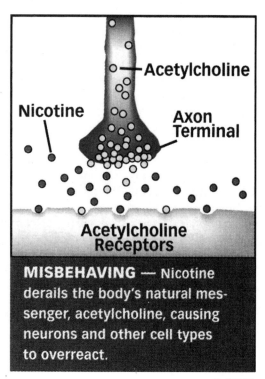

MISBEHAVING — Nicotine derails the body's natural messenger, acetylcholine, causing neurons and other cell types to overreact.

E. ROELL

short, leaving them with too little time to seal a wound before they conk out, he hypothesizes.

NOW WE'RE COOKING Nicotine's widespread effects result primarily from its imitating the natural stimulant acetylcholine. But a new study suggests that a derivative of the drug might also interact with the blood to literally fry proteins.

While poring over the chemical structure of nornicotine—a minor metabolite of nicotine—chemist Kim D. Janda of Scripps Research Institute in La Jolla, Calif., recognized that the compound has the potential to mangle proteins. The metabolite could spur the same chemical transformation that occurs when potatoes are fried, he suspected, a reaction familiar to food scientists as the browning effect. A similar reaction can occur without the high temperatures, Janda explains. Proteins altered

in this way have been implicated in diabetes, cancer, and normal aging.

In the laboratory, Janda and his colleagues added nornicotine to solutions of blood proteins. Nornicotine attached to the proteins, so that at the molecular level, the product looked like "Christmas trees with nornicotine lightbulbs on them," Janda says. when food browns, similar structures result.

In separate experiments on whole blood from smokers and nonsmokers, the team found that smokers' blood contains more such nornicotine-altered proteins than nonsmokers' blood does. The researchers reported their findings in the Nov. 12, 2002 *Proceedings of the National Academy of Sciences.*

"It's pretty shocking," says Janda. "Nornicotine can be involved in a chemical reaction no one had thought about." The team is now conducting studies to find out how common the nornicotine-blood reaction is in animals and people.

For people trying to kick the cigarette habit, gums, patches, lollipops, and lip balms that contain nicotine are often useful. High-dose nicotine replacements can deliver the stimulant at concentrations comparable to those in cigarettes while giving a person a more constant blood-nicotine concentration than smoking does and avoiding many of cigarettes' harmful components.

"It's still most important that people stop smoking—if they need [nicotine-replacement therapy] to do that, fine," says oncologist Dennis. "But nicotine itself might be harmful in the long term," he adds.

Some people use quitting aids for longer than the recommended few months. Ann N. Dapice, an educator at the addiction treatment center T. K. Wolf in Tulsa, Okla., says she's worked with people who have used nicotine patches and gums for years.

Although scientists don't know all of nicotine's long-term effects in people, emerging evidence makes a "whole new case" for the drug's potential to cause problems outside the nervous system, says oncologist John D. Minna of the University of Texas Southwestern Medical Center in Dallas.

And once scientists look closer, he adds, they might find disease connections to nicotine that haven't been considered yet.

From *Science News*, March 22, 2003, pp. 184-186 by Kendall Morgan. © 2003 by Science Service Inc. Reprinted by permission.

The Agony of Ecstasy

By Ria Romano, MA

On a raw winter day in 2001, 18-year-old Alexa Stevens returned to her dormitory, having just finished her mid-year exams at a prominent Boston-area college. The petite, young co-ed from a well-heeled family was packing to go home for the holiday break when several of her friends beckoned her to join them on the rooftop for some "X."

The languid high came on smoothly as she breathed in the fresh air off the Charles River. Thinking she had received a weak dose of Ecstasy, Alexa popped two more pastel-colored pills with the word "sex" engraved on them. Within minutes her heart began to race, terrified and confused she rushed down the stairwell—hair drenched in sweat—and dropped to her knees and convulsed. Twenty-four-hours later, after being admitted to a large University hospital, her condition deteriorated rapidly and doctors had to intubate. Forty-eight-hours later, discovering her liver was about to fail, they found a donor and grafted part of the donated organ. The liver graft failed, she slipped into a seizure, and her brain hemorrhaged. At that point, her family requested she be taken off life support.

The X files

Alexa died from a 90-year-old drug developed by the German company Merck in 1912. Contrary to Ecstasy's lore, Merck wasn't trying to develop a diet drug when it synthesized 3, 4-Methylenedioxymethamphetamine (MDMA) (see *What's in the Mix?*). Instead, the now pharmaceutical powerhouse thought it could be a promising "intermediary substance that might be used to help develop more advanced therapeutic drugs" (Cloud & Ratnesar, 2000). There is no evidence to support Merck employees ingested the drug at the time, and there are conflicting reports that Nazi soldiers used the drug to combat Posttraumatic Stress Disorder.

Yet MDMA virtually disappeared until 1953, when the U.S. Army funded a secret University of Michigan animal study of eight drugs, including MDMA (Cloud & Ratnesar, 2000). With the Cold War in high gear, the U.S. government was searching for potential chemical weapons, but MDMA didn't provide the necessary lethal results.

It wasn't until Alexander Shulgin, the Calvin Klein of designer drugs (ironically some Ecstasy pills have CK engraved on them), hit the scene that the pills resurfaced from obscurity. Shulgin began his career at Dow Chemical in the 1950s. In 1963 he took mescaline and never looked back. Shulgin had a particularly long leash at Dow Chemical due to the fact that he had helped create a successful insecticide. As a result, the young psychedelic chemist turned his attention to MDMA and became the stepfather of the "hug drug," publishing works that were eagerly read by several therapists (Cloud & Ratnesar, 2000). According to Shulgin, another therapist to whom he gave the drug in turn named it "Adam," and introduced it to more than 4,000 people.

However, among the therapist's patients were a few entrepreneurs. One of whom was based in Texas (and whose true identity is still unknown), hired a chemist, opened an MDMA lab, and promptly gave the drug a much more marketable name—Ecstasy. He began selling it to fashionable bars and clubs in the Dallas area, where bartenders sold it and charged patrons for the pills on their American Express cards (Cloud & Ratnesar, 2000). The then-legal stimulant had a very small place on the U.S. drug scene of the 1970s. The drug was not considered a controlled substance until 1985 and as one report put it, "that meant it was as legal as a scoop of Ben & Jerry's ice cream and only slightly more expensive" (Turney, 2001). However, the drug's streak of popularity in America did not occur until the mid-to-late 1980s when it began its symbiotic relationship with "raves."

From across the pond

Ecstasy came out of European clubs in resort locales such as Ibiza in the 1980s, and peaked in the 1990s when raves began to infiltrate nightlife. Raves originated in England as gatherings of thousands of young people revolved around "techno-music." They were traditionally held in large warehouses or open outdoor areas, and later moved into established clubs, where they were identified by police as "Drug Taking Festivals" (Keefe, 2001). In the late 1980s and early 1990s, the rave scene and techno-music migrated to the U.S. by way of promoters and entertainers. By the late 1990s, popularity had increased enough for the phenomena to be considered an established subculture. Although typical rave-goers are between 12 and 25 years old, and are generally from middle to upper-middle-class backgrounds, the drug has crossed over into America's heartland with ease (Keefe, 2001). According to the Drug Enforcement Agency (DEA), along with the new subculture's music and parties came a new drug empire.

MDMA is manufactured clandestinely in Western Europe, primarily in The Netherlands and Belgium (Keefe, 2001). Most often, the drug consumed in the U.S. is manufactured by Dutch chemists, and transported or distributed by various factions of Israeli and Russian Organized Crime groups. According to DEA reports, "The drug trafficking organizations involved in MDMA distribution are brought together by the enormous profit realized in these ventures. The cost of producing an MDMA tablet can run between $.50-$1.00.... Once the drug reaches the U.S., a domestic cell distributor will charge between $6-$8 per tablet. The MDMA retailer will, in turn, distribute the drug for $25-$40 per tablet.... Los Angeles, New York, and Miami are currently the major 'gateway cities' for the large influx of MDMA from abroad" (Keefe, 2001).

Supply and demand

At the American Academy of Pediatrics' annual meeting in October 2001, Dr. Peter D. Rogers, an associate professor of pediatrics at the Ohio State University College of Medicine and Public Health declared, "The use of Ecstasy is now an epidemic with teenagers. I've never seen a drug take off like this. The current popularity of Ecstasy could be the number-one public health problem in the United States" (Schorr, 2001).

Dr. Rogers' concern is supported by figures from the U.S. Customs Service. In 1999, Customs seized 3.5 million Ecstasy tablets. That figure jumped to 9.3 million tablets in 2000. By May 2001, Customs had seized more than 4 million tablets (at press time the total for 2001 was not available) (Winwood, 2001).

According to the latest results from a Monitoring the Future study based on 45,000 students in grades 8, 10, and 12, the use of Ecstasy has skyrocketed (The University of Michigan, 2000). The largest increase in the drug's use was among 12th-graders in the West, where 14 percent of the students reported using during the prior 12 months in 2000. That compares to nine percent in the Northeast, and six percent in the South and North Central regions. Although Stuart Gitlow, MD, medical director of Nantucket (Mass.) Behavioral Services, reportedly has seen a "huge" increase in the drug's use in the Northeast over the past two years (Landers, 2001). Dr. Gitlow says his patients tend to place Ecstasy in a different category from other illicit drugs: "When we question people about using drugs they say 'no,' but when we ask them if they are using Ecstasy, they immediately say 'yes'" (Landers, 2001).

Ecstasy was initially favored among males when studying the 12th grade population (measuring approximately five percent use in 1996), but was quickly adopted by females. Female

What's In the Mix?

MDMA is 3,4 methylenedioxymethaphetamine, a ring substituted derivative of phenethylamine, which is a close structural analog of amphetamine, methamphetamine, and 3, 4 methylenedioxyethylamphetamine (MDE: Eve)—and that's if you are lucky. Most pills kids are buying nowadays on the street have everything in them from aspirin, caffeine, heroin, LSD 2-CB, and ketamine, to more lethal substances such as atropine, 4-MTA, DXM (a cheap cough suppressant 13 times stronger than Robitussin that causes heat stroke), and Paramethoxyamphetamine (PMA). In the U.S., an organization called DanceSafe (www.dancesafe.org), which tests pills for anonymous users who send in samples from around the nation, found that 40 percent of the Ecstasy pills were fake.

While MDMA has analgesic and central stimulating effects (often known as the "six-hour orgasm"), it has been known to produce hyperthermia, memory loss, cognitive impairment, long-term neurochemical and brain cell damage, and most recently liver failure, kidney damage, brain seizures, and heart attacks. PMA, however, is similar in appearance to MDMA but is more toxic. Kids taking PMA may think they have received a "weaker" version of MDMA, and therefore take more pills. Doses over 50 milligrams can almost be guaranteed to produce cardiac arrhythmia and arrest, breathing problems, pulmonary congestsion, renal failure, hyperthermia, vomiting, convulsions, coma, and death.

Counselors looking for clues when questioining their patients' usage may want to call a dentist. Among the more bizarre effects of Ecstasy use is bruxism, or teeth grinding. One study reported on by SAMHSA at www.health.org showed 60 percent of Ecstasy users had warn their teeth through the enamel. Many of the kids constantly suck on baby pacifiers or lollipops to relieve the pain of grinding. Other physical side effects include eye spasms, vomiting, severe headaches, motor tics, extreme dehydration, as well as excessive, fast speech.

Sources: www.health.org, www.usdoj.gov, www.dea.gov, www.dancesafe.com

usage in 12th grade rose from approximately three percent in 1997 to over eight percent in 2000. African-American students showed considerably lower rates of use than white or Hispanic students in 2000. For example, past year use among African-American 12th-graders was 1.3 percent, compared to 7.6 percent for white 12th-graders, and 10.6 percent for Hispanics of the same age.

While in 1989 only 22 percent of 12th-graders said they could get Ecstasy very easily, that proportion rose over the following decade to 40 percent by 1999, before jumping to 51 percent in 2000 (The University of Michigan, 2000). This horrific jump in percentages is again supported by hospital emergency room data with the number of "club drug" episodes increasing dramatically between 1999 and 2000, from 6,964 to 10,212. Most of those episodes were due to Ecstasy (Family Research Council, 2001).

Invading the ranks

School counselors and parents aren't the only ones concerned about the club drug's use. The U.S. military is worried about the "skyrocketing" use of Ecstasy among its troops. Drug testing as of June 2001 by the Air Force, Army, and Navy indicates that usage is as much as 12 times what it was in 1999 (Moniz, 2001). In the year 2000, nearly 500 of the Air Force's 370,000 members either tested positive or admitted to investigators that they used the drug. That compares to 50 who were found to have used in 1998.

In the fall of 2000, five cadets at the Air Force Academy were charged with possession or use of Ecstasy. Two of them were sent to federal prison. Army statistics show the number of positive tests increased from 36 in 1998 to 440 in 2000, while the Navy had 238 positive tests in 2000, up from 34 in 1998. In most cases, those who tested positive were discharged from the military (Moniz, 2001).

Countering Ecstasy

To counter the club drug's use, the Air Force, which tests 70 percent of its personnel each year, is increasing random tests and weekend screenings. The Navy has formed a specialized task force to examine sailors' use of club drugs, and the Army expects to unveil a test that can better detect Ecstasy this year. Different levels of government are combating Ecstasy use as well. The Ecstasy Anti-Proliferation Act of 2000 (Public Law 106-310), was enacted by Congress in 2000, and directed the U.S. Sentencing Commission to provide for increased penalties for the manufacture, importation, exportation, and trafficking of MDMA (Keefe, 2001). U.S. Customs Service has taken several steps to try to control Ecstasy. Building on the theory that the best defense is less demand, Customs has established an Ecstasy Task Force in Washington, D.C. to lead investigative and counter-smuggling efforts. The Ecstasy Task Force is responsible for gathering daily intelligence on the drug's smuggling and coordinating Customs' response with other law enforcement agencies. Customs has also trained 106 drug-detecting dogs to respond to Ecstasy and stationed them at airports, mail, and cargo facilities across the country (Winwood, 2001).

In July 2001, the Ecstasy Prevention Act of 2001 was introduced to the Senate. The Bill to combat the trafficking, distribution, and abuse of Ecstasy asks for $15 million to combat the drug in high-trafficking areas; $7 million to institute a national youth anti-drug media campaign; $1.5 million to fund the National Institute on Drug Abuse report that evaluates the effects that MDMA use has on health; and $1 million to establish an interagency Ecstasy/Club Drug task force—all in fiscal year 2002 (Electronic Music Defense & Education Fund, 2001).

Soon to Be FDA Approved?

Sixteen years after Ecstasy was criminalized, the U.S. Food and Drug Administration has approved the first test of the substance as a treatment for people with posttraumatic stress disorder, according to a report in *The Wall Street Journal* on November 6, 2001.

The nonprofit group conducting the small pilot study on MDMA that is interested in developing it as a prescription drug, claims the wave of terrorism makes finding a treatment for PTSD more important than ever. The study's sponsor is Rick Doblin, founder and director of Multidisciplinary Association for Psychedelic Studies (MAPS), an organization that advocates using Ecstasy and other psychedelic drugs for therapy. The study includes 20 subjects, 12 of which will undergo MDMA-assisted therapy twice, each time taking a single 125-milligram capsule, and eight will receive a placebo. All sessions will be under the direct supervision of a husband-and-wife team of "psychedelic psychotherapists," according to *The Journal*. The hypothesis of the study is that Ecstasy reduces fear and anxiety, thus allowing sufferers to revisit a disabling trauma without being overwhelmed. Doblin has hopes of transforming MAPS into a nonprofit member-based psychedelic pharmaceutical company.

Marsha Rosenbaum, the director of The Lindesmith Center, Drug Policy Foundation San Francisco states, "We could, of course, continue to try (unsuccessfully) to scare teenagers into abstinence, as we have for two decades. But I believe that a more realistic, pragmatic approach to Ecstasy is 'harm reduction.' While, of course, we would rather they abstained completely, teens should have accurate information about Ecstasy to avoid serious mishaps. This may sound heretical, but safety should be the bottom line" (Rosenbaum, 2001).

Building upon the idea of harm reduction is DanceSafe (www.dancesafe.org)—a nonprofit, harm reduction organization promoting health and safety within the rave and nightclub community. They currently have local chapters in twenty-six cities throughout the U.S. and Canada, and by the middle of 2002, they expect to have at least a dozen more.

DanceSafe's local chapters consist of young people from within the dance culture itself who have a sincere interest in bettering their communities and educating themselves and their peers.

The organization trains volunteers to be health educators and drug abuse prevention counselors within their own communities, utilizing the principles and methods of harm reduction and popular education. DanceSafe's volunteers staff harm reduction booths at raves, nightclubs, and other dance events where they provide information on drugs, safer sex, and other health and safety issues concerning the electronic dance community (like driving home safely and protecting one's hearing).

One controversial aspect of the organization is the adulterant screening or pill testing services for Ecstasy users. A chemical called "Marquis reagent" changes color in the presence of certain drugs. It is believed that pill testing helps Ecstasy users avoid fake and adulterated tablets that often contain substances far more dangerous than real Ecstasy.

The founder, Emanuel Sferios, is a former social worker. He insists DanceSafe does not promote drug use, but attempts to make it safer. The organization's unconventional approach may prove useful when considering one 18-year-old's response regarding problematic brain changes attributed to Ecstasy.

"Oh yes," the youth smirks, "they told us about that with marijuana too. But none of us believes we have holes in our brains, so we just laugh at those messages" (Rosenbaum, 2001).

References

Cloud, J., Ratnesar, R. (2000). The Lure of Ecstasy. *Time Europe.* 04/17/2000, Vol. 156 No. 3. Retrieved October 27, 2001 from www.time.com/europe/magazine/2000/0717/ecstasy.html

Electronic Music Defense & Education Fund. (2001). *Pending Legislation: Ecstasy Prevention Act of 2001.* Retrieved on October 30, 2001 from www.emdef.org/billsus/S1208ISEcstasyPrevAct2001.html

Family Research Council. (2001). *Emergency Room Visits More Plentiful.* Retrieved October 30, 2001 from www.frc.org/get/df01h.cfm

Keefe, J. (2001). DEA *Congressional Testimony.* Retrieved October 29, 2001 from http://www.counselormagazine.com/www.dea.gov/pubs/cngrtest/ct073001.htm

Landers, S. (2001). Club drugs more agony than ecstasy for young patients. *American Medical News: The Newspaper for America's Physicians*, 08/13/2001. Retrieved October 30, 2001 from www.ama-assn.org/sci-pubs/amnews/pick_01/hlsc0813.htm

Moniz, D. (2001). Ecstasy Invading the Ranks. *USA Today*, 6/18/2001. Retrieved October 30, 2001 from www.usatoday.com/news/washdc/2001-04-15militaryecstasy.htm

Rosenbaum, M. (2001). *Convincing Research on Ecstasy Should Make Drug Users Wary.* Retrieved from www.drugpolicy.org/lindesmith/news/02_071Ecstasy2.html

Schorr, M. (2001). *Ecstasy Use Called 'Epidemic' Among Teens.* Retrieved October 30, 2001 from http://dailynews.yahoo.com/h/nm/20011022/ecstasy_2.html

Turney, L. (2001). *Ecstasy: Dancing with Mr. 'E.'* Retrieved October 28, 2001 from www.doitnow.org/pages/153.html

The University of Michigan. (2000). *"Ecstasy" use rises sharply among teens in 2000; use of many other drugs stay steady, but significant declines are reported for some. Retrieved October 30, 2001 from* www.monitoringthefuture.org

Winwood, C. (2001). *Ecstasy News.* Retrieved October 30, 2001 from www.customs.ustreas.gov/hot-new/pressrel/ecstasynews.htm

From The Counselor, February 2002, pp. 30-34. © 2002 by Health Communications Inc.

Afghanistan's opium:

A bumper crop

The fall of the Taliban has seen a big increase in poppy planting

KABUL

AT A seminar on drugs held recently in Nangarhar province, in south-eastern Afghanistan, 55-year old Khan Zaman, a farmer, puts it in a nutshell. "All our life depends on income from poppy, it is the best cash crop. If there are alternatives we will leave poppy. We accept the orders of the government, but there are problems for us." When asked about plans for this season's planting he says, "I will grow whatever the people cultivate; if it is poppy, if it is wheat."

This week, the United Nations Office for Drug Control and Crime Prevention (ODCCP) was due to release figures on this year's harvest. According to projections recently issued by Drug Scope, a British charity, output for 2002 is expected to be between 1,900 to 2,700 tonnes of opium resin, a huge rise on the 185 tonnes produced in 2001 during the Taliban regime's final year in power (though some may have been quietly hoarded).

In the future, the poppy problem will be a good indicator of President Hamid Karzai's hold over the country. At the height of their powers, the Taliban boasted a 94% reduction in output between their July 2000 decree banning poppy cultivation and last year's tiny harvest. It won them praise from the West, but that was swept away after September 11th.

With Afghan poppies accounting for around 80% of the supply of heroin in Europe, western leaders consider their reduction a priority. Under an agreement worked out by the G8 (the seven richest industrialised countries, plus Russia), efforts to improve drug control in Afghanistan are being led by Britain. It is working with both the Afghan government, which has just set up a National Security Council (NSC), and the ODCCP.

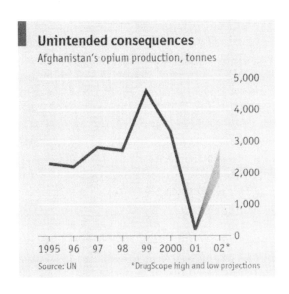

Unintended consequences
Afghanistan's opium production, tonnes

Source: UN   *DrugScope high and low projections

Part of the NSC's remit is to tackle the production and trafficking of heroin. But mechanisms are not yet in place at provincial level to achieve this. Even if they were, regional leaders, many of whom have benefited from opium trafficking in the past, are likely to object to any interference. The ODCCP aims to bring drug control into the mainstream of development assistance, focusing on law reform, the creation of an effective police force and, most important but most difficult of all, the development of alternative sources of income for Afghanistan's poppy farmers.

Finding money for all this is a problem. By last month, less than half of the $1.8 billion committed to the reconstruction of Afghanistan for 2002 had been disbursed, and most of that has been used to pay for emergency projects such as resettling refugees, rather than reconstruction. Little has been left for longer-term programmes, and nor are there institutions available to absorb it even if it were.

According to UN officials, there are obvious flaws in the existing schemes. A kilogram of opium is at today's prices worth around $300 to a farmer, so that with an average harvest of 50 kilos per hectare, he can expect to bring in around $15,000 per hectare, or $6,250 per acre. The cash scheme now in place offers a tenth of that.

The disincentives to growing alternative crops are formidable. Roads and irrigation channels need rebuilding, and Afghanistan's drought, now in its fourth year, makes the cultivation of crops needing more than minimal water, such as wheat, near-impossible. Wheat is also expensive to transport and to store. Poppies require little water to grow, and the harvested resin can be kept for years before being processed into heroin. Besides, the returns for wheat, at around $60 per hectare, are minuscule compared with poppy. That is a problem that is getting worse: as refugees return to their homes, there are growing pressures on land. So when planting is due to proceed in a few days, Khan Zaman, still concerned about putting food on the table for his children, may look to see what his neighbours are doing, and join them in planting poppies.

From *The Economist*, October 12, 2002, p. 42. © 2002 by The Economist, Ltd. Distributed by the New York Times Special Features. Reprinted by permission.

MODERN-DAY MOONSHINE

Appalachia's new cottage industry: meth

Locals are becoming addicted to both the drug and the production in
an area known for illicit stills.

By Patrik Jonsson
Special to The Christian Science Monitor

BENSON, N.C.—Known as a hard-working, Bible-thumping corner of North Carolina, Johnston County is also a patch of Appalachia: full of tool shops, tobacco plots, sawmills—and clandestine spirits.

Still one of the biggest bottlers of illicit "moonshine" whiskey in America, Johnston County now faces another sobering distinction: Over $300,000 worth of a methamphetamine known as "crystal meth" was seized here last year—the second-largest find in North Carolina.

But the stuff didn't come from big labs in California and Mexico. Using readily available ingredients like Red Devil lye, ephedrine, and phosphorous from match strikers, locals are now running thousands of so-called "Beavis and Butthead" operations—small labs set up in trailers, abandoned houses, even cars.

The thriving Appalachian trade feeds on a blustery independence that harks back to the days when Scotsmen first refused to pay the taxes on their stills. As it's raced from Ft. Payne, Ala., to Benson, N.C., locals are getting addicted not only to the all-five-senses rush of the drug, but also to the process of making it—or, as they call it, "hooked on the cook."

THE DRUG: Methamphetamine, or 'crystal meth,' is highly addictive.

"[Meth is] the moonshine of the 21st century, but 50 times worse," says US Rep. Zach Wamp (R), who represents eastern Tennessee.

Meth itself is hardly new. Known as "crank" and "tweak," it became popular more than 30 years ago among California biker gangs, and has spread steadily east. There's more of it in Oklahoma City than New York. In Fort Payne, Ala., where the jail population has tripled in the past two years and 60 percent of children in custody come from homes that made meth, the drug's grip has only tightened.

When a couple of West Coast chemists began a clandestine "how to" tour in the mountains six years ago, few realized how quickly it would find a home here along America's rough edge—a largely poor, white area, where illicit manufacturing has been part of life for hundreds of years.

As methmaking methods have simplified, the process today resembles a high school chemistry lab: a bunsen burner, some beakers, a Mason jar, and a handful of household chemicals. In short, a 21st century still.

"There's definitely a correlation [to moonshining]," says Van Shaw, a special agent with the State Bureau of Investigation (SBI) in Charlotte, N.C. "It's primarily being manufactured by folks from lower income brackets, who are using it as a means to make some money and provide for their habit."

Instead of finding a few people with a lot of meth, police are finding a lot with a little. To many, "tweaking" on meth is a balm for boredom. The main consumers, police say, are third-shift factory workers looking for a pick-me-up. And as with moonshine, the potential for making money in one of the nation's poorest regions has also fueled the drug's spread.

"They enjoy making it and producing it as much as they do taking the drug," says Chuck Phillips, a drug agent with the Jackson County Sheriff's Department in Scottsboro, Ala.

Potent smell requires isolation

The sparsely settled landscape has also fueled the meth explosion. "[Meth] is so volatile, and so smelly, that it works best in places that are isolated," says Pat Beaver, an anthropologist at Appalachian State University in Boone, N.C. But the acrid smell lingers, and police simply stumble on most of their arrests.

In North Carolina, police have made 30 busts already this year, up from a total of four in 1997. And in the past three years, police and social-worker caseload has increased 400 percent on

Alabama's Cumberland Plateau. The homemade drug is so pure and addictive that only about a quarter of users are able to quit.

Up on the side of Sand Mountain in northeastern Alabama, Brad Bewley knows what it's like to be "hooked on the cook": He admits he was once "the man" among meth producers.

A refrigerator repairman, Mr. Bewley enjoyed his hobby so much that he traveled across Alabama, Georgia, and Tennessee to watch others do it. The process could take from 20 minutes to two days, and he once watched a couple of "old-timers" in Georgia cook the raw product by leaving it foil-wrapped in a hot peanut field for a week.

"It just boosts all your senses at one time," Bewley recalls. "After that, then you're just trying to get that feeling back."

But as he followed the trade, he gave up fishing, hunting, and, finally, his family. Since being released from jail and preaching about the dangers of meth, Bewley has reunited with his wife and is winning local bass fishing tournaments.

In the end, the DEA broke down Bewley's door. But many meth producers are found when fire departments go out to extinguish a blaze.

Fighting back

In Tennessee, the picturesque Sequatchie Valley was, just a few years ago, littered with clandestine "tweaker labs" on hillsides, in trailers, and in motel rooms. Adherents, officials say, were turning $2,000 in raw materials into $20,000 in street profit.

But after several years of aggressive enforcement, helped by a grant from Washington, the East Tennessee Meth Taskforce has largely cleaned up the valley. The process has been difficult, though, and much of the action may have simply moved east to the mountains outside Knoxville, where officials have even found labs stuffed neatly into school book bags.

For now, government officials are training fire fighters and police in how to handle clandestine meth labs safely—and trying find a way to keep meth-makers from returning to their trade.

"Most of the guys who get out of jail for this get caught again," says Mr. Shaw of the SBI.

Heroin Hits Small Town America

'We're up to our eyeballs in it'

Chris Thomas, 52, rattles off the specific dates, seared in her memory, of devastating events in the family's war with heroin. The car accidents, multiple DUI charges, the credit card spending binges, the relapses into drug use, the days they threw their sons out, and last New Year's Eve—when they were arrested for possession of heroin—are recounted, sometimes by the time of day. The question "Is he alive?" has worked its way into the daily vernacular.

Tim Jones

A costly struggle against heroin rages in the comfy, cedar-paneled home on West Hanley Road, and everyone inside is losing.

The adult sons of Steve and Chris Thomas have stolen more than $50,000 from their parents' business to support their heroin addictions. The Thomas home is in a lockdown state, with money and other valuables that could be traded for drugs kept away from the boys. A bolt lock protects the master bedroom.

The Thomases now finance their vending machine business on low-interest introductory credit card offers, switching to new cards every 6 months.

Last week a Richland County judge arraigned Mark, 22, and Matt, 18, on felony drug possession charges. The next day Mark Thomas was caught by his parents using heroin again and, as has happened before, was thrown out of the house. It's a war with no victory in sight.

"I don't know what we're going to do," Chris Thomas said.

This is but one snapshot of a rising tide of small-town heroin abuse in the Midwest, occurring in tidy little communities with town squares, bicycles on front lawns and American flags flapping in the breeze. Hospitals and drug counselors note an alarming spike in overdoses, and overmatched police agencies are scrambling to address a drug onslaught once deemed the exclusive purview of big cities and longtime addicts.

In the northern Ohio railroad town of Willard, population 6,800, police are investigating five fatal heroin overdoses since December, two of them on a recent weekend.

"All of a sudden it blossomed," is how Capt. Robert McLaughlin of the Huron County Sheriff's Department described the arrival of heroin. "We're up to our eyeballs in it."

Although marijuana, sheltered among the tall stalks of cornfields, and crack cocaine, brought in from Detroit, had long been the mainstays in the tightly defined universe of illegal drug users, police officials and treatment experts say the heroin market has expanded beyond the predictable clientele.

More troubling, the price of heroin is dropping, the availability is increasing and the purity of the drug is rising. "It is much stronger than what abusers are used to," said Mansfield Police Chief Phil Messer, who leads a 10-county drug task force called METRICH.

This region of Ohio, described ruefully by one undercover police officer as "conveniently located" amid the inverted urban triangle of Detroit, Cleveland and Columbus, is especially susceptible to drug trafficking because of easy access to several major highways. Formerly isolated and exclusively rural communities are now primarily bedroom communities. It was often considered the "Crossroads of America," but many of Ohio's small towns have lost their insularity and are now part of interstate drug traffic.

Deb Kline, a nurse in rural Crestline, said the number of intravenous heroin addicts treated at Freedom Hall Treatment Center, about an hour north of Columbus, has quadrupled. Worse, Kline said, the universe of drug abusers is expanding from hardened addicts in their 40s and 50s to people in their early 20s.

"Kids who come from upper-middle class families, kids who had pretty decent high school careers," she said. "I wish I knew why."

Few people wonder more than the Thomases, who built their home 15 years ago amid the tall pines in rural Lexington, population 4,200. As Steve Thomas put it, they came to raise their boys "away from the bull-crap of the city." He was building what would become a thriving vending machine business.

"We're first-generation success," the 54-year-old Thomas likes to say, pointing to the 61-inch Sony TV in the living room. The TV is a symbol of achievement, he said. Leading by the example of hard work was the best teacher for his boys, Thomas believes.

Early signs of trouble

There were early signs of drug trouble with Mark, who started smoking marijuana at 14. Steve Thomas said he would occasionally smoke marijuana in front of his boys. "I knew when to stop and I expected the boys to be just as responsible with drugs as I was," he said.

They weren't.

Then teenagers, Mark and Matt would help their parents empty the coin trays from pop, cigarette, candy, pinball and other machines. Every night the Thomases would bring bags of coins home. They said they wanted to be home for their boys.

The skimming began at least two years ago—a few hundred here and there that would soon end up in the eager hands of heroin dealers on the east side of Columbus, about an hour away. Both boys had cars and every other day would make the run to Columbus.

"Steve would come home and wonder where the money was going," Chris Thomas said. "We never dreamed our kids would take it."

Their sons had stolen at least $50,000, but Round 2, the in-house war, had only begun. More thefts followed—money, alcohol, prescription drugs, keys to vending machines. After throwing the kids out of the house, they changed the locks. Mark and Matt crawled through the attic and dropped in through a ceiling entry.

"We don't keep any money here, and what we do have we hide. We don't keep keys to anything here," Steve Thomas said. "It's like the enemy living right beside you, right under your nose."

Chris Thomas, 52, rattles off the specific dates, seared in her memory, of devastating events in the family's war with heroin. The car accidents, multiple DUI charges, the credit card spending binges, the relapses into drug use, the days they threw their sons out, and last New Year's Eve—when they were arrested for possession of heroin—are recounted, sometimes by the time of day. The question "Is he alive?" has worked its way into the daily vernacular.

'I feel very betrayed'

Steve Thomas said he could shoot the person who turned Mark onto drugs, but he won't.

"I feel very betrayed, especially by my oldest son. They should give loyalty to their parents. They deceived me," he said. "I don't understand why my son doesn't have this hunger for knowledge and growth and achievement."

And he doesn't understand how anyone could take heroin.

"And you never will because you're not an addict," Chris Thomas said.

Their anger is mixed with guilt and second thoughts about all the long hours spent building a business. Chris Thomas clings to hope, however frail, and pulls the lyrics of music that Mark recently wrote, expressing remorse for his addiction:

"I was so numb and had no feeling to feel,
I was so dumb because I never realized this was real.
I still didn't care when you gave all you could give,
I just got around and got high with no reason to live."

That hope withered last week when she found a bag of heroin in Mark's room. Once again, Mark is out of the house. He is living temporarily in a family-owned apartment in nearby Mansfield, paying $20 a day to his parents. "I told him that was the last kind gesture," Chris Thomas said. "That was hard for me."

For now, Matt stays at home with his parents. He passed a milestone Friday. He has been drug-free for 90 days. That gives his mom cause for hope.

But neither parent expressed much confidence about their sons' future. They've been through too much to be optimistic. "I really get the feeling that Mark's never gonna quit," Steve Thomas said. "With Matt it can go either way.

"We just want the boys to get on with their lives so we can get on with ours," he said.

The nightmare for the Thomases reflects, in part, the new availability of illegal drugs. The reasons for the surge in heroin use vary—a poor economy, proximity to big cities and increased competition among dealers.

Sgt. Rick Sexton of the Willard Police Department said the annual influx into the region of migrant workers from Mexico, a country that is a major source of illegal drugs, is also a factor. Some police officials point to the post-9/11 obsession with terrorism, saying it has diverted attention from the drug fight.

Availability increasing

"The feds are claiming there are more drugs being seized at the border. But we haven't seen the effects of that locally. We haven't seen a spike in prices that would occur if interdiction efforts were working," Messer said.

"The availability is increasing. We're seeing a lot of young people—high school kids—using heroin," Messer said.

That analysis is confirmed by addicts, who were accustomed to dealing with older adults and driving an hour to get their fix.

"When I first started, I had to go to Cleveland or Columbus to get it," said a heroin addict who now does undercover drug buys for METRICH in Mansfield. "It's much easier to get now. I don't have to run all over the place to find it. Now it's just down the street.

"People figure they can deal drugs because of terrorism and the war. They figure everybody's got their minds on that," the addict said.

An old industrial city of 50,000, Mansfield offers a grim reminder of possible consequences of drug trafficking—three state penitentiaries and the now-abandoned gothic prison used in the movie "The Shawshank Redemption." At SCCI Hospital, emergency room doctors have a ringside seat to the effects of the drug trade.

"We see a ton of prescription drug abuse, and I've seen more heroin in the last two years than I've seen in the previous 10," said Dr. Anthony Midkiff.

To be sure, heroin is not the only drug threat in the region. In some rural counties, crystal meth is a bigger problem. In Richland County, it's crack cocaine.

Paul Jones, an investigator with the Richland County Coroner's Office, said drug users are mixing prescription drugs. When combined with heroin, the powerful pain reliever OxyContin or methamphetamine, an addictive stimulant, "it can be just enough to push them over the edge, and they don't realize it," Jones said.

UNIT 4

Other Trends in Drug Use

Unit Selections

Key Points to Consider

- How have the drug use increases of the 1990s suggested valid new worries about drug use by the young?

- What factors cause drug-related trends and patterns to change?

- How are drug-related patterns and trends related to specific subpopulations of Americans?

- How significant is socioeconomic class in influencing drug trends? Defend your answer.

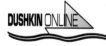 **Links: www.dushkin.com/online/**
These sites are annotated in the World Wide Web pages.

Marijuana as a Medicine
http://mojo.calyx.net/~olsen/

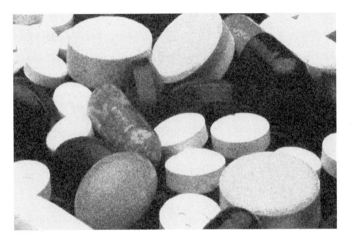

Rarely do drug-related patterns and trends lend themselves to precise definition. Identifying, measuring, and predicting the consequences of these trends is an inexact science, to say the least. It is, nevertheless, a very important process.

Some of the most valuable data produced by drug-related trend analysis is the identification of subpopulations whose vulnerability to certain drug phenomena is greater than that of the wider population. These identifications may forewarn of the implications for the general population. Trend analysis may produce specific information that may otherwise be lost or obscured by general statistical indications. For example, tobacco is probably the most prominent of gateway drugs, with repeated findings pointing to the correlation between the initial use of tobacco and the use of other drugs.

Currently, 19.5 million Americans report the use of illegal drugs. Marijuana remains as the most commonly used illegal drug with 14.6 million users. An estimated 2 million persons are current cocaine users, and an estimated 6.2 million are nonmedical users of prescription-type drugs. When reviewed by specific category, some interesting trends emerge. For example, 18–20 year olds report the highest rates of illicit drug use, at 20.2 percent. After the age of 26, illicit drug use falls to 5.8 percent. When race/ethnicity is examined, usage trends vary significantly. The highest rates of illicit drug use are by American Indians/Alaska Natives at 10.1 percent and persons reporting two or more races at 11.4 percent. Rates of illicit drug use are 8.5 percent for whites, 7.2 percent for Hispanics, 9.7 percent for blacks, and 3.5 percent for Asians. Additionally, current employment status is highly correlated with rates of illicit drug use. An estimated 17.4 percent of unemployed adults aged 18 or older were current users compared with 8.2 percent of those employed full time. Subsequently, the analysis of specific trends related to drug use is very important, as it provides a threshold from which educators, health care professionals, parents, and policy makers may respond to significant drug-related health threats and issues.

Historically popular depressant and stimulant drugs, such as alcohol, tobacco, heroin, and cocaine, produce statistics that identify the most visible and sometimes the most constant use patterns. Other drugs such as marijuana, LSD, ecstasy and other "club drugs" often produce patterns widely interpreted to be associated with cultural phenomena such as youth attitudes, popular music trends, and political climate. Still other drugs, such as methamphetamines, suggest use patterns of cocaine-like proportions.

One of two emerging drug trends that is expressing alarming consistencies concerns the use of club drugs such as MDMA (ecstasy), GHB (grievous bodily harm), Rohypnol (roofies, r-2, forget me drug), Ketamine (jet, special k, honey oil), PMA (death, mitsubishi double-stack), Nexus (venus, bromo, toonies), and PCP (angel dust, rocket fuel). Often, these drugs are perceived as less dangerous and less addictive as some mainstream drugs such as heroin and cocaine. Unfortunately, however, the quality of these drugs varies significantly and often substitute drugs are sold in their place. Because distribution networks associated with club drugs are unpredictable, users are subject to a constant menu of "look-alikes" or analogs. Rohypnol exists as one good example, as supplies are limited as a result of a significant government effort to curtail its availability. The government's Drug Abuse Warning Network (DAWN), which tracks drug-related emergency room visits, is reporting drastic increases in emergency room treatment for overdoses of ecstasy and GHB.

The other emerging and alarming trend concerns the abuse of prescription drugs. An estimated 6.2 million Americans a year are abusing prescription drugs—more than ever before. Opiate-related drugs such as codeine and Oxycontin, benzodiazepines such as Valium and Xanax, and stimulants such as Ritalin are repeated offenders. Some of the most alarming trends are reflected by the nonmedical use of these drugs by older Americans, adolescents, and women.

Information concerning drug-use patterns and trends obtained by means of a number of different investigative methods is available from a variety of sources. On the national level, the more prominent sources are the Substance Abuse and Mental Health Services Administration, the National Institute on Drug Abuse, the Drug Abuse Warning Network, the National Centers for Disease Control, the Justice Department, the Office of National Drug Control Policy, and the surgeon general. On the state level, various justice departments, including attorney generals' offices, the courts, state departments of social services, state universities and colleges, and public health offices, maintain data and conduct research. On local levels, criminal justice agencies, social service departments, public hospitals, and health departments provide information. On a private level, various research institutes and universities, professional organizations such as the American Medical Association and the American Cancer Society, hospitals, and treatment centers, as well as private corporations, are tracking drug-related trends. Surveys abound with no apparent lack of available data. As a result, the need for examination of research methods and findings for reliability and accuracy is self-evident.

The articles in this unit provide information about some drug-related trends occurring within certain subpopulations of Americans. While reading the articles, it is interesting to contemplate whether the trends and patterns described are confined to specific geographical areas.

Life or Meth?

It's being dubbed "Satan's drug." It's as addictive and destructive as heroin and crack cocaine. It's already destroyed the lives of thousands of Americans. It's called crystal meth, and its use is growing in the gay scene.

Imagine a dance club where the air is dark and sinister. A noise not unlike a cacophony of cement trucks blasts away at your eardrums as the aloof, detached crowd avoids eye contact, glancing at each other only to glare with empty, cold eyes and clenched jaws. There is no love, no laughter, no uplifting dance vibe; just grinding, dense negativity. This is the disturbing state of much of today's gay dance and circuit scene in America.

Methamphetamine (a.k.a. crystal meth, tina, ice, shabu, base, yaba, glass, crazy medicine) is a powerful highly noxious form of speed that ultimately wreaks havoc on the central nervous system, impairing the functioning of the brain and spinal cord. The drug was discovered in Japan in 1919 and developed by Nazi chemists during World War II to enable German soldiers to stay awake, alert and compulsively focused, while also rendering them emotionally sterile and quasi-psychotically aggressive.

These days 'crystal meth' is mostly mass-manufactured in illegal labs from an array of toxic substances including drain cleaner, lithium from camera batteries, antifreeze, ephedrine, red phosphorous and hydrochloric acid. Produced in concentrated crystal form and liquid, it is chemically concocted to artificially stimulate the brain's reward center inducing feelings of alertness and elation, giving the user a false sense of superhuman invincibility, control and power. Snorted, smoked or ingested, the effect is stronger than amphetamines like speed or cocaine, and the comedown—'crash'—significantly more intense.

Like heroin and crack cocaine, the first crystal meth hit delivers an almost instantaneous, euphoric high which locks seductively into the user's subconscious memory, enticing him to repeat the experience. Crystal meth preys on the addictive personality: the more the abuser consumes—chasing the high while delaying the onset of the crash—the less pleasurable the effect due to methamphetamine's ability to erode the brain's production of dopamine, the 'pleasure neurotransmitter' responsible for positive feelings. Job satisfaction, enjoyable social interactions, feelings of contentment, that life is meaningful and counts for something… all rely on dopamine transmission. Driven by his craving, crystal meth cynically zaps the abuser's dopamine and takes control, sucking him into a downward spiral of abuse and dependency.

Literally detached from all positive feelings, the abuser cannot experience or express love, happiness, joy or pleasure. Instead, crystal meth feeds on his fears and insecurities, turning him inward and causing him to react negatively to his environment. Unresolved painful issues from childhood may resurface to torment him and significantly intensify his growing psychological turmoil. Hitler himself was said to receive daily injections of methamphetamine from 1942, corrupting his judgment, undermining his health and, possibly, changing the course of World War II.

Physical symptoms—dry skin, sores, sweating, numbness, dilating pupils, dizziness, grinding of the teeth, impaired but incessant speech, ulcers, sleeplessness, nausea, exhaustion, vomiting, diarrhea, hypothermia, convulsions—manifest, and interest in the normal rewards of life fade as people, places and activities associated with using crystal meth take precedence. It also induces chronic loss of appetite and weight loss, satisfying the abuser in the early stages as fat is stripped away. But as crystal meth takes control his starved body starts feeding away at is own muscle tissue, resulting in a wasted, pallid appearance and ravaged facial features.

Crystal meth's toll is a tragically dehumanizing one. The abuser's deterioration into an 'empty shell' of his former self is likened to an internal light being snuffed out. He no longer even seems to be the same person, appearing 'wired'—nervous, depressed, irritable, fearful, anxious, compulsive, agitated, unpredictable, paranoid—and exhibiting signs of schizophrenia (panic, anger, repetitive behavior patterns, auditory and visual hallucinations). The abuser remains unaware or in denial of his erratic actions, believing himself to still be focused and in control and convinced that it is his external world that is going crazy.

The abuser's constant flow of anti-social behavior puts his career and financial security at risk, while love-based relationships and friendships are destroyed by his need to plug into, and drain any external sources of energy available to him. Relationships that persist become unhealthy co-dependent, fraught and abusive:

"Tina totally ruined a relationship I had with someone I loved very much," recalls Gary, a 37 year old New Yorker who was in a relationship of 13 years. "I can't tell you how I anguished over my lover and his addiction. It was as if I was watching someone drown. I tried so many times to throw him a lifeline, but he was unable or unwilling to grab it. In the end it was too much for me to bear and I had no choice but to leave. The simple face was that he was in love with someone else. Someone named Tina. And she was more important than me."

The abuser can't look others in the eye or at his own, gaunt reflection, and will resent anyone and anything that does not fit in with his addiction. If circumstances allow, he will isolate himself at home with the lights low and curtains drawn, sometimes too paranoid even to answer the phone or switch on the television or computer. Persistent denial and continued use will inevitably lead to destitution, poverty, despair and constant thoughts of suicide. Recorded suicide rates of gay male crystal meth abusers in America are rising dramatically and threaten to eventually outstrip deaths from AIDS, while murders triggered by acute paranoia have been directly attributed to the drug.

If he is lucky, the abuser's circumstances will force him to awaken to his problem and seek help medically or via a recovery and support program like Crystal Meth Anonymous (CMA). Methamphetamine abusers are among the hardest to treat of all drug users, often extremely resistant to any form of intervention, but acknowledging that they have a problem is a major first step toward recovery. The severe effects of withdrawal—drug craving, irritability, loss of energy, depression, fearfulness, insomnia, palpitations, sweating, hyperventilation—can last up to several weeks, but the 'wall' (craving) period continues six to

eight months for casual users and two to three years for addicts. The temptation to relapse is always strong, and there is growing concern in the medical field that some former abusers may never recover from irreversible damage to the brain, remaining dissatisfied with life and its rewards.

Significantly compounding the threat of crystal meth's influence on gay men is a heightened and compulsive desire to indulge in sex which, combined with sleeplessness—often lasting up to several days—and impaired judgement is often unsafe (the availability of protease inhibitors is typically cited as an excuse to engage in such activity). Although methamphetamine has been used as a 'dirty' recreational drug in the U.S. since the 80's, its use by gay men during most of that time was confined mainly to the AIDS-inflicted 'gay suburb' of West Hollywood in Los Angeles, and was largely non-sexual due to its constrictive effect on blood vessels, making erections difficult to sustain.

Crystal meth's use as a sexual aid was inadvertently popularized by the arrival, in 1998, of Viagra, which provided the solution to 'crystal dick'. Gay men, particularly on the 'party circuit', quickly discovered that crystal meth taken with Viagra simultaneously boosted sexual prowess and longevity. Like a time bomb waiting to explode, Viagra has fuelled crystal meth's use throughout other major U.S. cities; no longer was crystal meth just a drug for 'lost souls'. Alarmingly, this union also accelerated the risk of HIV transmission due to higher levels of unsafe sex induced by false feelings of invincibility. Even practiced safely there is a compounded risk of friction tears on the protective shield due to the significantly prolonged sexual duration crystal meth and Viagra together allow.

Viagra's arrival has coincided with the arrival of internet sex sites like 'Men-Men', specifically designed to make sex a commodity as easily available as home-delivered pizza. Today, a sizeable core group of users of these sites have emerged who remain online 24 hours a day in search of crystal-induced sex with fellow 'teachers', and who are upfront in their preference for unprotected 'bareback action'. 'Binge partying', where the abuser is typically awake for four straight days, crashes the following three and starts again, is driven by his compulsive desire for sex, which in turn is driven by his constant craving for crystal meth. Because crystal meth desensitizes, sex between abusers is rendered coldly 'mechanical', devoid of the usual free-flowing exchange of feelings and emotions. Where only one participant is an abuser he will, effectively, 'feed' off the other's higher energy levels, leaving the non-abuser feeling drained and listless.

Crystal meth is a very long-acting sympathomimetic and far more immunosuppressive than HIV, leaving someone immunosuppressed for days on end. This, combined with superhuman feelings of immunity to HIV, has triggered an epidemic of seroconversions in the USA. In Los Angeles alone over 75% of new HIV infections are now crystal meth related. Its ravaging of the body's immune system also hastens the onslaught of AIDS in HIV positive people, yet a recent U.S. study revealed that 47% of gay male crystal meth abusers were knowingly HIV-positive, with HIV rates high for casual users too. And in a report just published, a third of gay men surveyed in San Francisco reported using Viagra despite it being a prescription-only drug.

Crystal meth is ecstasy's complete antithesis, spawning an ugly new breed of insecure, sexually intense clubber, and transforming once uplifting dance environments into battlegrounds.

Combined with the alarming rise in crystal-induced HIV and syphilis infection over the last couple of years, much of the tireless work of America's safe sex campaigners since the start of the AIDS pandemic has been undone, with new rates of infection now higher than at any time since the early 90's. Little wonder that the marriage of crystal meth and Viagra is being referred to as 'the new gay plague'.

It is in some of the large dance clubs of major American cities and on the party circuit—lavish, decadent all-male dance events held throughout the States—where crystal meth's insidious influence is most evident. With the arrival of Viagra, club-goers have increasingly flocked from 'fun drugs' like ecstasy to crystal meth, enabling them to start the night with a buzz and stay awake, alert and 'hungry' for sex. Crystal meth's infiltration into social environments popular with abusers over the last couple of years has wreaked a devastating toll on the direction they have taken.

Over the last year alone in one of New York City's premier gay nightclubs, swelling numbers of crystal meth users have become abusers. Once fresh, vibrant faces are now etched in anger and paranoia as their dopamine levels progressively deplete, turning the venue palpably darker and more aggressive by the week. Alarmingly, this particular club is not alone in having adapted to this increasingly negative mindset; 'darker' forms of music are known to induce negative emotional responses, which explains why its DJ starts the night with uplifting tracks but, as the 'teachers' start to crash en masse, rapidly descends into a disharmonious, bass-heavy, discordant sound dubbed 'pots and pans'.

Where, just 18 months ago, this club was alive with people dancing and raising their spirits to uplifting deep house grooves and tribal rhythms, today the same environment resembles a swirling, dense 'no-man's land' driven by this sinister new sound seemingly tailored specifically for the crystal-addicted market. The crowd sways to and fro to the mind-numbing, soulless noise

in a detached, hollow-eyed, emotionless state. Even the occasional vocal track like 'I'm Addicted'—which provocatively repeats its title, mantra-like, over and over—seemingly serves to reinforce their dependency.

In just 18 months, an epidemic of crystal meth addiction has cut a vast, soul-destroying swathe through Manhattan's gay community, threatening to turn it in on itself as it did to the gay community of West Hollywood in the 90's. A walk along the Chelsea strip of 8th Avenue and in some of the more popular gay meeting places—including restaurants, cafes and gyms—indicate that the negative, hostile vibes that are the consequence of crystal meth addiction are not confined to the club scene. In just one year Manhattan's CMA meetings have exploded from one a week to almost daily, with attendance quadrupling from 15 to as many as 60 per class—a statistic that is all the harder to grasp in the wake of September 11, when New Yorker's generally united to rebuild their shattered city.

Circuit-goers, too, note with growing despair a palpably doom-laden vibe permeating their events, as Viagra and her twisted sister strengthen their destructive bond. Recalling a recent trip to Europe in the latest issue of the circuit bible, *Circuit Noize*, editor Steve Kammon lamented: "I felt like I'd been transported back to a happier time. People were really grooving on the music, dancing with abandon, and their faces were almost uniformly smiling—there was a really up, positive vibe… How different it seemed from so many of the all-night parties I'd been to this past year in Miami, Los Angeles and New York."

For all its negative press, in its 90's heyday, ecstasy connected people with their feelings, erased their barriers and, ultimately, brought them together in joy. Crystal meth is ecstasy's complete antithesis, spawning an ugly new breed of insecure, sexually intense clubber, and transforming once uplifting dance environments into battlegrounds of testosterone-fuelled masculinity. Ego and power play have always been an unfortunate aspect of gay club culture, not least in the U.S., but they are now becoming the dominant force. People just out for a fun time cannot express themselves in environments inflicted with crystal meth abuse. Their laughter and exchanges of affection are invariably met with bitter, resentful looks, even abuse, and the ensuing negativity forces them to leave earlier and earlier. Ultimately, they choose to stop clubbing altogether or are assimilated into the crystal herd, thereby perpetuating the cycle of abuse. People have been known to become addicted to meth while taking ecstasy because the pills can contain primarily methamphetamine.

American club and circuit promoters everywhere need to recognize their duty in placing the physical safety and mental well-being of their customers ahead of their profits, a responsibility they demonstrated with a widespread zero-tolerance policy towards GHB; a 'feel good' drug which, taken safely, has no lasting detrimental affect, but if overdosed rapidly sends a person into a deep sleep. If consumed in significant qualities with *any* amount of alcohol GHB can kill. Understandably, the unwholesome prospect of onsite paramedics tending to unconscious customers on their premises prompted this clampdown; yet agonizingly painful out-of-sight, out-of-mind crystal meth-induced deaths are significantly higher.

Many gay men drawn to the escapism of the gay dance scene have been playing Russian roulette with their lives for years now. Until we understand the impulses that drive us to indulge in self-destructive modes of behavior, and the reasons for our internalized homophobia which we project onto others, be it in the clubs, cafes, gyms, wherever, we will never shake free the shackles with which we allow mainstream society's narrow-minded, ignorant, views imprison us. Unless we say no now, then the horror that is crystal abuse will, like AIDS before it,

play into their hands, providing a weapon for them to attack us with, while we continue to tear ourselves apart. It is down to individual choice whether we allow crystal to control us, snuff out our light and provide our own weapon for fast-track self-annihilation. Or we can reject this cancer in favor of the very thing that crystal seeks to detach us from: love and respect, of ourselves and others.

Editor's Note

Again, I would like to remind our readers that we are offering this and other articles in [Outward Magazine, Volume 16, Issue 5, No. 236, March 13, 2003—March 27, 2003] as information. The views expressed are not necessarily those of this publication.

Alcohol, cigarette use declining

Ecstacy use declines as more teens recognize risks of drug

THE APPEAL OF THE ILLEGAL drug Ecstacy is wearing off among the nation's teens, with more youth recognizing that the drug is dangerous and disapproving of its use, a national survey released in December found.

The annual survey, which questioned 44,000 8th-, 10th- and 12th-graders, found that fewer teens have used Ecstacy, also known as MDMA, or methylenedioxymethamphetamine, during the past year. The decline came after several years of increasing Ecstacy use among teens.

"We have been saying for some time that the sharp rise in Ecstacy use would not turn around until young people began to see this drug as more dangerous," said Lloyd D. Johnston, PhD, program director and research scientist at the University of Michigan's Institute for Social Research, who served as the study's principal investigator. "Last year, more young people did report Ecstacy use as being dangerous, and the rise in use slowed."

The survey, Monitoring the Future, found that fewer teens reported using Ecstacy during the past month and year or during their lifetimes. Among high school seniors, annual use rates dropped by 24 percent, with just 7.4 percent reporting Ecstacy use in 2002.

The drop in use correlated with an increased awareness among youth about the dangers of the drug. In 2000, only 38 percent of 12th-graders agreed that there was a "great risk" in using Ecstacy once or twice. However, that percentage grew to 46 percent in 2001 and 52 percent in 2002. Among 8th-graders, 39 percent said there was a great risk in 2002, as did 44 percent of 10th-graders.

Johnston credited the "unusually rapid changes" in belief to both increased media coverage and educational campaigns by organizations such as the National Institute on Drug Abuse. Scientific findings showing a direct link between Ecstacy use and long-term brain damage have also been widely publicized in recent years, especially a 1999 study by Johns Hopkins University researchers that found four days of exposure to Ecstacy in monkeys caused brain damage that was evident seven years later.

More students in the 2002 survey said that they disapproved of using Ecstacy only once or twice. Additionally, fewer students said they believed that Ecstacy was fairly or very easy to obtain.

The annual survey also looked at use of alcohol and other drugs, finding that overall use of all illicit drugs was down. About 18 percent of 8th-graders reported using any illicit drug in the past year, as did 35 percent of 10th-graders and 41 percent of 12th-graders. About 25 percent of 8th-graders said they had used an illicit drug at least once during the course of their lifetimes, as did 45 percent of 10th-graders and 53 percent of 12th-graders.

Declines were also observed in alcohol and cigarette use. While more than a quarter of 8th-graders reported drinking alcohol during the past 30 days in 1996, only one-fifth reported the activity in 2002. There was also a decline among the percentage of younger students who had reported drinking alcohol in their lifetimes.

Teen use of cigarettes continued to drop from its peak rates reached in 1996 and 1997. The proportion of teens who said they had ever smoked cigarettes fell by four to five percentage points in each grade surveyed—more than in any other recent year.

Johnston linked much of the positive change in drug use and attitudes to a "cohort effect," in which behavior changes are reflected in a generation of individuals. For example, a resurgence of drug use in the 1990s was specific only to teens, and followed that group as they grew into young adults, he said.

"In more recent years, we seem to be seeing another cohort effect—a reversal of the first one—with the 8th-graders being the first to show declines in drug use, albeit very gradual ones," Johnston said. "To some degree, at least, those declines seem to be working their way up the spectrum, as the lower-using 8th-graders become the 10th- and, eventually, the 12th-graders."

Among the survey's other findings:

- Marijuana use declined for all grades surveyed, with 10th-graders showing the greatest decrease. About 30 percent of 10th-graders reported using marijuana in the past year, compared to 36 percent of 12th-graders.
- LSD use continued to decline significantly. Because perceived risk and disapproval did not change significantly, researchers said that the change may be due to drug users switching to Ecstacy.
- Use of inhalants continued to decline, with much of the improvement credited to the Partnership for a Drug-Free America's anti-inhalant drug campaign, which began at the same time as the decline.
- Methamphetamine use remained stable among 10th- and 12th-graders, but declined among 8th-graders.
- Use, perceived risk and disapproval held steady during 2002 for both heroin and steroid use.
- Use of Oxycontin and Vicotin, prescription narcotics that are sometimes abused, was tracked for the first time in this year's survey, with 1 percent to 4 percent of students reporting Oxycontin use and 3 percent to 10 percent reporting Vicotin use.

While most of the findings were positive, with "little remaining evidence of increases in illicit drug use among American teens," modest increases were measured in use of barbiturate sedatives and tranquilizers among 12th-graders.

Sponsored by NIDA and conducted by researchers at the University of Michigan, the Monitoring the Future survey has tracked drug use among 8th-, 10th- and 12th-graders for 12 years.

For more information, visit <http://www.monitoringthefuture.org> and <http://www.nida.nih.gov>.

A Worry for Ravers

One night of ecstasy could cause brain damage

BY MARY CARMICHAEL

Seven years ago Johns Hopkins neurologist George Ricaurte started a major battle in the war on drugs with a single image—a monkey brain on MDMA, the active ingredient in the drug ecstasy. The brain was shot through with holes where its neurons should have been busy making serotonin. The implications seemed obvious. If ecstasy could eat away at a monkey, it could do the same to us. The National Institute on Drug Abuse promptly put Ricaurte's brain scans at the core of its anti-ecstasy efforts. At least two groups weren't so quick to embrace Ricaurte's results: the club kids who keep the rave scene going and a faction of scientists led by Charles Grob. A UCLA psychiatrist, Grob became Ricaurte's foil, publicly attacking his experimental methods, subjects, even the wording of his press releases.

DOWNER: Ecstasy, a hit in clubs, may put even infrequent users at risk for Parkinson's

This week the two are at it again. Ricaurte has just published research in the journal Science indicating that one night's worth of ecstasy also kills the brain cells that produce dopamine, possibly putting even casual users at risk for Parkinson's disease later in life. Grob's response? "This just rein-forces my concerns." Ricaurte's new study simulates the effects of a rave, where partygoers may take several tabs of ecstasy. Injecting monkeys and baboons with small amounts of MDMA three times in nine hours, he produced the same effects he'd seen in his original study, which used more gradual doses. Ricaurte also found something new: two thirds of the dopamine neurons had frayed at the ends, possibly because the quick doses had poisoned the brain with too much MDMA at once. Dopamine deficiency is linked to cognitive and psychiatric problems, which may partially explain why users feel sad and sluggish after a night out. More troubling is the fact that Parkinson's is caused by the death of those same dopamine-producing neurons. "Obviously you can't compress 40 years of depletion into a week," says Ricaurte, noting that in Parkinson's more than 95 percent of the cells die. But in a few of his drugged-up monkeys, Ricaurte chemically simulated the decline in dopamine that comes with age. The animals, he says, became "slow."

If Ricaurte is right, Grob wonders, why don't more aging ravers have Parkinson's? "I am aware of only one report of a patient like that, and it's problematic," he says. Grob is also frustrated that Ricaurte's research coincides with the Senate's impending vote to crack down on rave promoters. "He's got a lot of money from NIDA and a very high profile," he says. "What I've got are the facts." But as the beat goes on, it's not clear if anyone really does.

new coke

It was the pill that helped hyper kids calm down, and millions of families signed on. Now Ritalin is the big, black-market drug on campus, for anybody who wants to work or party harder

By Harry Jaffe

On a warm spring night in March 2001, Vince Taylor and a buddy were cramming for two finals in his apartment on the campus of the University of Pennsylvania. Taylor, an A student with a double major in finance and political science, had put off studying until the night before the tests, as usual. His concentration was fading. The clock was about to strike 3 a.m. It was time for vitamin R.

The two juniors wanted to add a special touch to the occasion, so they took a few Ritalin pills down to the heart of the Penn campus, just west of downtown Philadelphia. They ducked under a massive Claes Oldenburg sculpture of a broken button, with a bronze Ben Franklin looking on benignly, crushed the pills on a small mirror, and snorted the powder through $20 bills.

Taylor looked at his friend, smiled, and said, "Put me in, Coach. I'm ready to play."

A generation of college kids and young professionals are getting in the game like never before. They're using Ritalin and its new relative, Adderall, to help them work harder, cram better, and party longer into the night. Their parents might have used Black Beauties and White Crosses—amphetamines that kept the beat and hippie generations going for two decades. But vitamin R, or Ritty, or New Coke, is much more widely available; it's also a much improved and refined stimulant.

"No jitters and better focus," says J.B., a student at Auburn University. "It's one of the most stimulating things. I take it and I can stay up all night, zipping through stuff."

J.B. was cramming hard before spring break this year. "Half of my friends use Ritty," he says. "Everybody's familiar with it, and it's real easy to get." [Names of users and some details have been changed; all quotes and school affiliations are accurate.]

Taylor, now in his senior year at Penn, used to pay $2 to $3 on the black market for the little yellow pills, but his new girlfriend has a prescription. "I guess I'm embarrassed about taking it," he says one night before spring break. "It's pretty sick, but it's real. Ritty got me through. You can quote me."

Says a former Wesleyan student: "Ritalin is the drug in the drawer."

An informal survey by *Men's Health* turned up testimony that—at least according to the kids themselves—large numbers of college students in top-rated schools are dropping or snorting Ritalin and Adderall. The students' own estimates place the number at 50 percent. Both drugs are classed as Schedule II stimulants by the U.S. Drug Enforcement Agency (DEA), grouping them with the most addictive drugs in medical use. Distributing them or using them without a prescription is a federal offense, but there is almost no enforcement. The DEA isn't conducting Ritty raids. And maybe with good reason: Overdoses are rare.

It is tempting to conclude that vitamin R is a harmless brother's little helper, an example of better brainpower through chemistry. But there is a downside. Like cocaine and other stimulants, Ritalin and Adderall increase dopamine levels in the brain. But exactly how they reduce the symptoms of ADD and ADHD remains a mystery. Potential long-term effects remain unknown. Snorting Ritalin and Adderall can send a potentially addictive jolt directly to the brain. At least three people have died from snorting the drugs.

But in a more subtle way, Ritalin and Adderall are gateway drugs, not to crack, but to the world of chemical dependency. Dan is a young lawyer who wakes up to a glass of water and an Adderall by his alarm clock every morning. "It helps me focus, but I sure don't love the fact that I have to take it every day."

Drugs that were designed to help fidgety elementary-school kids stay seated and learn how to spell have become

IwasonRittywhenIwrotethis.Canyoutell?Areyou doneyet?Now?Whatdoyouthink?Imeanreally…

Our author, under the influence of vitamin R

CALL ME LUCKY. I can get a decent buzz from a double espresso, but I needed a stronger push to write a big story about murder and mayhem in Washington. It was time to try vitamin R. I scored the usual way: off a kid. A friend had some leftovers from her son's old prescription.

First thing Sunday morning, I washed down a tiny yellow pill with cranberry juice. It was 5 milligrams, the smallest dose. I walked the dogs. I booted up the computer. An hour later, at 11 A.M., I was still waiting for liftoff. I took another little yellow pill. Fifteen minutes later, my fingers were dancing upon the keys, and the words were making plenty of sense. If you've got ADD, methylphenidate (sold under the brand names Ritalin and Concerta) fires up your brain's motivational circuits, leading to a calmer, more focused you. But if you've got the normal neural mess upstairs, it feels like speed. For me, it wasn't a body high. The steady rush was between my ears and behind my eyes. It came on and stayed on without giving me any jitters. Kind of a six-cup coffee jag without the bumpy stomach or clenching teeth. The story was writing itself.

Four hours later, I came down to the valley of the mild headaches. It felt as if my brain had shrunk inside my skull, and the soft tissue was banging against bone. By 9 p.m. I was back facing that blank computer screen, watching the moon rise over the Potomac River and in need of motivation. I took another yellow pill at 10. This time it landed and hit in minutes. I became a speed typist, and for 4 solid hours, the words flew from my fingers. When my brain ran out of ideas, vitamin R was still in control of my body. I shut down the computer and walked the dogs on the beach. I tried to yawn. I read. I hit the bed around 4 A.M. and finally slept, I think.

The next morning, as I brushed my teeth and tried to shake off a foggy hangover, the thought of taking another little Ritty popped into my mind. I was out. I could get more. How hard would I try to score? I contemplated the fine line between want and need and decided on an espresso. Those cute waitresses at the coffee bar always deliver.

—H. J.

---

the study aid and party drug of choice for suburban kids. The grand experiment to improve learning capabilities is mutating into a new speed culture on campuses and in offices everywhere. This phenomenon couldn't have happened without the willingness of doctors, who overprescribe the drugs; parents, who want to give their children an edge; and the kids themselves, who have seized that edge like a birthright, even if it happens to be illegal and potentially dangerous.

"That is the dirty little secret," says Eric Heiligenstein, M.D., clinical director of psychiatric services at the University of Wisconsin.

Gretchen Feussner first heard of methylphenidate in the late 1980s, when the drug was prescribed for a family member. Feussner, a pharmacologist, started gathering information and became fascinated with the drug. A few years later she joined the DEA and asked to work with the control of methylphenidate—sold under the brand name Ritalin. Now she's the agency's expert.

"When I started in 1991, the drug companies were making 2,955 kilos of methylphenidate a year," she says.

"This year they expect to make 15,946 kilos. It's a straight line going up."

A parallel line began in 1996, when Adderall—an amphetamine—joined the competition. In the 1990s, production of amphetamines rose 2,060 percent, from 417 kilos to 9,007. Eighty percent of this is used to treat hyperactive kids, and Adderall is the most popular.

Feussner began following Ritalin's rise just as the drug started to become the standard protocol for doctors treating children who were having trouble focusing. Their condition was dubbed attention-deficit hyperactivity disorder, and Ritalin was a godsend. Parents and teachers rejoiced at its calming effect. Though critics accused the medical establishment of drugging a whole generation and sapping the energy of naturally excitable children, Ritalin became a staple in schools across the country.

In 1998, more than three million kids were diagnosed with ADHD; the vast majority ended up with prescriptions in their hands.

For people with legitimate attention-deficit disorders, methylphenidate's molecules can have a soothing effect. But it's just plain speed for anyone who snorts, injects, or swallows more than the recommended dosage.

So it also became a drug teenagers used to get high, in schools and on the street.

"Methylphenidate is cocaine, pharmacologically," says Feussner. "They work the same way in the brain."

In 1995 the DEA's Office of Diversion Control began an extensive review of how the drug was being used and abused. "We already had anecdotal information that children who had legal prescriptions were selling it, giving it away, trading it," Feussner says. "But we didn't know how extensive the practices were." They fanned out to Wisconsin, South Carolina, and Indiana, visiting schools and pediatricians and emergency rooms. "We found that supplies of stimulants were poorly safeguarded and monitored," she says. "Students broke into school supplies. In one school a janitor was dispensing Ritalin. Kids were giving the medication away on the school bus or selling it to each other."

By 1998 the elementary-school students who'd started taking Ritalin in 1990 were going off to college.

"Many went with prescription in hand," Feussner says. "But the parental oversight was gone. They found themselves in a college culture of kids who knew that Ritalin and Adderall are potent stimulants. It was like cocaine, but you didn't need to go score on the streets." Ritalin was right there in the drawer. Or backpack.

In Austin, at the University of Texas, Justin says he used to pass out his Adderall like party favors when he had people over. "Everyone loves it," he says. "Anyone with a prescription has to guard it pretty carefully." Justin, an aspiring playwright, once took 40 milligrams of Adderall, locked himself in a motel room, and came out 17 hours later with a 100-page play. "The only ill effect is a little grinding of teeth on the way up, and a pretty noticeable rough ride down," he says. "I drink a beer to ease my way off."

A few days before spring break at the University of Virginia in Charlottesville, a friend popped his head into Robert Lender's room and asked, "Hey, anyone got an Adderall? I have a paper to write tonight." Says Robert, a varsity lacrosse player: "The fad for crushing it up and sniffing it has somewhat worn off. But it's pretty easy to get."

Bill Swain, a sophomore finance major at Georgetown University, never touches the stuff, but he knows when his roommate is blazing on Ritalin. "He sweats like crazy; he won't eat, but he can't stop talking. He's totally cranked." Swain did try it once. "I stayed up for 3 days. Never again."

On the West Coast, kids have the advantage of free trade across the border. Judy Trent, a UCLA graduate, says that Ritalin was a staple for studying and having a good time at her school. Students would slip into Tijuana or other Mexican towns, score Ritty by the 100s, and snort, sell, or save them for finals.

"I COULD SELL IT FOR $5 A POP IF I HAD EXTRAS. I HAD 60 [ADDERALL] PILLS STOLEN RECENTLY. IT'S LIKE ANY DRUG. PEOPLE ARE GOING TO GET IT ANY WAY THEY CAN."

Quinn Smith, a freshman at Tulane University in New Orleans, says the market for Adderall is "huge." Diagnosed with attention-deficit disorder in elementary school, Smith has a prescription for Adderall, but takes it only to study. "I could sell it for $5 a pop if I had extras," he says. Instead, he has to guard his supply. "I had 60 pills stolen recently. I filed a police report. It's very common. It's like any drug. People are going to get it any way they can."

At the University of Pennsylvania, Ritty can be used as currency or for barter.

"A girl called a few minutes ago," Vince Taylor tells me late one night. " 'Want to trade marijuana for Ritalin?' she asked. I said, 'Sure.' "

I asked Taylor if a dose of Ritalin had any positive effect on sex.

"Sure," he said. "It makes you focus on the booty."

A girl in the room heard the comment and said, "If you need it before sex, it means you're having bad sex."

"Typical Penn girl's answer," Taylor said. "It's always the guy's fault."

Given Taylor's admission that he snorts Ritalin, is he worried about becoming addicted to it? "I don't see it," he says. "We do it, but we just don't do it that often. We don't need it. We just like it."

As the Ritalin generation started going to college, Gretchen Feussner could understand why it was becoming so ingrained in the culture of some schools.

"These kids in college remembered their friends back in grade school who were taking Ritalin on a daily basis," she says. "They figured if a 50-pound kid could take it with no ill effects, where was the problem? The fear factor was minimal."

Even the drug companies knew there could be fearsome consequences for some who misuse Ritalin and Adderall. Manufacturers cautioned physicians about a range of adverse side effects, such as nervousness and insomnia; nausea, vomiting, and loss of appetite; dizziness, palpitations, headaches, skin rashes, and itching; digestive problems; toxic psychosis; drug-dependence syndrome; and severe depression upon withdrawal. Consequences of abusing high doses of methylphenidate can include paranoia, hallucinations, delusions, and formication—a sensation of bugs crawling under the skin.

But students in dorms weren't reading the labels. "Besides," says Feussner, "they think they're invincible."

And even some of the country's top experts on Ritalin and its "nonmedical" use are soft on its ill effects.

"Pharmacologically, these are very safe drugs," says Dr. Heiligenstein, a Ritalin authority who's studied its extracurricular use at the University of Wisconsin. "You can't say it's a terrible drug. You can't moralize that it will destroy your self-control. You would have to take a lot to wind up in the E.R."

Indeed, there were only 1,487 people who mentioned methylphenidate as their reason for going to emergency rooms in 2000, according to data gathered by the Substance Abuse and Mental Health Services Administration. In the same year, 174,881 people mentioned cocaine.

According to Nora Volkow, M.D., a psychiatrist and imaging expert at the Brookhaven National Lab, if Ritalin is swallowed, it takes longer than cocaine to raise dopamine levels in the brain. It doesn't jolt the synapses, so its effect is like "cocaine dripped through molasses," according to an article in the *Journal of the American Medical Association*. That may limit its addictive qualities. Still, the article on Dr. Volkow's work included this statement: "The long-term dopamine effects of taking methylphenidate for years, as many do, are another unknown." Two epidemiological studies examining how long-term use of Ritalin influences future drug addiction came up with conflicting results. If they were to stamp a warning label on the bottle, it would have to say, "Get back to us in a few years and we'll let you know how big a problem this is."

Beyond addiction, researchers are just beginning to explore the ways that methylphenidate alters brain chemistry. Joan Baizer, Ph.D., a physiologist with the University of Buffalo, told the Society of Neuroscience last year, "Our research… suggests that it has the potential for altering gene expression in the brain, which might lead to long-lasting changes in the nerve-cell structure and function." In essence, doctors and parents have been plying children with Ritalin for more than a decade, while, back in the lab, scientists are still trying to determine its long-term effects on the brain. Another uncertainty for the warning label.

According to Dr. Heiligenstein, everybody agrees that the potential for physical damage and addiction goes up when students snort Ritalin. "The more-rapid absorption makes the drug more like cocaine," he says, "but we have very little information. It's a more recent phenomenon."

Anecdotal reports from a number of campuses would indicate that snorting is one popular option. "There definitely are a lot of people who snort it at Tulane," says Quinn Smith. "It works quicker if you want to study. But I know people who bump it before they go out to party."

Yet the comparisons with deadly and addictive illegal drugs go only so far. Vitamin R is not caught up in a criminal network. It's not smuggled in like cocaine or cooked up in garages like crystal methedrine or diverted for mass-market distribution like OxyContin, the prescription painkiller. Ritalin seeps legally into the lives of middle-class and upper-class families and flows easily from the kitchen table to the college dorm. No Mafia, no Colombian cartels, no gangs—just Junior with pill bottles from the family stash. Serious drug users consider Ritalin a "sissy drug," the "poor-man's cocaine."

TWO DORMS IN WHICH GRADES WERE EXCEEDINGLY HIGH WERE KNOWN AS THE RITALIN DORMS, SAYS ONE DEA AGENT. "IT WAS SAID THAT THE KIDS WERE USING RITALIN AS A STUDY AID. IT WAS A BIG JOKE."

But in the late 1990s, Feussner became alarmed as the nonmedical use of methylphenidate started exploding at colleges, particularly the University of Pennsylvania.

"Two dorms in which the GPAs were exceedingly high were known as the Ritalin dorms," she says. "It was said that the kids in those dorms were using Ritalin as a study aid. It was a big joke."

Chances are, Vince Taylor—or his drug-vending brethren on other campuses—will never be busted for selling Ritalin and Adderall on the Penn campus. Brittany, a junior at Penn, has a theory about why this is the case.

"The college police have no interest in busting anyone for drugs," she says. "It gives the university a bad name."

Officially, Penn is clueless. "I've never heard anyone voice any concern about this," says Ron Ozio, Penn's media-relations manager. After consulting with the student health service, he said, "No cases of anyone abusing those two drugs have been brought to anyone's attention."

Let's face it: The most popular recreational substances at colleges are still alcohol and marijuana, with Ecstasy coming in a distant third. Ritalin and Adderall are simply blips on the radar screen of campus cops, and the feds, for that matter.

"DEA does not have the manpower to go to colleges and universities and enforce the use of a legitimate pharmaceutical drug," says Feussner. "We do, however, provide education and confer with local and state police."

Beyond enforcement, colleges do have some control over the delivery of these drugs. At George Washington University, in Washington, D.C., Ritalin and Adderall prescribed by the student health service are closely monitored. "We allow only one prescription a month," says Isabel Goldenberg, M.D., director of the health service for the past 22 years. "If a student comes to us and says his prescription was stolen, he has to report it to the university police before we will refill it. No report, no refill."

But Dr. Goldenberg knows she can control only prescriptions dispensed from her office.

"I have seen a huge number of students who are prescribed these medications—every year, more and more,"

The Quicker Picker-Upper

Swallow Ritalin, and it's a wake-up call. Snort it, and it's apocalypse, now

LEAVE IT TO THE COLLEGE KIDS to take a good drug and push it right to the edge. Snorting Ritalin, one favored delivery option, is "like a sledgehammer on the brain," says Xavier Castellanos, M.D., director of the Institute for Pediatric Neuroscience at NYU's Child Studies Center. Seconds after the drug disappears up the nose, it enters the bloodstream and from there, the brain, where it enhances dopamine processing (the source of the high). Snort enough and the blood vessels in your nose may tighten, break, and bleed.

Still, even snorted Ritalin takes about 90 minutes to leach back out of the brain, far longer than cocaine. So while coke fiends can get high hit after hit, bingeing on Ritalin doesn't have the same effect, and this dulls the risk of addiction. "Ritalin can be abused, but it never has the addictive potential of cocaine," according to Nora Volkow, M.D., a psychiatrist at the Brookhaven National Lab. "It will not allow you to go into a binge."

The effects of long-term medical use are less clear. Two large studies of addiction in kids with ADHD conflict on whether use of Ritalin is linked to tobacco or cocaine use later in life. One, released in 1998, implicated childhood use of Ritalin and other drugs in later drug dependence, but a study published the next year reached the opposite conclusion. "I don't think the question is a trivial one," says Dr. Castellanos. "These clearly are powerful drugs."

—BRIAN REID

she says. "We have no data, but we know it's used. Amphetamines enhance student performance when they're crashing for finals. Since that many students have the medications, we figure some will give them to friends."

At least a few campus professionals are aware of Ritalin's seductive allure. Not so the doctors who prescribe all those kilos of Ritalin and Adderall.

"I am not aware there's a problem," says Brenda Craine, director of media for the American Medical Association, which represents the doctors. "Why is Ritalin being used by college kids?"

To study or party into the night, I explain.

"I haven't heard any discussion of it."

Neither had the American Academy of Pediatrics, when I called.

After following methylphenidate for more than a decade, Feussner has concluded that the use and misuse of vitamin R in its various forms has its roots in the current culture.

"We want our children to succeed," she says, "and that pressure creates a certain acceptance of the means. I feel sorry for the kids. I feel sorry for the parents. They need to better understand the pros and cons of taking these medications. They need to be sure that they're necessary. Ritalin is not a One-a-Day vitamin."

Dr. Heiligenstein, at the University of Wisconsin, also recognizes the societal pressure. "People can't afford not to do well in college," he says. Which brings him to his "dirty little secret" of the doctors who are aiding and abetting students who want that educational edge. "We see some ADHD students come to campus with 4 months of medication," he says. "When you have hundreds of pills in a bottle, it's easier to feel you have plenty to hand out to friends or to misuse yourself.

"More control is needed," he says. "No one would write a 90-day prescription for morphine for the convenience of the patient."

And, according to the Health Insurance Association of America, nobody should be getting more than a 30-day supply of Ritalin or Adderall by prescription. But clearly, a lot of college kids are.

Dr. Heiligenstein also believes that using vitamin R is a subtle form of cheating.

"It probably gives some students an unfair advantage," he says. "They can procrastinate for weeks, go on a 3-day Ritalin bender, and potentially make up the work. What's the difference between that and an Olympic athlete who's a great runner but will take blood-doping medication for that extra edge?"

One difference is that students are using vitamin R for an edge beyond the classroom. Take Vince Taylor, who recently started snorting Ritalin before going out to party. "When you drink on it," he says, "you can drink more, and it feels a lot better."

So maybe it's time to sell the Starbucks stock. Generations X, Y, and beyond are embracing a whole new wake-up call.

Clicking for a Fix: Drugs Online

**The U.N. fears the Internet is providing a haven for drug dealers.
But how easy is it, really, to find narcotics on the Web?**

By Jessica Reaves

Wednesday, Feb. 27, 2002

How easy is it to buy illegal drugs on the Internet?

Pretty darn easy, according to a new study by the United Nation's International Narcotics Control Board. The report, issued Wednesday, warns that drug traffickers are finding myriad ways to conduct their illegal transactions in cyberspace—leaving law enforcement officers struggling to keep up.

The INCB study details the ways traffickers communicate with each other and with their clients, often commandeering unrelated chat rooms to set up deals, or using Web courier services to transport their contraband packages.

Even without the examples offered by the INCB, it's not hard to imagine that for professional drug dealers, the Internet is a virtual playground. It's incredibly difficult, if not impossible, to control and censor; it has no borders, and, unlike in the physical world, criminals can change identities and locations in the time it takes to switch on a new computer.

But what about the rest of us? Is it really so very easy to track down drugs on a whim, just by opening a browser? In the interest of journalism, I set out to answer my own question, and found a very different world than what's described in the U.N. report. The U.N., of course, is a venerable institution with many resources, and I am just one small person—so perhaps it's not surprising that I could find no evidence of said hard-core Internet drug culture.

Before recounting my online experiences, I want to issue the following disclaimers: One, many of the drugs discussed here are illegal and it's extraordinarily stupid to use them. Two, I spent a limited time (several hours) conducting this research; I'm sure I missed many sites, but as we've all come to realize (and my editor keeps reminding me), it's impossible to search the entire Internet.

Cocaine: It's not just for soft drinks any more

My search for "cocaine" came up with thousands of entries, most of them anti-drug sites sponsored by federal or local government agencies. (I also tried "buying cocaine," and "cocaine sources" but had less luck.) Sprinkled among the "just say no" messages, however, there were a few oddball sites—some of which took me by surprise.

A few sold booklets purporting to show exactly how to combine "everyday household products" to make cocaine—these booklets, of course, are "for law enforcement officials only." How do these vendors check your credentials? They don't.

Then, there are sites that actually spell out how to make cocaine in your very own (very well-equipped) kitchen. True, the recipes require a Ph.D-level understanding of pharmacology and tools such as space-age thermometers, but hey, if you're really hooked, I'm sure you'll find a way to overcome these minor speed bumps.

If you're interested, you can also trace the history of cocaine through the ages, from its beginnings as a treat for the royalty of the Andean Indians to its role as a "wonder drug" and its infamous inclusion in the formula for Coca-Cola.

Heroin: A little taste of history

Again, plenty of opportunities to manufacture or grow your own stuff, but nowhere to buy it straight from a dealer. Also lots of paeans to the wondrous effects of heroin, most dating back to the 19th century, when opium was all the rage, and when kids were given heroin in the form of cough syrup. You can also read horrific addiction stories by people who've fallen in love with heroin and lived to tell about it. Support groups for addicts abound as well, as do contact numbers for needle exchange centers.

Perhaps the dearth of opportunities to buy heroin online is directly traceable to the spectacular popularity and widespread availability of Oxycontin, an even more addictive opiate pain-killer which, until very recently, was barely regulated.

Marijuana: Easy as pie. Mmmm… pie.

You want to buy, sell, grow, cultivate or just talk about marijuana? You're in luck—the Internet is a veritable treasure trove of pot-related sites. You can read stories written by stoned people, stories about stoned people, stories about how much better life is when enjoyed in a stoned state, and even a smattering of stories detailing how incredibly screwed up people's lives have gotten because they've spent all their time getting stoned.

You can also learn more than you (probably) ever wanted to know about different ways of getting stoned, and various ways to escape detection. This last category includes my favorite find, a site called UrineLuck.com, a service that promises to help you pass any drug test—guaranteed. Hmmmm.

Prescription medications: No doctor's visit necessary!

This is where the Internet drug trade lives. First off, let's be perfectly honest: if you're truly desperate for the hard stuff, of course, it's undoubtedly faster to personally investigate local dealers than to wait around for UPS to deliver a fix. But if you're willing to wait a few days and are loath to leave the comfort of your home, your computer can provide a few options.

Online "pharmacies" are everywhere; the domestic operations offer a limited number of relatively harmless prescription medications (including Viagra and the hair-loss drug Propecia), others (primarily Mexican) providing a larger selection, ranging from antidepressants to highly addictive opiates such as Oxycontin. Other big sellers: methadone, codeine, testosterone and anabolic steriods. It's breathtakingly easy to log on, pick a drug and place an order—all without the pesky inconvenience of a doctor's appointment. I quickly discovered that if I were interested, I could order thousands of dollars' worth of addictive opiates and see them land on my doorstep in less than 24 hours.

Payment options are equally varied: you can pay $20 extra for priority mail, or you can have everything shipped UPS. Scrolling through the (minimal) shipping guidelines, some sites make it hard to ignore flashing disclaimers: "Some of our suppliers will send you drugs even though they violate the laws of your country. It is your responsibility to consult with your physician before taking any medication, and know the laws concerning the importation of scheduled drugs to your location."

There it is, in black and white (or bright, undulating yellow): Ordering and/or possessing these drugs may be illegal. Does that stop you? It depends on your tolerance for risk.

"This is a very fuzzy area of the law," says Dr. Frank Palumbo, director of the University of Maryland Center on Drugs and Public Policy in Baltimore. "I could see law enforcement going after you, because you're in possession of a controlled substance without a valid prescription."

Let's say you do have a prescription, written by one of the kindly docs employed by the offshore pharmacies. They asked you a few questions when you logged on, and dashed off a cyber "scrip" on the spot. Does that make your case any stronger, if, say, a customs agent opens your package of opiates en route from Mexico? Maybe, says Palumbo, and maybe not. "The Controlled Substance Act in the U.S. says a prescription must be written for a legitimate medical purpose, but the feds generally don't go after patients ordering drugs for themselves." Of course, he adds, if you're caught selling the drugs you've ordered, you're in deep trouble.

What's the government doing to keep offshore pharmacies in check? Everything they can—which, quite frankly, isn't a whole lot. "The FDA has a major effort going on with regard to offshore pharmacies," says Dr. Palumbo. "They're really trying to keep a handle on all this," but they're stuck with fairly ineffectual techniques, like issuing email warnings. "They don't have jurisdiction over the countries where these pharmacies are located, and they can't flex the muscle of the U.S. government, so instead they try to work in cooperation with local governments."

The Orphan Drug Backlash

The Orphan Drug Act of 1983 was supposed to provide incentives for private industry to develop needed, but unprofitable, drugs to treat rare diseases. It has done so, but not without eliciting controversy

By Thomas Maeder

IN JUNE 1989 AMGEN, A SMALL BIOTECHNOLOGY COMPANY IN Thousand Oaks, Calif., gained U.S. Food and Drug Administration approval to market its first product, epoetin alfa (Epogen), to treat the anemia that accompanies end-stage kidney failure. Because the number of patients with this condition was not large—only around 78,000 at the time—it seemed unlikely that Amgen could make a profit or even recover the development costs of the drug. But it sought FDA approval for the agent anyway, in part because of incentives it was deemed eligible to receive under a law called the Orphan Drug Act. The act, which encompasses a set of laws that went into effect in 1983, provides benefits to encourage private industry to develop treatments for rare diseases. Treatments with such modest markets would otherwise remain "orphans," with no one to sponsor them through FDA scrutiny.

Once on the market, Epogen proved useful for other, more common purposes: restoring red blood cells in people suffering from bone marrow suppression as a result of taking AIDS drugs or cancer chemotherapy, and reducing the need for transfusions in surgery patients. It wasn't long before the company started to earn tremendous profits on the drug. Outraged legislators and consumer groups cried foul, accusing Amgen and a few other companies of parlaying government largesse into private fortunes. By 2001, Epogen and Procrit, the latter a version of epoetin alfa made by Ortho Biotech in Raritan, N.J., were the sixth and seventh best-selling drugs in America, respectively, together generating more than $5 billion in revenues a year. Based on the drugs' success, people began to ask: Had the Orphan Drug Act been co-opted as a Biotechnology Promotion Act? And if so, shouldn't something be done to curb potential abuses in the future?

A Look Back

THESE ARE REASONABLE questions, best answered by first recalling some of the act's history. Before 1983, even when treatments for rare diseases had been discovered, drug companies often did not want to make them. Although rare diseases collectively affect 25 million Americans—a huge constituency in aggregate—they are an unattractive market because they are subdivided into more than 6,000 subpopulations ranging in size from a

Overview/*Orphan Drugs*

- "Orphan" drugs are those for which the markets are so small that they are unlikely to be produced by a for-profit drug company. The U.S. Food and Drug Administration defines an orphan drug as one that is anticipated to treat fewer than 200,000 people.

- The 1983 Orphan Drug Act offers incentives for pharmaceutical and biotechnology companies to develop drugs for rare disorders. The act provides tax credits and seven years of market exclusivity to a company willing to make an orphan drug.

- Several orphan drugs—notably epoetin alfa, which builds up red blood cells—have now become blockbusters, leading critics to question whether drug companies are abusing the Orphan Drug Act.

- But advocates say the act has worked well: 229 orphan drugs that together treat 11 million patients, most with serious or life-threatening diseases, are now on the market.

handful of patients to a couple hundred thousand. Development costs for drugs are incredibly steep (the pharmaceutical industry routinely claims that it costs $800 million to get a new drug to market), so large pharmaceutical companies have historically concentrated on top-selling products, especially those to treat relatively common, chronic disorders such as hypertension, depression and arthritis.

ACTORS JACK KLUGMAN and Robert Ito testified before a fake Congress in an episode of the television drama *Quincy, M.E.*, that focused on the dearth of treatments for rare disorders. Five days after the show aired, Klugman appeared before the real Congress and offered testimony that aided the passage of the 1983 Orphan Drug Act, which offers incentives to drugmakers.

In the late 1970s individual patients and volunteer health organizations began agitating for legislation to encourage the development of needed therapies that basic research had already identified but that were unavailable commercially. A company scrapped plans to make pimozide for Tourette syndrome, for instance, even though it was the only drug that helped many sufferers. Penicillamine for Wilson disease, 5-hydroxytryptophan for myoclonus, gamma-hydroxybutyrate for narcolepsy, sodium valproate for certain forms of epilepsy, and cysteamine to treat children with cystinosis [*see glossary*] were also quietly dropped when they proved more costly than their meager sales projections warranted. Patients had to smuggle supplies from abroad, concoct illegal home brews or simply do without. The challenge was

how to motivate the powerful drug industry to respond to desperate needs—how to make the unprofitable profitable. Orphan drugs "are like children who have no parents," says Representative Henry A. Waxman of California, "and they require special effort."

Early orphan drug legislation failed because it lacked the necessary economic incentives, yet it focused industry, government and popular attention on the problem and galvanized patient advocacy groups into action. One of the most influential events was a curious case of life imitating art imitating life: actor Jack Klugman, who played a strident medical examiner on the television show *Quincy, M.E.*, was inspired to create an episode focusing on rare diseases after reading a newspaper article about the plight of a Tourette patient and of someone with myoclonus. In the show, which aired in 1981, Quincy testified before Congress about the shameful lack of drugs for rare diseases. Later, Klugman reenacted his fictitious TV testimony in front of the real Congress. Finally, in January 1983, President Ronald Reagan signed the Orphan Drug Act into law. It was subsequently modified several times and now allows companies to take a 50 percent tax credit on all clinical trial costs, exempts them from paying the so-called user fee (currently $533,400) that the FDA usually charges drug sponsors, and bars other firms from obtaining FDA approval for the same drug for seven years.

Cornering the Market

THE SEVEN-YEAR MARKET exclusivity clause has been key to the effectiveness of the act. The FDA can approve the same drug made by a prospective competitor only if it is "clinically superior"—if the product is safer, more effective or easier to take. The original act defined orphan drugs as those that could not reasonably be expected to recover their cost of development through sales in the U.S. But the complexity of making such projected economic analyses at first deterred companies with orphan drug candidates, and the initial industry response was discouraging. A 1984 amendment clarified matters by stipulating that drugs for conditions with fewer than 200,000 American sufferers would be presumed to be unprofitable and would therefore automatically qualify for orphan drug designation.

The Orphan Drug Act was needed not only to provide financial incentives to companies but also to allow drugmakers more leeway in designing studies to prove that a drug candidate is safe and effective. The standard set of human clinical trials can take years and involve thousands of patients at multiple sites. The entire patient population with a rare disease, on the other hand, may be smaller than the number of subjects in most ordinary trials, so testing cannot follow the usual protocols. Only 12 children in the U.S. suffered from adenosine deaminase (ADA) deficiency, a cause of severe combined immunodeficiency disease (SCID), for example, when a company was developing a drug for it. Similarly, sacrosidase, for a congenital enzyme disorder (sucrase-isomaltase deficiency), was approved on the basis of two trials that had a grand total of 41 patients.

Because of such special circumstances, interactions between the FDA and companies working on orphan drugs tend to be more collegial than the usual arm's-length relationships the agency typically maintains with drug sponsors. Marlene E. Haffner—director of the Office of Orphan Products Development at the FDA, and the self-styled "mother of orphan drugs"—is adamant that the role of her office is both to regulate new drugs for rare disorders and to help get safe and effective ones on the market. To this end, her agency administers a grants program to assist researchers working on drugs eligible for orphan status. Since 1983 the FDA has awarded 370 such grants, totaling more than $150 million. It also assists orphan drug sponsors in designing statistically meaningful clinical trials, a tricky undertaking for rare disorders.

Grateful Orphans

BUT RESEARCH into rare disorders has sometimes yielded disproportionately fruitful results. This effect, which has much to recommend it, also occasionally leads to windfalls for drugmakers and, in turn, to some seriously raised eyebrows.

Rare diseases often result from a specific genetic defect, such as a single mutation, so their symptoms may reveal the normal function of a particular gene. Alpha-1-antitrypsin deficiency, for instance, produces emphysema in young people—a tragedy for those with the underlying mutation but an opportunity for researchers to study the causes of the disease without the confounding effects of smoking and age. In the case of thrombotic thrombocytopenic purpura, blood clots caused by the absence of an enzyme that normally cleaves a blood protein may highlight a possible contributor to heart attack and stroke.

Indeed, rare diseases and orphan drugs have been boons to applied pharmaceutical research, although no one anticipated that the Orphan Drug Act would end up kick-starting the nascent biotech industry. Unlike conventional pharmaceutical companies, which mostly manufacture drugs composed of small molecules, biotech firms at the time tended to be start-ups and to focus on producing proteins needed to replace those that were defective or missing in unlucky people. And biotech firms made the proteins using recombinant DNA technology, which was first introduced in the 1970s. They would isolate, or clone, the gene encoding a human protein and splice it into bacteria or mammalian cells grown in laboratory culture dishes to produce the protein in quantity.

Many rare diseases, it turned out, were ideally suited to treatment with biotech products. Serious or life-threatening hereditary disorders, such as enzyme deficiencies stemming from a single defect in the enzyme's genetic blueprint, were both rare and potentially treatable with recombinantly produced replacement proteins—mole-

GLOSSARY OF SELECTED RARE DISORDERS

CYSTINOSIS: A buildup of the amino acid cystine, a constituent of proteins, causing organ damage [particularly in the kidneys and eyes]. Affects roughly 400 people in the U.S.

GAUCHER DISEASE: An accumulation of a fatty compound, especially in the bone marrow, spleen, lungs and liver, resulting from a deficiency in glucocerebrosidase. Symptoms, afflicting fewer than 10,000 people worldwide, include enlarged liver and spleen, anemia, low levels of blood-clotting platelets, and skeletal abnormalities.

HEREDITARY TYROSINEMIA TYPE 1: A deficiency in the enzyme that normally breaks down the amino acid tyrosine. It can result in severe liver and kidney disease among the 100 individuals who have it in the U.S.

MYOCLONUS: A neurological disorder characterized by sudden, involuntary muscle contractions and relaxations. Strikes roughly nine of every 100,000 individuals.

SUCRASE-ISOMALTASE DEFICIENCY: The lack of the enzymes sucrase and isomaltase, leading to the inability to digest sugars and starches properly. Experienced by 0.2 percent of North Americans.

THROMBOTIC THROMBOCYTOPENIC PURPURA: Abnormally low platelet counts and shortened red blood cell survival time, resulting in a tendency to bleed excessively into the skin or mucous membranes. There are 15,000 to 22,000 U.S. sufferers.

TOURETTE SYNDROME: Muscle and vocal tics that can take the form of involuntary movements of the extremities and face, accompanied by uncontrollable sounds or socially inappropriate words. Roughly 100,000 Americans have the disorder.

WILSON DISEASE: A buildup of copper in various body tissues, particularly in the liver, brain and corneas. Can lead to liver failure and central nervous system dysfunction in the 30,000 people affected worldwide.

cules that were too difficult and expensive for conventional pharmaceutical companies to manufacture and often costly and hard to extract from human or animal tissues. When the act went into effect, it motivated small biotech companies to develop these recombinant proteins into drugs even if they couldn't patent them—a particularly acute worry in the early days of biotechnology, when the U.S. Patent and Trademark Office was still struggling to figure out how best to provide patent protection to naturally occurring molecules.

People began to ask: Had the Orphan Drug Act been co-opted as a BIOTECHNOLOGY PROMOTION ACT?

A recent study by the Tufts Center for the Study of Drug Development found that from 1983 to 1992 the biotech industry secured 19 percent of all orphan drug approvals; 76 percent of such approvals went to pharmaceutical companies. By 2001 biotech's share had grown to 41 percent. Of the 10 best-selling biotech drugs

TOP 10 BIOTECH DRUGS AND THEIR ORPHAN DRUG STATUS

RANK	TRADE NAME	GENERIC NAME	MAJOR INDICATION	2001 SALES WORLDWIDE (in U.S. millions)	ORIGINAL U.S. DEVELOPER	ORIGINAL U.S. APPROVAL DATE
1	Epogen Procrit Eprex	Epoetin alfa	Anemia	$5,588	Amgen	June 1989
2	Intron A PEG-Intron Rebetron	Interferon-alpha 2b	Hepatitis C	$1,447	Schering-Plough	November 1988
3	Neupogen	Filgrastim	Neutropenia (low white blood cell count)	$1,300	Amgen	February 1991
4	Humulin	Human insulin	Diabetes	$1,061	Genentech	October 1982
5	Avonex	Interferon-beta 1a	Multiple sclerosis	$972	Biogen	May 1996
6	Rituxan	Rituximab	Non-Hodgkin's lymphoma	$819	IDEC Pharmaceuticals	November 1997
7	Protropin Nutropin Genotropin Humatrope	Somatropin	Growth disorders	$771	Genentech	October 1985
8	Enbrel	Etanercept	Arthritis	$762	Amgen (formerly Immunex)	November 1998
9	Remicade	Infliximab	Crohn's disease	$721	Centocor	August 1998
10	Synagis	Palivizumab	Pediatric respiratory disease	$516	Medimmune	June 1998

Ranks 1, 5, 6, 7 and **9** were originally approved as an orphan drug

Ranks 2, 3, 8 were not originally approved as an orphan drug but now granted orphan drug status for one or more subsets of disorders

Ranks 4 and **10** were never designated an orphan drug.

SOURCES: Nature Reviews: Drug Discovery, Vol. 1, No. 11, page 846; November 2002; FDA

worldwide in 2001, five were originally approved as orphan drugs, and three more were approved for orphan indications in addition to their original use, which afforded their developers seven years of marketing exclusivity [*see table*, "Top 10 Biotech Drugs"]. Indeed, the biggest moneymaking orphan products helped to launch some of the major players in the biotech industry, including Amgen and Genentech.

A striking example of an orphan drug technology that blossomed into more widespread use is pegylation, the process of adding to a protein a waxy substance called polyethylene glycol (PEG), which slows the drug's clearance from the blood stream and masks it from attack by the immune system. Pegylation debuted in 1990 in Enzon's orphan drug Adagen for the treatment of ADA-SCID. Although only a few dozen children worldwide suffer from this condition, pegylation technology is now used in PEG-Intron, part of a combination treatment for hepatitis C, and has tremendous potential in other therapeutic applications.

Even aside from serendipitous blockbusters, one can make money on orphan drugs. In 1988 Lars-Uno Larsson,

a former Bristol-Myers Squibb executive, founded Swedish Orphan International in Stockholm on the belief that the Orphan Drug Act made it possible to earn modest but sufficient returns on drugs for rare diseases. Now with affiliates around the world, Swedish Orphan has developed a number of products and inspired others to establish similar companies. "The financial markets look on smaller products and say, 'How can you make money with a $10-million product?'" observes John Bullion, a former venture capitalist and now the CEO of Orphan Medical, a Minnesota-based company with half a dozen approved orphan products. "Well, you can make very good money with a $10-million product, but you need several of them," he says.

People with rare diseases are usually treated by a handful of doctors who have experience in the disease and often join patient education or advocacy groups to share information and to lobby for more research on their disorder. This combination makes finding patients to participate in clinical trials and to buy the drugs relatively easy and cost-effective. According to a recent industry

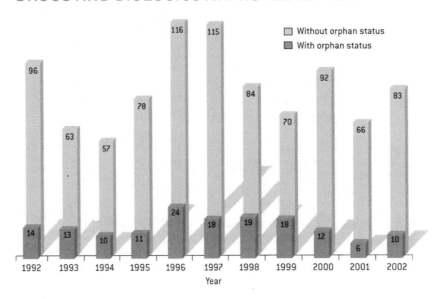

DRUGS AND BIOLOGICS APPROVED BY FDA

ORPHAN DRUGS account for 17 percent of all drugs and biologics (therapeutics derived from living sources) approved for sale in the U.S. over the past 10 years.

analysis, it costs about one fourth as much to develop a drug for a rare disease as one for high blood pressure, and annual marketing costs are one seventh as high.

Rich Orphans

BUT SOME OF THE ABUSES of the Orphan Drug Act have been glaring—and it's not only Amgen's epoetin alfa that has hit the jackpot. When they were first introduced, Genentech's human growth hormone (hGH) and Glaxo-SmithKline's AZT were approved for rare disorders (hGH deficiency and AIDS, respectively), but they subsequently earned billions when physicians began to prescribe hGH for many short-statured children and when the AIDS epidemic ballooned. Some critics suggest that orphan drugs that make profits no longer need help and should forfeit the act's benefits. The European Union recently enacted a law that would strip orphan status from a drug that becomes "extraordinarily profitable" after five years, but similar measures have been rejected repeatedly by American legislators under the lobbying pressure of the U.S. pharmaceutical industry. It is too early to tell whether Europe's law will prevent drug companies from abusing orphan drug designation; national health plans that exert controls on drug prices will also make the law's effects hard to assess.

A notable case of pricing and profits, according to some, is Genzyme's imiglucerase (Cerezyme). The drug—and enzyme-replacement therapy for Gaucher disease, which afflicts 2,000 Americans—is the world's most expensive medicine. Genzyme reportedly earns close to half a billion dollars a year from this treatment by charging patients between $100,000 and $400,000 a year for it, de-pending on whether the patient is a child or an adult. And the company did not lower the price when it switched from extracting the substance from human placentas to using the less expensive recombinant method of production. Patients, some of whom must spend their way into poverty to qualify for Medicaid to afford Cerezyme, are angry about the price but grateful for their lives.

"To know whether [an orphan drug] is excessively PROFITABLE, you have to look at [the company's] books. And how would you define 'unreasonably profitable'?"

Abbey S. Meyers, president of the National Organization for Rare Disorders (NORD)—the fiercest defender of those with rare diseases—is weary of answering the question of whether companies should be barred from making unreasonable profits on orphan drugs. "To know whether something is excessively profitable, you have to be able to look at their books, and they won't let you do that," she states. "And how would you define 'unreasonably profitable' anyway?"

Companies defend their crushingly expensive prices by citing their need to survive and to fund future research. And they point out that in some cases, they could charge much more than they do. Rare Disease Therapeutics, a Tennessee affiliate of Swedish Orphan, priced Orfadin, its recently approved treatment of hereditary tyrosinemia type 1, by making it $80,000 cheaper than a liver transplant, the only other therapy for the disorder. (Company officials say they arrived at the price by computing their costs.) The firm—which is not publicly held and therefore not under profit pressure from Wall Street—could easily have gotten twice as much for the only drug that keeps these children alive.

That's small comfort to patients. Happily, though, patient-advocate Meyers can think of no one with a rare disease who has been unable to obtain an FDA-approved drug because he or she could not pay for it. Most companies that produce orphan drugs have formal or informal programs for providing drugs free to indigent patients, but they hardly ever make public the number of patients they accommodate or what such patients must do to qualify. State and federal plans also exist for helping those with various rare disorders, especially hemophiliacs, some of whom must spend $100,000 or more each year for a blood-clotting protein called Factor VIII.

But only selected disorders are covered by such corporate and government programs, a policy that "leaves the rest of us out in the cold," Meyers comments. And many families have sold their houses or spent their life savings to qualify for the support. Even those with insurance are unprotected when treatment costs either exceed their plans' lifetime cap or drive premiums unaffordably high, she explains: One man who worked as an accountant for a small company resigned because payments for his son's human growth hormone drove his employer's insurance rates through the roof and affected fellow employees. He went to work as a manual laborer in a factory with a workforce large enough to distribute the cost.

No one has been able to offer an acceptable solution to the problem of unseemly profits. Haffner accepts it as the way things are in a free-market society. Meyers, the most obvious person to protest, is grateful for what populations with rare diseases have won. "Pricing is something we can't do anything about. As long as we can make sure that patients have access, it's great. If they don't, *then* it should be on the front page of the newspapers," she asserts. She worries that efforts to fine-tune the delicate structure might bring the whole system down. "We use all of our energy trying to keep the Orphan Drug Act the same," she says. "When the drug companies want to fight, they can hire a lobbyist for every member of Congress, while we have a bunch of mothers wandering around with sick babies."

In the end, the high cost of orphan drugs probably has to be addressed as part of the bigger problem of high drug costs in general. The FDA itself is in no position to insist that costs come down for orphan drugs or any others. It has no authority over pricing, only over which, if any, uses can be claimed for a given drug. All it can do to influence profits is to decide whether a compound said to target a rare disease is truly likely to have an extremely limited market and thus deserves the protection of the act.

Salami Slicing

BESIDES ALLOWING companies to retain orphan status for drugs that end up with an unusually large market, the act has been used to favor corporate bottom lines in another way that critics are protesting. The FDA permits companies to parse diseases into "medically plausible subsets," a term that it does not define clearly. The agency's orphan products office has tried to fight such "salami slicing," but some firms still try to define one stage or manifestation of a disease as a distinct entity entitled to orphan drug benefits if it affects fewer than 200,000 people.

This issue will inevitably grow more complex with the advent of pharmacogenomics and personalized medicine—the possibility of targeting treatments more accurately, and thus more safely and effectively, at subpopulations and even at individuals by determining through genetic profiles who would respond best and who would be least likely to suffer adverse reactions to a given drug. This prospect could benefit patients, but it is also expected to challenge the pharmaceutical industry, which has hitherto relied on mass sales of identical drugs to large, poorly differentiated patient populations. In the next decade a multitude of diseases may be broken down into diagnostically and therapeutically distinct populations that meet the threshold requirement of medically plausible subsets. Then society may find that many or all drugs are orphans, and policymakers will need to revisit the question of how to stimulate research for truly rare diseases.

Twenty years after the passage of the Orphan Drug Act, many believe that it has exceeded its original expectations. During the decade before its appearance, 34 orphan products went on the market, 10 of them developed by the pharmaceutical industry and the other 24 by federally funded efforts. In the two decades since, 229 orphan drugs that together treat 11 million patients, most with serious or life-threatening diseases, have entered the market, and the FDA has granted orphan status to nearly 1,000 other drugs. "The Orphan Drug Act works fabulously well," Meyers concludes. "We have treatments we never imagined we would." Existing pharmaceutical and biotech companies have been induced to develop orphan products, and new companies have been founded for the exclusive purpose of addressing unmet needs.

In a more subjective measure of the act's success, it has been copied almost verbatim by the European Union, Australia, Japan and several other Asian countries. And the U.S. Department of Homeland Security is even considering it as a model for how to steer efforts toward developing vaccines and antidotes for possible biological warfare agents.

The act certainly has it warts, but in a free-market economy, it is the best model devised so far to ensure that those with rare diseases can get the treatments they so desperately need.

MORE TO EXPLORE

Two Decades of Orphan Product Development. Marlene E. Haffner, Janet Whitley and Marie Moses in *Nature Reviews: Drug Discovery,* Vol. 1, No. 10, pages 821–825; October 2002.

The U.S. Food and Drug Administration Office of Orphan Products Development Web site includes complete information on the Orphan Drug Act and amendments, procedural guidelines, and lists of all orphan drug designations, approvals and grants: **www.fda.gov/orphan**

The National Organization for Rare Disorders [NORD] is a source of comprehensive information on rare diseases, support groups and news: **www.rarediseases.org**

Orphanet is a multilingual European orphan drug/disease database: **orphanet.infobiogen.fr**

THOMAS MAEDER is senior adviser for scientific strategies at the Georgetown University Medical Center. He is the author of numerous books, including *Adverse Reactions,* about modern drug regulation as seen through the tragic story of chloramphenicol, which caused a fatal blood disorder. He has done graduate work in neurobiology at the University of Pennsylvania and was previously senior science writer at *Red Herring* magazine.

Use Caution with Pain Relievers

Acetaminophen is a safe and effective pain reliever that benefits millions of consumers. However, taking too much could lead to serious liver damage. The drug is sold under brand names such as Tylenol and Datril, but it is also available in many cough and cold products and sleep aids, and is an ingredient in many prescription pain relievers.

In September 2002, the FDA Non-Prescription Drugs Advisory Committee discussed safety issues related to the use of pain relievers sold over-the-counter (OTC), including acetaminophen, aspirin, ibuprofen and naproxen.

Acetaminophen can cause liver injury through the production of a toxic metabolite. The body eliminates acetaminophen by changing it into substances (metabolites) that the body can easily eliminate in the stool or urine. Under certain circumstances, particularly when more acetaminophen is ingested than is recommended on the label, more of the harmful metabolite is produced than the body can easily eliminate. This harmful metabolite can seriously damage the liver.

The signs of liver disease include abnormally yellow skin and eyes (jaundice), dark urine, light-colored stools, nausea, vomiting, and loss of appetite. The signs can be similar to flu symptoms and may go unnoticed for several days if consumers believe their symptoms are related to their initial illness. Serious cases of liver disease may lead to mental confusion, coma, and death.

To avoid accidental overdosing, it's very important not to take more than the recommended dose on the label. Also, you should not take acetaminophen for more days than recommended, or take more than one drug product that contains acetaminophen at the same time. Consumers should be aware that taking more than the recommended dose will not provide more relief.

If you're taking a prescription pain medicine, check with your doctor first before taking OTC acetaminophen. The prescription pain medicine may also contain acetaminophen. Acetaminophen is also available in combination with other OTC drug ingredients. So, you need to check the labels of other OTC drug products for the ingredient. In some cases of accidental acetaminophen overdose, it appears that consumers used two or more acetaminophen-containing products at the same time.

Some individuals appear to be more susceptible to acetaminophen-induced liver toxicity than others.

People who use alcohol regularly may be at increased risk for toxicity, particularly if they use more than the recommended dose. Further research needs to be conducted in alcohol users to determine what factors make some alcohol users more susceptible to liver injury than others.

Parents should be cautious when giving acetaminophen to children. For example, the infant drop formula is three times more concentrated than the children's suspension. It's important to read drug labels every time you use a drug and to know what dosage strength you are using.

Improvements to labeling and consumer information for acetaminophen are among the recommendations made by the FDA's Nonprescription Drugs Advisory Committee. The committee recommended including the word "acetaminophen" in bold type on the labels for all drug products containing the ingredient and a warning about acetaminophen's potential to cause liver damage.

The committee also recommended that labeling for aspirin and other non-steroidal anti-inflammatory drugs (NSAIDs) such as ibuprofen and naproxen include warnings about the potential for gastrointestinal bleeding that may be associated with use of these products. Aspirin is sold under brand names such as Bayer and St. Joseph's. Ibuprofen is sold under names such as Advil and Motrin. Naproxen is sold under the name Aleve. There are generic versions available for all of these products, as well.

The risk for bleeding is low for those who take these products intermittently. For those who take the products on a daily or regular basis, the risk is increased, particularly for those over 65 years of age or those who take corticosteriods (such as prednisone). Those who use hormone therapy (estrogens and progestins) for postmenopausal symptoms or birth control do not have an increased risk for bleeding.

In addition, the committee recommended adding labeling language that urges consumers to ask health care providers about NSAID use if they have kidney disease or are taking diuretics (fluid pills).

The FDA is evaluating the committee's advice and working to complete rulemaking for these OTC pain relievers/fever reducers.

'I Felt Like I Wanted To Hurt People'

Emergency rooms report the violent return of PCP

BY SUZANNE SMALLEY AND
DEBRA ROSENBERG

Mike is hardly a seasoned drug user. When the shy 16-year-old bought marijuana in the bathroom of his suburban Hartford, Conn., high school, he didn't know what it was supposed to smell like. The stuff gave off such a strong chemical stench that Mike hid it in the attic insulation at home. The pot seemed more potent than he'd expected, too. The next day, when most people would feel normal, I would still have trouble walking, says Mike, clad in frayed-bottom khakis and a red Nike T shirt. "I felt like I wanted to hurt people. I felt like everybody was after me." When Mike's parents finally discovered some of the stash in his reeking bedroom, they knew it wasn't the marijuana they remembered from the '70s. Turns out Mike's pot was "wet-laced" with the hallucinogen PCP and, for an extra kick, embalming fluid.

Known as angel dust in the 1970s, PCP, or phencyclidine, gave users superhuman strength and a numbing calm. But the addictive, psychedelic drug also made many paranoid, violent and completely out of touch with reality; they leapt off roofs and broke out of handcuffs with their bare hands. Police cracked down, and eventually the drug got such a bad reputation that even junkies wouldn't touch it. But now there are signs that the disco-era scourge is quietly gaining a new following—often among unwitting users like Mike. PCP is cheap and relatively easy to make in the lab, and boosts the effects of other drugs. PCP seizures by the Drug Enforcement Administration shot up 24 percent from 2000 to 2001 (not counting a big Texas bust that drove the numbers through the roof). Nationally, PCP-related visits to the emergency room jumped 48 percent from 1999 to 2000 and were still on the rise in the first half of 2001, the latest year for which figures are available. To be sure, PCP is still a small part of the nation's drug problem: the 2000 National Household Survey on Drug Abuse found that 264,000 Americans fessed up to PCP use in the previous year—a fraction of the million who said they'd tried methamphetamines. But given PCP's nasty history, drug experts worry about the smallest uptick. "PCP can make users so delusional that they become like a hand grenade with the pin missing," says Jim Parker of the Do It Now Foundation, a drug-education group. "Any increase is cause for alarm."

It's easy to see why. In April, aspiring rapper Antron Singleton was arrested after Los Angeles police found him standing in the street, naked and covered in blood. Prosecutors say he brutally murdered his 21-year-old roommate—she had bite marks on her face, a slashed cheek and a lung that appeared to have been gnawed on. Singleton's defense? He was smoking PCP the morning before the killing. In Phoenix, a man bit off and swallowed the thumb of his 2-year-old son in a wigged-out attempt to mix their DNA. (Later, while telling police he'd taken several hits of PCP, the man regurgitated the thumb.) In Pittsburgh last month, a man who said he was on PCP shot a pregnant woman and her parents before beating, stabbing and shooting their 12-year-old son who somehow lived to testify against the alleged killer.

Many of today's PCP users are too young to remember the havoc the drug caused the last time round. At Ben Taub Hospital, Houston's busiest emergency room, Dr. Janice Zimmerman treats from one to five PCP patients every day—most of them 17 to 25. Cynthia Hepler, admissions manager at a Houston drug-treatment center, estimates that 40 percent of her admissions are now young PCP users. "Wet started being used in the inner city, but it is hitting the suburbs," says Hepler.

And that counts only those who knowingly try the drug. In addition to soaking pot in it, dealers have been mixing PCP with ecstasy—upping the potency while lowering the price. "Most people using PCP have no idea they are using," says Dr. Barry Spiegel of the Rosecrance Treatment Center in Rockford, Ill. It was certainly a shock to Mike, who's now in treatment and has sworn off smoking any more mysterious substances. "I never want to do PCP again," Mike says. A lesson learned the hard way: it's just not worth the risk.

GHB's Deadly Allure

Growth hormone releaser or lethal drug?

BY BRIAN ROWLEY, MS

A firestorm of controversy has surrounded GHB (gamma-hydroxybutyrate) ever since it was banned by the U.S. Food and Drug Administration in 1990, pulled from health food store shelves in 1991 and put on the schedule 1 list in 2000, joining heroine and cocaine. Since then, partygoers, insomniacs and a minority of hardcore bodybuilders have lobbied for its return. For bodybuilders, the allure is growth hormone (GH) release, and the claim that GHB boosts muscle recovery by inducing a deep sleep. Nonetheless, government scientists and emergency physicians alike have denounced GHB as an addictive and dangerous drug. What's the truth about GHB, and what are the alternatives?

GHB & Bodybuilders

Most people take GHB as a sleep aid and to improve mood. Curiously, while a low dose of GHB may have a mild euphoric effect, a bigger dose knocks a person out for about four hours, after which time he or she suddenly awakens (hopefully) fully alert. The effect is related to the buildup and release of dopamine, a brain chemical involved in pleasure, motivation, sex drive and addiction.

In the hardest of hardcore bodybuilding circles, the most talked-about claim for GHB is that it causes release of growth hormone. A study of eight healthy young men found that 3 grams of GHB nearly doubled GH release and caused a deepening of slow wave sleep, both of which could theoretically improve a bodybuilder's recovery and muscle growth.[1] However, no GH-releasing effect and no gains in muscle mass were found when a similar dose was given to recovering alcoholics for a full six months.[2] The evidence for an anabolic effect for GHB is therefore somewhat mixed, and the drug doesn't seem to work well over the long term.

Alternatives

As a result, the search began for legal alternatives. Although GHB was banned from commercial sale in 1990, the Dietary Supplement Health and Education Act of 1994 made it legal to sell GHB precursors as dietary supple-

ments. These precursors are chemicals the body can convert into GHB for a similar effect. In particular, gamma-butyrolactone (GBL) and 1,4-butanediol (BD) started cropping up in health food stores and on the Internet under a variety of guises. Some partygoers would drink GBL straight, occasionally suffering seizures and/or violent regurgitation. Yet basement chemists more commonly use GBL to synthesize GHB, either for personal use or for illegal sales over the Internet. Also, GBL is easier to get than GHB because of its widespread use as a paint stripper and industrial grease-remover.

The "fun" ended when GBL was made a List 1 chemical on Feb. 18, 2000, as part of the Date-Rape Prohibition Act, so anyone planning to buy or sell GBL or GHB as a dietary supplement is risking severe legal trouble. As a result, those looking for an anabolic hormone-releasing effect at night are really better off with 10 or so grams of glutamine and/or three capsules of ZMA before bed. They're safer than GHB (see "Toxicity") and less likely to land you in the clink for drug possession.

Clip Notes: GHB

What is it? Gamma-hydroxybutyrate, a drug banned by the FDA.
Uses: Party drug, date-rape drug, supposed sleep enhancer, purported GH enhancer.
Effectiveness: Risks outweigh any benefits for sleep enhancement and GH release.
Possible consequences: Death, coma, addiction, breathing difficulty, arrest.
The better alternative: For growth-hormone stimulation, glutamine or ZMA.

Toxicity

Although GHB has been tested as a possible treatment for narcolepsy and insomnia in the elderly, its risks outweigh its benefits where bodybuilders and other athletes are concerned. GBL, BD and GHB can all cause head jerks and addiction, and none are safe enough to justify using even if they were legal. Unfortunately, the drugs increase the sedative effects of alcohol and may eventually cause inopportune seizures or "absences," which could be disastrous if you're driving a car or bench pressing a 250-pound barbell.

GHB can also cause breathing trouble, coma and death. As of November 2000, the Drug Enforcement Agency documented 71 deaths from GHB misuse, and the drug's popularity among partygoers is increasing.[3] Nowadays, GHB causes more emergency room visits than Ecstasy, a number that quadrupled between 1998 and 2000.

Even relatively low doses may cause dizziness, drowsiness, nausea and visual disturbances, and the effects can be unpredictable, especially in combination with other sedatives. For example, the body breaks down GHB less well during the night, so a dose that's safe in the daytime may not be safe at night. An overdose often requires emergency room treatment, including intensive care for difficulty breathing and coma. More recently, GHB's addictive potential has come to light due to the emergence of a number of GHB-dependent users.

References

1. Van Cauter, E., et al. Simultaneous stimulation of slow-wave sleep and growth hormone secretion by gamma-hydroxybutyrate in normal young men. Journal of Clinical Investigations 100(3):745–753, 1997.

2. Addolorato, G., et al. Long-term administration of GHB does not affect muscular mass in alcoholics. Life Sciences 65(14):PL191-196, 1999.

3. U.S. Department of Justice website: MACROBUTTON HtmlResAnchor http://www.usdoj.gov/dea,/pubs/intel,101026/.

Brian Rowley has a bachelor's degree in dietetics, a master's in neuromuscular physiology and pharmacology, and has done doctoral work in biochemistry.

Ban Ephedra Now!

Momentum builds to get this lethal herb off the market

By Paul Solotaroff

Ten months ago, I wrote for this magazine about an exceptional ex-soldier named Todd Weger. A decorated war veteran and one of the more remarkable physical specimens in the 82nd Airborne, Weger suffered a stroke at age 28 that later necessitated the removal of half his brain in order to accommodate swelling. An hour before he collapsed, he'd mixed a glass of Ultimate Orange, an amphetamine-like powder containing ephedra. This happened in 1998, before the ephedra-related deaths of star college athletes Devaughn Darling and Rashidi Wheeler (and the death, suspected to have been ephedra-related, of Minnesota Viking Korey Stringer), but emergency rooms were already seeing more users of the herb. Like Weger, these victims had succumbed to marketers' promises of rapid weight loss and explosive energy, and to the premise that their best wasn't good enough, that the only way to compete for a girl, a medal, or a spot on a team was to join the chemical arms race.

WIN AT ANY COST: Steve Bechler's death this winter focused attention on the prevalence of ephedra use in baseball.

Steve Bechler, the 23-year-old Baltimore Orioles reliever who died this February in Fort Lauderdale, was, it seems, a believer in that notion. Bechler, an end-of-the-roster type with a lousy medical history, a barstool belly, and a desperate need to impress his manager fast, appears to have rolled the dice on a crash dose of Xenadrine RFA-1. He was hoping to burn off extra weight; instead, he cooked from the inside out, his body temperature rising to 108. In so doing, he reflected heat on one of baseball's dirtiest secrets: the pervasive use of ephedra and other stimulants. Outfielders who daydream during double-headers have been popping "beans" since the early sixties, as have portly pitchers who turn spring training into a nutritional game of chicken. David Wells, the Falstaffian

lefty, was taken to the hospital with an irregular heartbeat seven years ago after downing Ripped Fuel ephedra. Bill Pulsipher, of the New York Mets, had a similar episode after taking Xenadrine.

No Free Ride Just because a dietary supplement comes in an "ephedra-free" version doesn't mean it's safe. Products like Bio Burn, NoPhedra, Ripped Fuel, and Fat Busters all contain citrus aurantium, or bitter orange, a stimulant that can cause the same deadly side effects.

In the wake of Bechler's death, Major League Baseball's commissioner, Bud Selig, called on Congress to remove ephedra from retail shelves and banned its use in the nonunionized minor leagues. The powerful major league players' union defended its members' right to take any legal substances they want but urged them to "be extremely reluctant" to use ephedra. As for Wells, he still uses ephedra, though like the consummate pro he is, he's switched brands.

Since MJ's Weger story ran, there has been some progress. Suffolk County, on eastern Long Island, became the nation's first jurisdiction to halt the sale of products containing ephedra. The state of California passed a law in January forbidding sales to minors. And a recent *Annals of Internal Medicine* study found that ephedra, which accounts for 1 percent of all supplements sales in the U.S., triggered 64 percent of the complaints filed with poison-control centers. Even the timid Food and Drug Administration, still handcuffed by a lenient, industry-supported 1994 regulatory bill, is now proposing labels warning that ephedra use can be deadly.

The most telling development has come from Weger himself. Four surgeries later, he has reenrolled in college and is one semester away from getting his bachelor's degree. His left hand, once clenched in a fist, has relaxed enough to let him scoop up his house keys or drink a soda. But just as he declared himself to be in the clear, Weger suffered a cerebral clot and was raced to a hospital in February. Although blood thinners prevented a stroke, Weger was shattered by his flash relapse. "How long do I have to keep on paying the price for a fool mistake I made five years ago?" he says. "And how many players are going to have to drop dead before I can read the sports page in peace?"

Prescription Drug Abuse: FDA and SAMHSA Join Forces

By Michelle Meadows

Kyle Moores, 19, of Manassas, Va., says he knew he needed help when his abuse of the pain reliever OxyContin (oxycodone) left him drowning in debt and unable to hold a job. "It put me basically in a zombie mode for a year and a half," says Moores, who crushed and snorted the drug. "I finally realized I was losing my life."

Moores was successfully treated at an addiction facility in Richmond, Va. He spoke about his journey to recovery in January at a media event to kick off a joint public education program on the dangers of prescription drug abuse.

The program, sponsored by the Food and Drug Administration and the Substance Abuse and Mental Health Services Administration (SAMHSA) includes posters, public service announcements, and brochures featuring the slogans "The Buzz Takes Your Breath Away… Permanently" and "It's To Die For." The messages target people ages 14 to 25, but they

are relevant to anyone who abuses prescription drugs.

John Jenkins, M.D., director of the FDA's Office of New Drugs, says the FDA is especially concerned about the misuse of single ingredient, controlled-release formulations of opiates, such as OxyContin. "Abuse and misuse of these products is particularly dangerous because they contain higher doses of the drug and are designed to release the drug slowly over a 12- or 24-hour, or longer, period of time for sustained relief of pain," Jenkins says. "Damaging the controlled-release mechanism for these products, such as crushing an OxyContin tablet, can result in immediate release of the high dose of drug, which can be fatal."

In 2001, almost 3 million youths ages 12 to 17 and almost 7 million young adults between 18 and 25 reported using prescription medications non-medically at least once in their lifetimes, according

to the National Household Survey on Drug Abuse conducted by SAMHSA.

Data provided by SAMHSA's Drug Abuse Warning Network indicates that visits to hospital emergency departments related to narcotic prescription pain relievers increased significantly from 1994 to 2001. The highest increases were seen with oxycodone, methadone, morphine, and hydrocodone. Narcotic pain relievers, also known as opiates, are the most commonly abused prescription drugs.

The FDA is working with manufacturers of controlled-release opiates to implement risk-management plans aimed at minimizing abuse while still keeping the products available for people with a legitimate medical need. "In many cases, prescription opiate pain relievers are the most effective treatments available to help patients control their pain and lead productive lives," Jenkins says. But they also have potentially serious side effects,

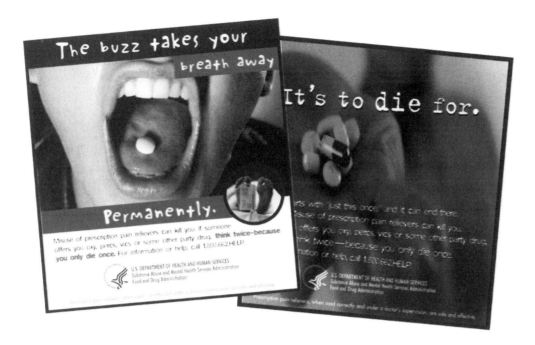

the most serious of which is the risk of respiratory failure.

"While addiction occurs after repeated use, death can occur after a single dose," Jenkins says. "So the first time that someone decides to abuse or misuse a prescription opiate pain reliever may be their last decision."

H. Westley Clark, M.D., J.D., director of SAMHSA's Center for Substance Abuse Treatment, wants people who are abusing prescription drugs to know that effective addiction treatment is available. Clark says that primary care physicians play a critical role in screening, assessing, and referring people with potential substance abuse problems.

According to Clark, "The recent approval by the FDA of buprenorphine to treat prescription drug abuse, and the office-based use of other addiction medications likely to be approved in the years ahead, makes the role of primary care physicians more vital than ever." In October 2002, the FDA approved Subutex (buprenorphine) and Suboxone (bu-

prenorphine and naloxone)--the first narcotic drugs available to treat opiate dependence that can be prescribed in an office setting.

To contact SAMHSA's substance abuse treatment 24-hour helpline, call 1-800-662-HELP (1-800-662-4357) or visit www.findtreatment.samhsa.gov

From *FDA Consumer*, March/April 2003, p. 36. © 2003 by FDA Consumer, the magazine of the U.S. Food and Drug Administration.

UNIT 5
Drugs and Crime

Unit Selections

Key Points to Consider

- What role does the media play in influencing drug-related crime?

- Explain why you believe that drug-related crime is either overrepresented or underrepresented.

- Survey your class to determine what percentage have been victims of crime. Determine what percentage of those were victims of drug-related crime.

- Consider the costs of drug-related crime on the criminal justice, health care, and educational systems in your community.

- How is the fear of crime continuing to change the way we live?

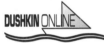 **Links: www.dushkin.com/online/**
These sites are annotated in the World Wide Web pages.

Drug Enforcement Administration
http://www.usdoj.gov/dea/
The November Coalition
http://www.november.org
TRAC DEA Site
http://trac.syr.edu/tracdea/index.html

Crime is intrinsic to the world of illegal drugs. The relationship is strong and enduring. The type of crime associated with this world varies according to the type of drugs involved and certain environmental factors associated with them. For example, patterns of violent crime consistently accompany the trafficking of cocaine, methamphetamine, and marijuana. The lucrative nature of the market, the fierce competition it generates, and the tendency for street dealers to be users of the product all serve to perpetuate violence. British Columbian marijuana, for example, sells for $1,500 a pound in Vancouver, but transported to Washington it brings $3,000. Transported to California or New York City, the same pound commands a price of $6,000 and $8,000 respectively. Canadian and U.S. authorities are confronting a new wave of violence associated with this trend. Almost all research that examines behavior associated with using, trafficking, or being present at locations where illegal drugs are sold or used produces relationships between that behavior and various levels of violence.

The use and abuse of legal drugs, although not as publicly sensational, also generate a significant relationship with crime. Most notable is alcohol, which studies repeatedly connect to crimes ranging in severity from shoplifting to rape, homicide, and child abuse. The high percentage of perpetrators as well as victims using alcohol before and during the offense is a long-established criminological phenomenon. One study reported that violence was 10 times more likely to occur during the commission of a crime if the offender had been drinking. Another recent study suggested that alcohol-related deaths of young people occur at rates 6.5 times higher than those caused by all illegal drugs combined. The best evidence suggests that the relationship between drugs and crime is developmental rather than causal and varies by the nature and intensity of drug use.

Ample evidence exists supporting the strong relationship between drug use, criminal activity, and being arrested. Over half of the crime in this country occurs by persons under the influence of drugs. Research suggests that 80 percent of men and women behind bars in the United States are seriously involved with alcohol and other drugs. Crime increases as drug use increases. Criminal activity is reported to be two to three times higher among frequent users of heroin and cocaine as compared to the criminal activity of irregular users. In most cities surveyed, over 68 percent of arrestees reported recently using drugs. Three out of four arrestees reported drug use in their lifetime. Among the 1.8 million adults on parole or other supervised release from prison during the past year, 29.1 percent were current illicit drug users compared with 7.7 percent among adults not on parole or supervised release. Among the estimated 4.8 million adults on probation at some time during the past year, 28.7 percent reported current drug use as compared with 7.4 percent of adults not on probation.

Another different but remarkable dimension of the drugs/crime relationship concerns the expanding relationship between drug use and sexual assault. More than 430,000 sexual assaults occur annually in the United States, and many of these involve drug and alcohol use on the part of the victim as well as the offender. In the mid- and late 1990s, however, an alarming phe-

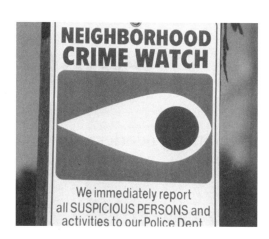

nomenon involving new rape-facilitating drugs became distinctly apparent in reports to police and rape crisis centers. The primary drug culprits identified in these attacks are Rohypnol, a benzodiazepine, and GHB, a drug most commonly used in Europe as an adjunct to anesthesia, and derivatives of GHB, most commonly, GBL and 1,4 butanediol (1,4,BD). The secret administration of one of these drugs into the drink of a victim can create a situation in which assailants do not have to overcome resistance, use force, make threats, or attract attention. These drugs immobilize and silence the victim. The drugs may also produce amnesia preventing recall and disqualifying victims' statements in court. In September of 2002, U.S. and Canadian investigators arrested 115 persons in 84 cities in the United States and Canada in the largest Internet trafficking network of these drugs ever discovered.

It is an error, however, to limit the discussion of drug use and crime to suspects and perpetrators. Sexual assault, domestic violence, and child abuse have long established the relationship between drug use and victimization. One must remain aware of how the use and abuse of drugs have often caused disproportionate tolls on specific populations of people.

Currently, no discussion of large-scale drug-related crime and trafficking is possible without recognizing the emergence of powerful Mexican cartels. In addition to purchasing cocaine and heroin directly from Colombian traffickers for sale in the United States, Mexican traffickers now manage the largest methamphetamine manufacturing and distribution network in the hemisphere. The "Kingpin Act," designed to frustrate trafficking by targeting business transactions of all entities associated with traffickers, has been recently credited with crippling some major Mexican syndicates. Similar sanctions have been applied successfully to Colombian traffickers. However, it is estimated that the rebel organization FARC, which drives much of the Colombian cocaine trade, still nets profits of more than $300 million per year.

The articles in unit 5 help illustrate the wide range of criminal activity associated with the manufacture, trafficking, and use of some illicit drugs. As you read, consider the significance of drugs as they relate to the most pervasive fear in this country—the fear of crime.

'The Perfect Crime'

GHB is colorless, odorless, leaves the body within hours—
and is fueling a growing number of rapes

BY SUZANNE SMALLEY

AFTER TWO WHISKY AND COKES, Patricia White decided to call it a night. The 47-year-old mother of three had been talked into helping her boss, Lorenzo Feal, celebrate his birthday with several colleagues. As she was leaving, Feal handed White a bottle of water, she says. She took a big gulp and spit the rest out because it tasted salty. Three hours later, White woke up in Feal's bed, naked and nauseated: she'd been drugged and raped.

White fled and called the police from her cell phone. Doctors found traces of gamma hydroxybutyric acid (GHB)—a recreational drug that is fueling a growing number of rapes—in her system. She's one of the lucky ones. Most women don't have proof that they've been dosed with GHB—because it exits the body within six to 12 hours. "Sexual predators are hunting with GHB," says prosecutor Christopher Frisco, who convicted Feal of using an anesthetic substance in carrying out White's rape. (Feal claimed the sex was consensual.) "It's ideal for predators and tough for prosecutors." Another prosecutor, Timothy Walsh, calls GHB-fueled sex assaults the "perfect crime" since the liquid poison is colorless, odorless and frighteningly easy to use. And without toxicological evidence, it can be difficult to prove that the rape victim didn't willingly consent to sex. GHB, long popular among club goers, has been illegal since 2000, but it can be manufactured in the kitchen sink using commonly available chemicals. Most victims wake up hours later with little or no memory of what has happened.

GHB's use has been growing for almost a decade, but recently doctors, advocates for rape victims, and toxicologists called in to testify in sex-assault cases have seen a large surge in reports of GHB-fueled sex assaults. In just the past couple of weeks, both coasts have featured sensational GHB cases. In San Diego, Andrew Luster, a Max Factor cosmetics heir, went on the lam in the midst of his trial for multiple rapes; prosecution tapes show Luster having sex with snoring girls. And in New York, a Hofstra University student pleaded guilty to the 2001 murder of another student who was doped on GHB at the time of his death. As recently as 1994—when the drug was still relatively new—there were only 56 GHB-related emergency-room visits nationwide. By 2001 that number had spiked to 3,340, according to the Substance Abuse and Mental Health Services Administration.

Alarmed, colleges are taking an active role in protecting women. More than 40 universities and thousands of bars have ordered coasters that detect the drug by turning blue when exposed to GHB (women splash their drink onto "test spots"). But activists are already warning women not to rely solely on the coasters, since they don't test for increasingly popular, easy-to-obtain—and still legal—GHB knockoffs like GBL and 1,4BD.

The DEA is so concerned about the rise in GHB-facilitated sexual assaults that officials have been meeting with representatives from the Rape, Abuse & Incest National Network (RAINN) to heighten awareness of GHB and other "predatory" drugs—an unusual move for an agency typically focused on interdiction. In November, the DEA announced that it will double the number of predatory-drug investigations it undertakes. Perhaps the agency was inspired by a recent success: in September authorities announced the arrests of 115 people in 84 cities for peddling GHB on the Internet.

The DEA's attention to the problem couldn't come at a better time. Some RAINN centers are reporting as much as a 50 percent uptick in GHB-fueled rapes in the past year. Trinka Porrata, a 25-year veteran of the Los Angeles Police Department and founder of Project GHB, has been flooded with messages from flummoxed cops trying to learn how to investigate rapes featuring this quickly vanishing drug.

And victims are helping to spread awareness. "You don't get over rape," White tells NEWSWEEK. She now counsels victims and says she is talking publicly so that others know what she didn't about GHB. With this drug, the more you know the safer you are.

Harder times for meth makers

Canada, anti-terror efforts have an impact.

By Steve Wiegand
BEE STAFF WRITER

A new law in Canada and heightened anti-terrorism security may be putting the squeeze on methamphetamine manufacturing in the Central Valley, law enforcement officials say— and squeezing it into neighboring countries.

Federal and state drug agency sources also say there is increasing evidence of links between meth trafficking in California and the financing of Middle Eastern terrorist organizations.

The Canadian law, which went into effect in January after more than a decade of discussion, requires licenses for people who import, export, buy or sell pseudoephedrine. The synthetic chemical compound is used mainly in cold and allergy medicines and is a key ingredient in the production of meth.

Pseudoephedrine is heavily regulated in the United States. Before January, however, and much to the chagrin of American police, it was relatively easy to obtain in Canada.

Smuggling rings based in Michigan and other parts of the Midwest regularly moved tractor-trailers full of pseudoephedrine pills from Canada into the United States and sold them to meth producers in California.

A case of 75,000 pills might sell for $18,000 and produce eight pounds of meth that might sell for $48,000 wholesale.

But law enforcement agents say the new law has combined with tighter border controls spurred by terrorism threats to make it tougher to smuggle the "precursor" chemicals to clandestine California labs.

"Before, they were literally crossing the border with tractor-trailer loads of pseudoephedrine in tons," said Bill Ruzzamenti, a federal Drug Enforcement Administration agent who directs the nine-county Central Valley High Intensity Drug Trafficking Area (HIDTA) program. "Now, we are seeing the Federal Express-type shipment of maybe a hundred pounds."

In response, however, outlaw motorcycle gangs in British Columbia and sophisticated "poly-drug" groups in Mexico are making meth in those countries, where it is still easier to obtain the ingredients than in the United States. The meth is then smuggled into the vast U.S. market.

The meth money pyramid

Here's the economic pyramid for a pound of methamphetamine in the Central Valley. Although these are typical prices, meth costs vary from day to day, depending on supply and demand.

Amount	Price
1. 9,375 pseudoephedrine tablets	$2,250
Enough to make 1 pound of meth at 80 percent to 90 percent purity	
2. One pound of meth	$4,000 - $6,000
3. The meth is "stepped on," or diluted, to double the previous amount	
32 ounces	$12,800 - $19,200
at $400-$600 an ounce	
4. The meth is diluted again to double the previous amount:	
1,792 grams	$71,680 - $179,200
at $40-$100 a gram	

Source: Central Valley High Intensity Drug Trafficking Area program
Sacramento Bee/Sheldon Carpenter

"Ten pounds of meth is easier to get in than 100 pounds of pseudoephedrine," Ruzzamenti said.

"We're seeing more and more 'finished' meth coming in from across the borders. It's too early to tell how big or how much that will take away from the market here in Central California, but I think it's a harbinger of things to come," he said.

For more than a decade, California, especially the Central Valley, has been the mother lode for making meth, a drug that can be intensely addictive, trigger intense paranoia and shattering violence in its users, and cause irreparable brain damage.

Because production of the drug is a relatively simple process, thousands of amateur chemists set up small operations often referred to by cops as "Beavis & Butt-head labs," a reference to the moronic cartoon characters.

Those labs are dwarfed in production by "super labs" controlled by organized crime groups. Those groups are believed to be dominated by Mexican nationals who are based in California and ship meth all over the country.

The combined result has been a Valley pandemic of meth-related crime and environmental messes caused by the dumping of the toxic wastes that are byproducts of meth production.

Government efforts to stem the flood have escalated in the past two years, with more funding, the creation of specialized law enforcement groups and several major international sweeps of precursor smuggling rings.

Three weeks ago, U.S. and Canadian drug agents culminated an 18-month investigation by arresting 67 suspects around the country and confiscating 34,000 pounds of pseudoephedrine. The busts, called "Operation Northern Star," grew out of another major sweep in January 2002 that resulted in more than 100 arrests and the seizure of 60,000 pounds of pseudoephedrine.

The sweeps have had some impact on the street, officials said, driving up meth prices. They've also driven down the drug's "purity" because meth makers "step on," or dilute their product to make it stretch further. A favorite dilution agent is MSM, a substance primarily used to increase joint flexibility in horses.

But the meth industry is nothing if not flexible.

In the past year, Valley drug cops say, meth labs have become smaller and more streamlined. Manufacturers are compartmentalizing various stages of the production process at different sites, lessening chances of detection and of losing all of the inventory in the event of a raid.

Dealers are also diversifying.

"What's really different around here is that even the small-quantity sellers will have two, three, four different varieties of crank at different purity levels, which they're selling at different price ranges," said Sacramento County Sheriff's Sgt. Bob Risedorph, who is with the California Multi-Jurisdictional Methamphetamine Enforcement Team (Cal-MMET).

"I guess the longer you sell something, the more variations you need to have."

The post-Sept. 11 scrutiny of terrorist activity has put more of a spotlight on pseudoephedrine smuggling groups with connections to the Middle East.

For years, small Central Valley markets were sources of pseudoephedrine. Law enforcement agents said some grocers, many of them with Middle Eastern roots, sold large quantities of cold pills literally out the back door to meth makers.

When new state and federal laws helped crack down on the practice, according to Ed Manavian of the state Justice Department's California Anti-Terrorism Information Center, some of the same grocers formed groups with friends and relations in the Midwest to smuggle pseudoephedrine in from Canada.

An analysis by the center of 74 major meth-related investigations in California in 2000 and 2001 found the primary pseudoephedrine trafficking groups were Yemeni, Jordanian or Palestinian.

Many of the groups have used the same financial networks used by terrorist organizations to funnel and launder money. The networks, called "hawalahs" (Arabic for "word of mouth"), rely on oral agreements to honor each other's financial obligations without leaving a paper trail.

The Office of National Drug Control Policy says it has identified at least 12 foreign terrorist organizations with links to drug trafficking.

Manavian declined to say whether there is evidence the drug groups were subgroups of terrorist organizations, or whether they were just showing their political sympathies by making contributions to the cause.

"What I can say is that we know that money from the illegal trafficking of drugs in California is making its way back to the Middle East to support terrorist activities," he said.

That stance has been disputed by attorneys for some of those arrested in the national meth sweeps of the past two years.

"There is no evidence to that; it's pure speculation," said Mark Werksman, a former federal prosecutor in Los Angeles who is representing a Chicago resident accused of conspiracy to sell pseudoephedrine to California customers. "No defendant has admitted to it in court or out of court to my knowledge."

No matter how Valley meth makers manufacture the drug and where they make it, or what they do with the money, law enforcement officials say the one sad constant is the abundance of customers.

"Except for marijuana, which everyone on drugs uses, meth is still the drug of choice here," said Risedorph, of the Sheriff's Department. "We still see plenty of cocaine, plenty of heroin, but meth dominates."

The Bee's Steve Wiegand can be reached at (916) 321-1076 or swiegand@sacbee.com.

Combating Methamphetamine Laboratories and Abuse:
Strategies for Success

"It is critical that agencies tailor responses to local circumstances and that each response be justified based on reliable problem analysis. In most cases, an effective strategy will involve implementing several different responses. Law enforcement responses alone are seldom effective in solving the problem."

Michael S. Scott
Author of Problem-Oriented Guides for Police Series:
Clandestine Drug Labs

The Methamphetamine Problem

Methamphetamine is a highly addictive central nervous system stimulant. It can be injected, snorted, smoked, or ingested orally. Commonly used street names for methamphetamine include meth, crank, crystal meth, speed, and ice. Methamphetamine can be relatively easily manufactured through storebought materials, and according to the Office of National Drug Control Policy, is the most prevalent synthetic drug produced in the United States.

Methamphetamine is frequently produced in clandestine laboratories. These labs can result in serious physical injury from explosions, fires, chemical burns, and toxic fumes, produce environmental hazards, pose clean-up problems, and endanger the lives and health of children. There are generally two types of clandestine drug labs, "super labs" and "mom and pop labs." According to the U.S. Drug Enforcement Administration, "super" labs are highly organized and account for approximately 80% of all methamphetamine produced. "Mom and pop: labs are more common and typically manufacture a much smaller amount of methamphetamine often only producing enough drugs for their own and close associates' use. Although these labs account for a much smaller portion of all methamphetamine produced, they account for far more explosions, fires, hazardous waste dumping, and child endangerment.

During the year 2000, approximately 8.8 million people in the U.S. reported trying methamphetamine at least once in their lifetime and over a quarter of high school seniors indicated that it was "fairly easy" or "very easy" to obtain "crystal meth."[1] The effects of methamphetamine intake include decreased appetite, increased activity and sense of well being. The negative effects of methamphetamine use can include physical addiction, psychotic behavioral episodes, and brain damage. Chronic methamphetamine use can cause anxiety, confusion, insomnia,

paranoia, and delusions. According to a report by the National Institute on Drug Abuse, the damage caused to the brain by methamphetamine can be similar to that caused by Alzheimer's disease, stroke, and epilepsy.[2]

Methamphetamine abuse is a serious problem across the nation, but has been particularly prevalent in the West and Midwest. Police officials, public health officers, policymakers, state legislatures, the U.S. Congress, and the media have all warned that methamphetamine is dangerous to those who manufacture, possess, and use it. Methamphetamine is also a serious health hazard to anyone who comes into reasonable contact with the chemicals used to produce it; notably, these include children, residents who live near meth labs and first responders to the scene of a clandestine laboratory—emergency medical teams, fire fighters, and police officers.

Local police are faced with the challenge of disrupting a drug market where much of the buying, selling, and cooking happens in private residences or rural locations, and among people who are often familiar with one another. In addition, due to the various chemicals used in the cooking process and the inexperience of many cooks, there is also a high potential for fires, explosions, or chemical spills. First responders are faced with an extraordinarily dangerous situation, especially if they are unaware of the presence of a methamphetamine laboratory at the scene.

COPS Funding to Combat Methamphetamine

From 1998–2002, the U.S. Department of Justice, Office of Community Oriented Policing Services (COPS) has provided approximately $137 million in funding to more than 100 state and local law enforcement agencies to combat the production, distribution, and use of methamphetamine. COPS methamphetamine grants encourage law enforcement agencies to use advanced technologies and creative problem-solving strategies to implement resourceful solutions to persistent crime and disorder problems. Consistent with community policing approaches to methamphetamine reduction, law enforcement agencies were encouraged to develop partnerships with other local government agencies and community groups to enhance the effectiveness and sustainability of programs. Agencies were also encouraged to craft innovative strategies (to move beyond mere enforcement) and to track and evaluate implementation efforts. COPS has also provided $64 million to the DEA for lab clean up efforts and training. Training funds allow state and

Partnerships can be developed with:

Emergency Response Agencies (Fire and Medical)

Neighboring Law Enforcement Agencies

City Prosecutors/District Attorneys (increase penalties and prosecution)

Parks Departments

Departments of Public Safety

Environmental Protection Agencies

Agencies or Businesses Involved in Hazardous Chemical Clean-up

Local Health Departments (enforce nuisance laws and conduct clean-up efforts)

Child Welfare Agencies

Youth and Family Service Agencies (to assist endangered children and families)

Neighborhood Watch Groups

Hotel/Motel Staff/Gas Service Employees (to assist in lab identification)

Local Retailers of Precursor Chemicals

Drug Courts

Treatment Centers

Drug Enforcement Administration (DEA)

U.S. Attorneys' Offices

Partnering with such agencies provides a vast array of previously untapped resources. It can assist in getting more methamphetamine-involved individuals into treatment, being better prepared to handle children exposed to methamphetamine, providing appropriate resources to help families recover from the effects of methamphetamine abuse, and coordinating with other law enforcement entities to share intelligence about methamphetamine-related activity.

local law enforcement officers to become OSHA qualified in lab identification, enforcement, and dismantling strategies. Additionally, COPS has provided a series of regional training conferences that allow grantees to share information with one another and learn about methamphetamine problems and solutions from experts in the field.

The COPS Methamphetamine National Evaluation

In 1998, the first year of the program, the COPS Office provided approximately $750,000 each to six carefully selected agencies. Through a competitive process, the Institute for Law and Justice (ILJ)(www.ilj.org) in partnership with 21st Century Solutions, Inc. received a grant to conduct an evaluation of this initial program. The evaluation focused on the history of the methamphetamine problem in these sites and developed a detailed process evaluation of their implementation. Researchers conducted interviews, collected data from police, observed clandestine lab seizures and other interventions, surveyed partners about their roles and responsibilities, examined newspaper articles, and made use of existing national databases to augment their findings. This document provides a brief summary of the findings of this National Evaluation and, based on other COPS-funded research, provides suggestions for how agencies can better deal with their own methamphetamine problems. Readers are encouraged to review the entire evaluation report that can be found on the COPS Web site (www.cops.usdoj.gov).

Overall Findings and Recommendations

In part, the National Evaluation found that:

- Educating police officials about methamphetamine, precursor chemicals, and clandestine labs led to increased lab identification and helped prevent on-scene injuries to officers. This is essential given the serious health and safety problems that methamphetamine laboratories can create and the difficulty in identifying possible lab locations.
- Training public works and hotel/motel staff proved successful. Given that they are frequently the first individuals to come across a lab or a contaminated space, educating these workers about how to identify methamphetamine, precursor chemicals, and lab equipment can prevent injury and promote quick reporting of illegal activity.
- Community education via public awareness campaigns provided invaluable information on methamphetamine-related issues and increased awareness about the prevalence of the problem. Community members were better able to identify methamphetamine-related activity and were more likely to contact police about suspicious activity in their neighborhoods.
- Drug courts could be a beneficial option for offenders, primarily because it immediately exposes methamphetamine-addicted individuals to treatment and provides a rigid structure with little tolerance for infractions. This is particularly important because methamphetamine users are often multi-drug users and because of the highly addictive nature of the drug.
- One of the major successes of the Methamphetamine Initiative was the partnerships that were formed as a result of the program. Given that methamphetamine presents a number of

serious problems in a community (e.g., dirty houses, environmental hazards, chemical contamination, endangered children), partnerships among police departments and other local agencies as well as with community members are essential to successfully reduce the problem.

A brief description of each of the six agencies included in the National Evaluation is provided below.

Phoenix Police Department, Arizona used a non-traditional media campaign and increased enforcement and officer training as part of their overall methamphetamine reduction efforts. The media campaign involved educating the public about the dangers and consequences of methamphetamine use and production and how to identify possible methamphetamine activity. The campaign used a video, presentations to community groups (including hotel/motel workers), billboards, postcards, and announcements on grocery store bags. Officer training involved the identification of possible methamphetamine activity. There was an increase in reported methamphetamine activity by both officers and citizens, many of the additional reports were directly attributed to this increased training. There was also an upsurge in methamphetamine investigations at hotels and motels as training efforts at these locations appeared to be effective.

" *Public attitudes about drug abuse need to be addressed. Too many people believe abuse is only the users' problem as well as their prerogative. The media could take greater responsibility to educate the community, but generally report only sensational events, e.g., labs blowing up. Similarly, the educational efforts should be reality-based, focusing on the health hazards of meth production and effects of long term use on the brain.* "

**Anonymous Respondent, Phoenix
ILJ Methamphetamine Evaluation 2002.**

Oklahoma City Police Department, Oklahoma focused on increased enforcement, training, a public education campaign and a partnership with a drug court to deal with methamphetamine problems. Officers used undercover buys, knock and talks, confidential informants, surveillance, and assistance from patrol officers making traffic stops to apprehend methamphetamine users and distributors. A 70% increase in methamphetamine labs seized occurred in the first year of the grant program. City-wide citizen training in methamphetamine abuse and identification was also conducted. Part of this training was focused on hotel/motel associations and natural gas employees. Gas company employees respond annually to over 600,000 service calls in Oklahoma City and service technicians perform a variety of inspections both inside and outside residences and businesses. Thus, they have wide-spread and frequent access to properties and may be particularly effective at identifying possible lab locations.

Dallas Police Department, Texas engaged in public education campaigns, drug court treatment programs aimed at reducing recidivism, training on the identification of precursor chemical suppliers for citizens and officers, and enforcement. Specific criteria were developed for admission to and for participation in the drug court program. The fact that these criteria were strictly enforced helped to increase the program's success rate. During the grant period, the department increased the number of clandestine lab seizures and arrests for methamphetamine. Identification of precursor chemical suppliers was hampered by the state's lack of laws restricting the purchase of these chemicals in large quantities.

" *Before, I would have walked through an apartment and had no clue what all that glassware meant. It would have just been harmless junk. Now I realize that it is a potential health and public safety hazard.* "

**Dallas Police Department Officer, Dallas
ILJ Methamphetamine Evaluation 2002.**

Little Rock Police Department, Arkansas focused on increased enforcement and training of all sworn officers regarding methamphetamine identification and response. These training efforts have also been extended to the public. The initiative has established a telephone hotline which citizens are encouraged to call if they suspect methamphetamine activity is taking place. An information campaign was also developed for retailers or precursor chemicals. The lack of laws restricting access to precursor chemicals limited the ability of police to reduce large purchases of these items. However, reports from retailers increased dramatically providing the police with invaluable information including the license plate numbers of large quantity purchasers. The majority of lab seizures over the course of the program were the direct result of citizen or informant information. This exemplifies the closed nature of the methamphetamine market and why citizen/retailer training in methamphetamine identification is crucial for success. In addition, interviews with jail detainees regarding methamphetamine abuse and manufacturing were useful to better understand the methamphetamine market. Perhaps most importantly, the program increased the local police department's understanding of the nature and extent of the methamphetamine problem.

Salt Lake City Police Department, Utah took a multidisciplinary and interagency approach to combating the methamphetamine problem. These efforts involved the use of enhanced enforcement and prosecution, child endangerment laws and service providers, civil remedies to reduce neighborhood impacts, public awareness campaigns, and the formation of a methamphetamine training team. More than thirty city, county, and federal agencies were recruited to participate. These partnerships were organized into regularly meeting committees and subcommittees and formed the basis of this comprehensive prevention, intervention and enforcement program. This demonstrates

Equipment and Chemicals Commonly Used for Methamphetamine Cooking

Household Equipment	Chemicals (Source)
Tempered Glass Baking Dishes	Ephedrine (Cold and Allergy Medicine)
Glass Pie Dishes	Pseudoephedrine (Cold and Allergy Medicine)
Glass or Plastic Jugs	Alcohol (Rubbing/Gasoline Additive)
Bottles	Toluene (Brake Cleaner)
Measuring Cups	Ether (Engine Starter)
Turkey Baster	Sulfuric Acid (Drain Cleaner)
Glass Jars	Methanol (Gasoline Additive)
Funnels	Lithium (Camera Batteries)
Coffee Filter	Trichloroethane (Gun Scrubber)
Blender	Anhydrous Ammonia (Farm Fertilizer)
Rubber Tubing	Sodium Hydroxide (Lye)
Paper Towels	Red Phosphorous (Matches)
Rubber Gloves	Iodine (Veterinarian Products)
Gasoline Can	Sodium Metal (Made from Lye)
Plastic Tote Box	MSM (Animal Food Supplement)
Tape	Table Salt/Rock Salt
Clamps	Kerosene
Hotplate	Gasoline
Strainer	Muriatic Acid
Aluminum Foil	Campfire Fuel
Propane Cylinder (20-lb.)	Paint Thinner
	Acetone

Source: www.streetdrugs.org

how a large-scale project involving multiple agencies can create effective partnerships and interventions to combat methamphetamine problems. Having a committed project coordinator was central to the success of the partnerships and programs.

> " *This initiative has brought several organizations together where little contact or understanding existed before. The result has been outstanding cooperation and some real successes in dealing with various different aspects of the problem.* "
>
> **Anonymous Respondent, Salt Lake City
> ILJ Methamphetamine Evaluation 2002.**

Minneapolis Police Department, Minnesota focused on impeding the flow of methamphetamine before it became a serious problem and preparing for the likely increase in its manufacture, distribution, and use. The department first engaged in comprehensive data collection to obtain information on the extent and nature of the drug problem. Interviews with probationers and drug court clients were conducted and were helpful in developing a program. For example, this analysis confirmed police suspicions that, when compared to users of other drugs, methamphetamine users were more likely to be white and employed. They also primarily purchased methamphetamine from residences as opposed to the street. The methamphetamine initiative also helped to improve the relationship among local law enforcement agencies. Key law enforcement players were regularly brought together to share information and effective communication occurred among them. Comprehensive training materials were developed including a general training video on lab identification and a video dealing specifically with methamphetamine identification at traffic stops. The department also developed resource guides for businesses and neighborhoods. The department trained community groups, officers, transit, housing sanitation, and park employees who may come into contact with clandestine methamphetamine labs.

What Can Be Done About Clandestine Drug Labs?

The COPS Office has produced a series of Problem-Oriented Guides for Police to assist police in identifying potential factors and underlying causes of specific problems, identifying known responses to each problem, and providing measures to assess the effectiveness of the responses. One of these guides focuses on the problem of clandestine drug labs (by Michael Scott, 2002). A variety of illicit drugs are produced in such labs, including methamphetamine, amphetamines, MDMA (ecstasy), methcathinone, PCP, LSD, and fentanyl, although methamphetamine typically accounts for 80 to 90 percent of the labs' total drug production. Thus, the problem of clandestine drug labs is closely tied with the problems associated with methamphetamine abuse. A brief summary of the major findings of this publication, titled *Problem-Oriented Guides for Police: Clandestine Drug Labs,* are discussed below; however, it is recommended that readers obtain the entire guide which can be found online at the COPS Web site (www.cops.usdoj.gov) or can be ordered by calling the U.S. Department of Justice Response Center at 800.421.6770.

The *Problem-Oriented Guides for Police: Clandestine Drug Labs* publication offers a series of critical questions that police agencies should ask in analyzing their particular drug lab problem. Although answers may not always be readily available to these questions, they are important because they will help agencies choose the most appropriate response to their particular methamphetamine problem. The guide includes lists of questions on the characteristics of drug labs, the victims of drug labs, offenders, chemical supplies, and current responses. It also offers a series of possible responses to clandestine drug labs and details some of the issues surrounding each option.

For example, with respect to "Finding and Seizing Labs" as a response, the author notes that although this is a common response, in the long term this may not be the most effective or efficient strategy for dealing with the problem. Smaller labs are easy to set up and nearly impossible to find. In addition, because seizing labs is time consuming and costly, police agencies may exhaust all of their resources on this single response, leaving no resources for other responses.

A more effective approach may be "Controlling the Sale of Precursor Chemicals." This strategy requires efforts at all levels of government (in terms of enforcement and enacting regulatory laws). Laws can be enacted that limit the purchase of large quantities of precursor chemicals and cash registers can be programmed to flag suspicious purchases. Even in the absence of such laws, local police can be involved in education efforts for chemical manufacturers and distributors (including local retailers), deliverers, and other regulators that may lead to increased offender identification. These groups can improve record keeping, container labeling, and engage in large quantity purchasing customer identification. In addition, laws can be enacted to encourage the safe storage of anhydrous ammonia (used in methamphetamine production) that is frequently stolen from such places as farmers' storage tanks.

Police departments cannot effectively fight a methamphetamine problem through enforcement alone. As the author states, "It is critical that agencies tailor responses to local circumstances and that each response can be justified based on reliable problem analysis. In most cases, an effective strategy will involve implementing several different responses. Police responses alone are seldom effective in solving the problem."

Possible Responses to Clandestine Drug Labs:

- Finding and Seizing Labs
- Arresting and Prosecuting Lab Operators
- Seizing Lab Operator Assets
- Enforcing EPA Laws Against Operators
- Filing Civil Actions Against Properties Used for Labs
- Controlling the Sale of Precursor Chemicals.
- Training Citizens to Report Suspected Labs
- Training Sales Clerks to Report Suspicious Purchases

- Training First Responders in Lab Identification and Clean-up
- Providing Child Protective Services to Children Exposed to Labs
- Providing Adequate Treatment Resources for Users

Notes

1. Substance Abuse and Mental Health Services Administration, Summary Findings from the 2000 National Household Survey on Drug Abuse, September 2001. www.samhsa.gov
2. National Institute on Drug Abuse, Methamphetamine Linked to Long-Term Damage to Brain Cells, March 2000. www.nida.nih.gov

Additional Resources

To receive a copy of *Problem-Oriented Guides for Police: Clandestine Drug Labs* please contact the U.S. Department of Justice Response Center at 800.421.6770. To download any of the Problem-Oriented Guides for Police or ILJ's complete *National Evaluation of the COPS Methamphetamine Initiative* please visit COPS online www.cops.usdoj.gov.

Other useful web sites include:
Office of National Drug Control Policy
www.whitehousedrugpolicy.gov
Substance Abuse and Mental Health Services Administration
www.samhsa.gov
National Institute on Drug Abuse www.nida.nih.gov

Authors: Matthew C. Scheider (Office of Community Oriented Policing Services), Michael S. Scott (Center for Problem-Oriented Policing, Inc.), Tom McEwen (Institute for Law and Justice), Craig D. Uchida (21st Century Solutions), Thomas C. Castellano, Edmund McGarrell, Stacy L. Osnick, Susan Pennell, Carol A. Putnam, and Kip Schlegel (Project Staff) 2002.

From *COPS Innovations*, March 29, 2003, pp. 1-13. © 2003 by COPS Innovations.

About Face Program Turns Lives Around

By Mary Baldwin Kennedy

The About Face Program, operated by the Orleans Parish Criminal Sheriff's Office in New Orleans, provides an innovative approach toward helping the region's male inmates learn how to redirect their lives. Sheriff Charles C. Foti Jr. developed the program in 1986 as the nation's first regimented life-changing program operated at the parish/county level. "Although initially intrigued by the boot camp concept, we soon realized that to have a permanent impact on an individual, we would have to provide more than just short-term discipline," he explains. "As the name implies, the About Face Program seeks to turn lives around completely." Today, with more than 500 inmates in its various phases, the About Face Program has become one of the largest jail-based therapeutic communities in the country.

During the past 10 years, the program has changed to better meet the needs of its participants. At its inception, the About Face Program was primarily a boot camp designed to last six months. However, with the addition of a drug treatment component in the early 1990s, the term has been extended to nine to 12 months or longer, depending on the length of an inmate's sentence. Between 1996 and 2002, more than 2,500 inmates completed the program.

Currently, the About Face Program consists of three basic segments, each 12 weeks in length. A new class begins every 45 days. The initial phase operates within a strict boot camp environment that places heavy emphasis on self-discipline, responsibility for one's actions, education and some physical activity. All inmates are tested at entry to determine their educational level, the average of which for both reading and mathematics is fifth grade. Classes are divided into three levels: literacy (below the sixth-grade level), adult basic education or intermediate, and the GED preparation class (above the ninth-grade level). The goal for each inmate is that he attain his GED. While this is not realistic for some, in 2000, one out of every four GEDs earned in New Orleans was by a participant in this jail system. The figures for 2001 are consistent with those of 2000.

The second and third phases of the program operate according to a modified therapeutic community modality of substance abuse treatment. During these phases, individuals learn about addictions of all forms and are encouraged to confront the behaviors that led to their criminal activity. They are taught that alternatives exist and are urged to use these when faced with problematic situations that could lead them back into destructive behaviors. Emphasis on education, self-discipline and some physical activity continues, and a work skills component is added when inmates approach the end of their sentence. After completion of the body of the program (the first three segments), inmates may first move to the re-entry phase, in which emphasis is on honing skills necessary for successful re-entry into society while maintaining the basic structure of the program. At the end of their incarceration, inmates may be eligible to move to a work tier in which they are taught a skill they can use to attain gainful employment such as various food service jobs, auto mechanics and body repair, horticulture, and electrical and plumbing repair. Inmates, however, must continue to work in their program and attend GED classes, if applicable.

Some of the men housed on the work tier are eligible for enrollment in a program sponsored by a local industrialist that attempts to train inmates about to be released in construction, home building/repair and related carpentry skills. These men go through an intensive training program, both in the classroom and on the job, and are guaranteed job placement in a related field after their release. The participants, with the direction and aid of professionals, have built new homes for low-income families in the New Orleans area. This program, which is supported by a grant from Louisiana, has been recognized as a model for its use of inmate skills in the redevelopment of housing in blighted areas.

Networks have been established in the community to ease offenders' transition back into life outside of the jail setting.

Networks have been established in the community to ease offenders' transition back into life outside of the jail setting. For some inmates with little or no support network, placement in a halfway house is recommended. Graduates are encouraged to return to the nightly group meetings held at the jail to continue their own recovery and give back to the therapeutic community their successes and struggles in remaining drug-free as they re-enter society.

In addition, the About Face Program also provides an aftercare program for its graduates in which they attend weekly drug and/or alcohol treatment meetings with a member of the counseling staff at a facility not affiliated with the jail system. This group has grown dramatically, and it is currently seeking a new home for its meetings as its numbers far exceed the space provided. Finally, the counseling staff welcome calls for assistance from graduates who have been released, and they are eager to provide whatever support is needed. "This long-term approach is what sets the About Face Program apart and makes it successful," Foti says.

Acceptance Process

Admission to the About Face Program begins with a referral. Judges may recommend that an individual be placed in the program at sentencing, inmates may self-refer at any time after conviction, family members or attorneys can request that an individual be evaluated or the jail administration may place an inmate in the program. Inmates are never removed from the program for misbehavior. After admission, there is a strict code of conduct to which inmates must adhere. Failure to comply with the rules in any phase of the program will result in immediate disciplinary action but will not be accepted as a mechanism to allow the inmate to avoid the rigors of the program. Both positive and negative reinforcement, when appropriate, are used to ensure that each individual receives everything the program has to offer. In certain cases, successful completion by offenders sentenced by the court may prompt the judge to re-evaluate and amend their sentence. The parole board also recognizes the value of this training for the inmates who come before it and often bases its decision for early release upon the inmate's successful program completion.

Upon referral, potential participants must meet certain screening criteria, the most important of which is a review of their criminal record for violent offenses. Charges or convictions for arson, kidnapping, armed robbery (more than one charge), sex offenses of any kind, homicide, escape, crimes against juveniles or any other charge that places the individual in a high-security category make applicants ineligible. In addition, applicants cannot have any out-of-parish or out-of-state warrants, or open state charges.

Most participants enter the program shortly after they are sentenced. Sentence length should allow for completion of the three main phases of the program, but not be so long that inmates grow frustrated with the daily routine of meetings and group sessions. However, individual attention is given by counseling staff to individuals who will be released from jail prior to the end of the third phase, but who actively seek the help. Inmates will stay in the About Face Program until they are released from custody, as a return to general population could cause them to revert and lose the focus developed during the course of their participation.

Following a criminal history review, potential participants are screened for any medical conditions that might preclude their being able to successfully complete the physical aspects of the program. An effort will be made by program staff to work with individuals who have limitations, but who are motivated and willing to make the effort necessary for completion. The primary focus of this program is in behavior modification for the individuals, not their physical fitness.

There are no age restrictions in the About Face Program, and it is the staff's belief that a cross-section of ages and backgrounds is preferable because it better-replicates free society. One About Face cohort of note had a 16-year-old (the age of majority in Louisiana is 17) who had been "waived up" and tried as an adult, as well as a 63-year-old. When young and old inmates go through the process together, they are generally better-equipped to deal with age-related issues after their release.

Core Curriculum

There is a strict code of discipline as well as many demands—mental, physical, intellectual and spiritual—made on the participants. After graduation from the boot camp phase, inmates move into the first of two drug treatment phases. Although some inmates have never used drugs or alcohol, they are addicted to the money that the sale of these substances provides; this addiction is just as powerful. In the first phase, the orientation, inmates learn to live in a therapeutic community setting and accept the responsibility placed on them for "their brothers'" recovery, as well as their own. The group, now known as the "family," moves through the program as a unit, much like the cohort effect seen in educational systems. There is a special language composed of terms such as learning experience, push up and pull up, which is used during group meetings and during the course of daily living in the therapeutic community. This modality emphasizes that the "family" must adopt a new set of standards to live by 24 hours a day, not just during group meetings. Using the tenets of Alcoholics Anonymous, Narcotics Anonymous and Cocaine Anonymous, intensive work is conducted on the effects of drug and alcohol use on the body, mind, spirit and community.

After completion of this phase, inmates move to the second drug treatment phase—main treatment—in which they work on their own personal addictions using the 12 steps of AA as their guide. All participants are required to change and to grow. Some, however, will be reluctant to take the risks and face the rigorous discipline and self-examination essential to this process—they will require more time and attention. Graduation from one phase to the next is not guaranteed, but must be earned based on successful completion of core curriculum in that phase.

While there is no structured input from the inmates' friends and families, they are encouraged to be supportive of the inmates' progress and be sympathetic to the pain they must endure to address their particular problems and situations and to make an honest commitment to change. The inmates are told that to be successful, they must change "their people, places and things"; families and other members of their support group have to work with them to make this possible.

In 2001, a female component was added that attempts to mirror the basic concepts of the male program. Because females represent less than 10 percent of the inmate population (rated capacity of 7,250 inmates), the actual structure of the female program had to be modified. Emphasis is placed on parenting and family management skills, preparation for work training, GED education, self-discipline, behavior modification and drug education/treatment. Group and individual counseling replaces the therapeutic community approach employed with the men.

Summary

With more than 500 inmates in the various phases, the About Face Program has become one of the largest jail-based therapeutic communities in the country. Its success can be attributed to the sheriff's foresight and his eagerness to have this program grow with the needs of his department and the community as a whole.

Last summer, a graduate of the program called and left the following message: "This is H. C. I was an inmate in the About Face Program about a year ago.... I was in the boot camp program. I want to thank you for allowing me to enter your program. It has changed my life a lot and I'm doing just fine. Tell Mr. M and the counselors that I say thank you.... God bless you and have a nice day, and remember—one day at a time. Peace."

In the 17 years since its inception, more than 2,500 men and 11 women have completed the About Face Program. It has shown them that they have options and choices in the lifestyles they choose. Some of them avail themselves of the options they have been shown in the About Face Program and many are successful in turning their lives around. A formal study of the program's recidivism rate is difficult due to problems with developing a control group to compare with its graduates. However, an informal study completed in the late 1990s showed that less than 10 percent of the program's participants returned to jail within the first six months after their release. For more information about this program, contact the Orleans Parish Criminal Sheriff's Office, 2800 Gravier St., New Orleans, LA 70119; (504) 827-8501; or visit www.opcso.org.

Mary Baldwin Kennedy is director of the About Face Program at the Orleans Parish Criminal Sheriff's Office in New Orleans.

Congress Stiffens Requirements For Drug Treatment In Prisons And Jails

Congress approved a revision of the drug grant program for prisons by stiffening requirements and mandating inmates must be drug-free before release.

The new program in HR 2215 replaces the incentive grants of the 1994 Omnibus Crime Act with "bonus" grants and would be effective through fiscal 2004.

To qualify for drug care funding, correctional facilities must have a certified treatment program that continually monitors inmates and assures they are drug-free at completion.

Adult and juvenile facilities are eligible to compete for bonus grants provided they have established within 18 months after application a drug-free program or policy.

The policy would require:

- Zero-tolerance for drug use or presence, random and routine sweeps and inspections for drugs, random and routine drug tests of inmates, and improved screening for drugs and other contraband of prison visitors and prisoner mail;
- Establishment and enforcement of penalties, including prison disciplinary actions and criminal prosecution for the introduction, possession, or use of drugs in any prison or jail;
- Implementation of residential drug treatment programs that are effective and science-based; and

- Drug testing of inmates upon intake and upon release from incarceration as appropriate; and incentives for prisoners to participate in drug treatment and drug-free wings with greater privileges.

The bill, which went to the White House for enactment, sets up a separate program for jails. To be eligible for bonus grants, the jail would have to offer three months of substance treatment for nonviolent adult and juvenile offenders as well as after-care.

Local jails would be eligible for 10 percent of any grants made to a state. All states that qualify would be eligible for at least 0.75 percent of the total nationwide appropriation. The amount will be set in separate legislation since the bill is only an authorization for funding.

Congress would give preference to local jails that offer after-care to assure that the offender remains in treatment and drug-free following release.

The jail could cooperate with human service and rehabilitation organizations in implementing after-care. Eligible partners would include educational and job training programs, parole boards, halfway houses, self-help and peer groups.

The drug treatment provisions are contained in the 21st Century Justice Department Appropriations Authorization Act, the first overhaul of justice programs in three decades. The measure

provides $3.5 billion in new annual funding through fiscal 2007.

BILL EXPANDS POWERS OF DRUG PROSECUTORS

Congress in the 21st Century Justice Department Act gave new powers to state and local prosecutors dealing with substance abuse crimes.

The reform bill, HR 2215, expands the role of drug courts and sets up a new pilot program to award grants for treatment as an alternative to incarceration for offenders.

The pilot grants for fiscal 2003 and 2004 could be used for developing, implementing or expanding drug treatment alternatives.

The reform measure also calls for a study of the effectiveness of drug courts to determine whether Congress should expand grants for a specialized judiciary.

The program for prosecutors would provide federal funds for up to 75 percent of the cost of operating a program.

The measure gives prosecutors complete discretion as to the participants, but requires the prosecutors to have a monitoring system in place and mandates imprisonment for participants that violate the conditions of treatment.

The prison alternative program also allows jails and prisons to compete for grants to support rehabilitation of drug abusers. Funds could be used during an offender's incarceration and for continuing the program after release.

The measure bars participants that have been convicted of felonies or drug trafficking.

JUVENILES WILL FACE GRADUATED SANCTIONS

Congress has approved an overhaul of juvenile justice that repeals some grants, mandates graduated sanctions, and creates a new class of prosecutors to pursue gun crimes and grants for juvenile facilities in adult prisons.

The Juvenile Justice and Delinquency Prevention Act (JJDPA), HR 2215, reauthorizes block grants to states and assures funding programs through fiscal 2007.

One program under Truth-in-Sentencing would provide funding for states and localities to create separate prison facilities for juveniles convicted as adults.

The sanctions provisions, known as the Consequences for Juvenile Offenders Act, provides $350 million in annual grants through fiscal 2004 for states and localities that adopt escalating penalties laws.

The bill also authorizes 94 new assistant U.S. attorneys under Project Safe Neighborhoods to assist in targeting juveniles who obtain weapons and commit violent crimes, as well as the adults who place firearms in the hands of juveniles.

The juvenile provisions are part of the 21st Century Justice Department Appropriations Authorization Act that provides $3.5 billion in new annual funding through fiscal 2007. The bill strengthens protection for girls and women but leaves funding for School Resource Officers to the discretion of the attorney general.

The bill, when acted, would repeal six programs in the 1994 law—national programs, gangs, state challenge activities,

juvenile offenders who are victims of child abuse, mentoring and boot camps.

There is a new grant program, Part E, for prevention initiatives.

JJDPA REFORM BILL HIGHLIGHTS

- Create 94 assistant U.S. attorneys to prosecute gun crimes involving juveniles under Project Safe Neighborhoods.
- Award grants to states to establish separate facilities for youths convicted as adults and serving time in adult jails.
- Reauthorize Juvenile Justice Block Grants.
- Reauthorize youth grants for tribal organizations.
- $350 million in grants for states and localities that adopt graduated sanctions that increase penalties for subsequent offenses.
- Repeal six grant programs from the 1994 Crime Control Act.

From *Corrections Digest*, October 18, 2002, pp. 1-2. © 2002 by Corrections Digest.

As Drug Use Drops in Big Cities, Small Towns Confront Upsurge

By Fox Butterfield

The trophy houses, with wrought-iron gates and grand-columned entryways, keep popping up on little country roads here, in clearings in the piney woods and near doublewide trailers. Sometimes there is a Mercedes or two in the driveway.

In the affluent suburbs of Boston, New York or Dallas, these fake chateaus might belong to successful doctors, lawyers or software company owners. But Prentiss, a small town in south-central Mississippi, has no industry or affluent professional class in the conventional sense. The last sizable factory moved to Mexico three years ago, leaving an unemployment rate of 25 percent.

Instead, the police say, many of these houses belong to drug dealers, made rich by a flourishing business in crack, methamphetamine, marijuana and OxyContin, the prescription painkiller. They are the most visible manifestation of an explosion of rural drugs and crime that is overwhelming local law enforcement agencies and bringing the sort of violence normally associated with poor neighborhoods of big cities.

The upsurge has been felt across the nation, from Maine to Oregon and from Georgia to Texas, even as drug use in most cities has been declining.

In December, for example, Ron Jones, one of five members of the Prentiss Police Department and the son of the police chief, was shot to death as he entered an apartment to serve a search warrant for drugs.

It was the most recent of 14 homicides in the last two years in Jefferson Davis County, which has 14,000 residents, giving the county a homicide rate of 50 per 100,000.

That is higher than the rates of Detroit, Washington or New Orleans, cities that regularly have the highest homicide rates in the nation.

Nationwide, while the rate of arrests in drug crimes has fallen 11.2 percent in cities with more than 250,000 residents over the last five years, it has risen 10.5 percent in rural areas, according to the Federal Bureau of Investigation.

Even more striking, from 1990 to 1999, the last year for which figures are available, the percentage of drug-related homicides tripled in rural areas but fell by almost half in big cities.

To measure the problem another way, a continuing survey of drug use among junior high and high school students by the University of Michigan has found that crack is now more widely used among 8th, 10th and 12th graders in rural areas than among those in metropolitan areas. Methamphetamine use is now highest in rural areas among all three grades and heroin use is about equal in urban and rural areas, the survey found.

The spread of drugs in the countryside is uneven, the experts say, with heavy concentrations of certain drugs in some counties.

In Washington County, for instance, at the far northeastern corner of Maine, prosecutions in crimes involving OxyContin are 10 times what they were in 1998, say law enforcement officials, who estimate that at least 1,000 of the county's 35,000 residents are addicts.

"It's gone beyond the epidemic stage," Sheriff Joe Tibbetts said. "I can't think of a family in Washington County that hasn't been scathed by it in some way."

His officers' families are among those who have been affected, Sheriff Tibbetts said.

In Dawson County in western Nebraska, the problem is methamphetamine. "The percentage of meth-related crimes is through the roof," said Paul Schwarz, an investigator with the county sheriff's office. He repeated two local sayings: "You're either stealing or dealing" and "If you're not using, you're a cop."

In the state as a whole, officials discovered 38 methamphetamine laboratories in 1999; last year they discovered 179.

"If there is a battle going on out there," Mr. Schwarz said, "we're honestly not winning it."

Similarly, in Douglas County, a vast timber, farming and fishing area in southwestern Oregon, Lt. Mike Nores of the sheriff's department estimates that 12 percent to 14 percent of the 103,000 residents are making, selling or using drugs, particularly methamphetamine and marijuana. Drug use and trafficking now account for 80 percent of all crime in the county, including killings, Lieutenant Nores said.

One reason for the growth in rural drug problems, federal officials say, is that aggressive prosecution in cities has led dealers to seek safety in the farms and forests of rural counties, which have far fewer law enforcement officers.

"We've seen drugs and crime migrate to the rural areas in the past several years to get away from law enforcement," said Tony Soto, director of the Gulf Coast High Intensity Drug Trafficking Area in New Orleans, a task force of federal, state and local law enforcement authorities established by the White House Office of Drug Policy Control. "It's happening all around the United States, as the dealers and gangs go deeper into rural areas."

In Jefferson Davis County in Mississippi, Sheriff Henry McCullum said: "It's gotten so bad, drugs have become our major industry. Almost every person living in this community is profiting from the escalating drugs, directly or indirectly."

Drug money, Sheriff McCullum explained, is helping contractors, building supply stores and grocery stores stay in business.

By his estimate about half the young men in the county have been to prison by the time they reach the age of 21, with almost all their crimes related to drugs.

Even Sheriff McCullum's brother-in-law, Billy Ray Barnes, is in the sheriff's jail, charged with robbing a bank to get money for crack. In an interview in the sheriff's office, Mr. Barnes, 34, said it would take him only five minutes after walking out of jail to find more crack.

"It's everywhere," he said. "The county is infested."

To spend a day with the sheriff is to hear the toll drugs are taking in Jefferson Davis County. A high school teacher calls, warning that drug-dealing students are threatening to shoot each other in a classroom. An elderly woman reports that a drug dealer is coming to her home to shoot her crack-addicted son.

Sheriff McCullum takes these calls seriously. Last year a 13-year-old, Brendan McCullum (no relation to the sheriff), was fatally shot as he stood inside his house when a drug dealer drove by looking for Brendan's older brother, with whom the dealer had had a quarrel.

"Brendan was a good boy, an honor roll student, a kid who went to Sunday school," said his older sister, Ressie Davis. At the time of the shooting, Ms. Davis was in state prison for shoplifting, something she admitted doing to support her crack addiction. She was later released but is now back in the local jail for not reporting to her parole officer.

As bad as the drug problem is here, "It is pretty typical for all of rural Mississippi," said Charlie Brown Jr., the assistant special agent in charge of Mississippi for the Drug Enforcement Administration.

"You've got counties where there are no jobs and the income is below poverty level, so you have groups trafficking in drugs who take advantage of that, and you have local sheriffs and small-town police chiefs who have very limited resources," Mr. Brown said. "Everybody in the community knows who is dealing, but because of their limited manpower, there is very little law enforcement can do."

Experts in rural crime agree that the reasons Mr. Brown cited are some of the basic causes of the growth in rural drug use and crime.

"You have many rural areas that are persistent poverty areas, in essence rural ghettos," said Joseph Donnermeyer, professor of rural sociology at Ohio State University. "They were once isolated and were protected by that, with lower crime, but now better communications have broken down that buffer so they begin to resemble poor neighborhoods of big cities, where people are segregated by poverty."

Asa Hutchinson, the administrator of the Drug Enforcement Administration and a former federal prosecutor and congressman from Arkansas, said the movement of drug dealers to rural areas was "absolutely something I am aware of."

Mr. Hutchinson said the problem was difficult to combat because of a gap in law enforcement. Federal drug prosecutions have tended to focus on the largest dealers, usually in cities, and county sheriffs and small-town police forces lack the manpower or experience to combat them.

One other theory was offered by Henry Donaldson, Brendan McCullum's stepfather. Mr. Donaldson attributes the spread of drugs in part to the number of young people who have moved to Mississippi from Chicago, many of them sent by parents, originally from the state, to escape the urban drug problems.

The lack of law enforcement resources is glaring in Jefferson Davis County. Sheriff McCullum has five deputies to patrol a county of almost 600 square miles. In practice, this means that he normally has only one deputy on duty at a time. The budget of Sheriff McCullum's office is so meager that when he was elected two years ago, he did not have a fingerprint kit, a camera to photograph suspects or a video camera. Nor do his deputies have bulletproof vests or computer terminals for their patrol cars, which are common in big-city police cruisers to call up information on suspects.

"How are we going to do an undercover operation?" Sheriff McCullum asked. "We can't. Everybody here knows everybody else. Besides, we don't have the money to make a buy."

Three men awaiting trial for murder in Jefferson Davis County recently escaped from the county jail.

On a drive around the county's back roads, the sheriff pointed to new house after new house, some with mansard roofs, some with Palladian windows, that he said were built with drug profits. Some dealers, Sheriff McCullum said, truck drugs from El Paso on the Mexican border to the county, hiding the drug-loaded trucks in barns before selling the narcotics to other dealers.

The sheriff pointed to one house, a new gray stone structure with twin brick gates, a high black wrought-iron fence and security cameras. It belongs to Glenn Russell, Sheriff McCullum said, adding that Mr. Russell is awaiting trial on federal drug charges after being arrested in Texas with $150,000 worth of drugs.

It may be impossible to compare the ravages of the new wave of rural drugs with the crack epidemic in big cities in the late 1980's and early 1990's. But experts say the small populations of rural counties often magnify the impact, making it more personal.

On Dec. 26, in Prentiss, Officer Ron Jones, 29, called his father, Ronald N. Jones, the police chief, for permission to get a search warrant for an apartment where an informer had told him there was crack. An hour later, as Officer Jones led a team into the apartment, he was shot in the abdomen. The suspect in the shooting, Cory Maye, has been charged with capital murder.

"The hardest thing for me is that I'm the one who gave him the approval," Chief Jones said.

His son had been taking classes in drug enforcement and was the town's K-9 officer.

"He thought he could clean Prentiss up," Chief Jones said. "He honestly gave his life trying to make a difference."

UNIT 6

Measuring the Social Cost of Drugs

Unit Selections

Key Points to Consider

• What do you believe to be the greatest drug-related threat facing our nation? Explain.

• How do drug-related threats and impacts differ from city to city and state to state? Why?

• It is often argued that Americans overreact and overemphasize the harm from illegal drugs while ignoring or underrepresenting the harm from legal drugs, namely alcohol and nicotine. Do you agree or disagree with this argument, and why?

• Has there been a significant shift in public concern over the abuse of legal drugs? Support your answer.

• Explain whether or not the harmful impacts from the abuse of drugs are greater today than they were a decade ago.

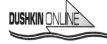 **Links: www.dushkin.com/online/**
These sites are annotated in the World Wide Web pages.

DrugText
http://www.drugtext.org

The National Organization on Fetal Alcohol Syndrome (NOFAS)
http://www.nofas.org

National NORML Homepage
http://www.norml.org/

The most devastating effect of drug use in America is the magnitude with which it affects the way we live. Much of its influence is not measurable. What is the cost of a son or daughter lost, a parent imprisoned, a life lived in a constant state of fear? The emotional costs alone are incomprehensible.

The social legacy of this country's drug crisis could easily be the subject of this entire book. The purpose here, however, can only be a cursory portrayal of drugs' tremendous costs. More than one American president has stated that drug use threatens our national security and personal well-being. The financial costs of maintaining the federal apparatus devoted to drug interdiction, enforcement, and treatment are staggering. Although yearly expenditures vary due to changes in political influence, strategy, and tactics, examples of the tremendous effects of drugs on government and the economy abound. The federal budget for drug control exceeds $11.7 billion and includes more than $731 million for the Andean Counter Drug initiative and $141 million for Colombia alone. The Department of Justice commits more than $2.5 billion to antidrug efforts, the Department of Health and Human Services over $3.5 billion, the Department of Defense almost $1 billion, and the Department of Homeland Security over $2 billion. More than $20 million is committed to state and local authorities to clean up toxic methamphetamine labs. Drugs are the business of the criminal justice system. The United States incarcerates more of its citizens than almost any other nation, and the financial costs are staggering. Doing drugs and serving time produce an inescapable nexus, and it does not end with prison. More than 36 percent of adults on parole or supervised release are classified with dependence on or abuse of a substance. Some argue that these numbers represent that Americans have come to rely on the criminal justice system as an unprecedented way of responding to social problems. Regardless of the way one chooses to view various relationships, the resulting picture is numbing.

In addition to the highly visible criminal justice–related costs, numerous other institutions are affected. Housing, welfare, education, and health care provide excellent examples of critical institutions struggling to overcome the strain of drug-related impacts. In addition, annual loss of productivity in the workplace exceeds well over $160 billion per year. Alcoholism alone causes 500 million lost workdays each year. Add to this demographic shifts caused by people fleeing drug-impacted neighborhoods, schools, and businesses, and one soon realizes that there is no victimless public or private institution. Last year, 3.5 million Americans (1.5 percent of the population) received some kind of treatment related to the abuse of alcohol or other drugs. The number of persons needing treatment for an illicit drug problem was 7.7 million, and the number of persons needing treatment for alcohol abuse was 18.6 million. Add 60,000 infants born each year who suffer irreversible forms of fetal alcohol syndrome, and no amount of debating, arguing, or denying the specific cause-and-effect relationships really amounts to much in the face of reality. Add injured, drug-related accident and crime victims, along with demands produced by a growing population of intravenous-drug users infected with AIDS, and a failing health care system frighteningly appears. A universally afford-

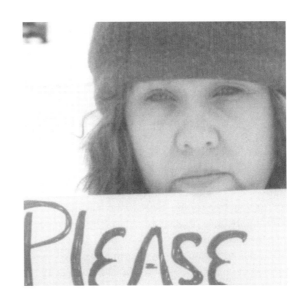

able health care plan capable of addressing drug-related impacts of such vast medical consequences may not be possible. Health care costs from drug-related ills are overwhelming. Drugs cost the economy $13 billion in health care costs alone.

It should be emphasized that the social costs exacted by drug use infiltrate every aspect of public and private life. The implications for thousands of families struggling with the adverse effects of drug-related woes may prove the greatest and most tragic of social costs. Children who lack emotional support, self-esteem, role models, a safe and secure environment, economic opportunity, and an education because of a parent on drugs suggest costs difficult to comprehend.

As you read the following articles, consider the costs associated with legal and illegal drugs. However, before joining the debate on which is the greater harbinger of pain and suffering, consider the diversity of impacts to which legal and illegal drugs contribute. Combining pharmacological, environmental, legal, and the multitude of other factors influencing drug-related impacts with cause-and-effect propositions soon produces a quagmire of major proportions. Although it is tempting to generalize while considering and lamenting the impacts of drug use on our society, it seldom produces the most salient observations. An incremental approach to assessing drug-related impacts and costs may produce a greater understanding of how to measure social costs than an attempt to make a case for a combination of impacts generated because of issues such as the legal status of a drug.

Lastly, as you read and think about the different articles in this unit, keep in mind the pervasiveness of drug-related impacts affecting American families. Subsequent reflection reveals that we do not just "change schools," "move to a different town," or flee drug-related issues, and that the most critical component of defense against drug ills, the family, is the most mercilessly pursued target. Most people recognize that the world's most powerful institutions merely buy time in hopes that family institutions will come together, endure, and prevail against drugs.

Beware the dark side of pharmacy life

One for you, two for me. Selfish, but harmless child's play, right? Wrong. It's one of many ruses used by pharmacists when they dispense drugs in order to satisfy their drug addiction.

While drug addiction among pharmacists is certainly not a new phenomenon, experts report that the number of pharmacists in treatment has increased. Why are R.Ph.s turning to drugs? Which drugs are they abusing? What are the telltale signs of addiction? What rehabilitation programs are available to help impaired pharmacists recover and return to work?

Dave Marley, Pharm.D., RAS (registered addiction specialist), executive director of the North Carolina Pharmacist Recovery Network Inc., Winston-Salem, said that the program has treated 135 pharmacists for addiction since 1995. "Our case load has consistently increased—from five in '95 to 25 in '98 to 30 a year since 2001," said Marley.

Tim Benedict, R.Ph., assistant executive director, Ohio State Board of Pharmacy, has seen a surge in the past 10 years in the number of R.Ph.s in Ohio who have drug addiction problems. "I spent the early '80s in the field and investigated six or seven pharmacists with addiction problems," he said. In 1986, when he became compliance and enforcement administrator for the board, he investigated a couple of cases a year.

"We now investigate 20 to 30 pharmacists a year in Ohio for drug addiction problems, and that doesn't include drug trafficking and doesn't count technicians," said Benedict. "We're doing at least as many cases with techs in the past few years as we are with pharmacists. Some of the technicians are addicted, but most are stealing for resale in the streets."

Merrill Norton, R.Ph., NCAC-II (Nationally Certified Addictions Counselor), CCS (Certified Clinical Supervisor), is director of the Recovering Pharmacists Program at the Talbott Recovery Campus, a private facility in Atlanta. "We have treated close to 1,000 pharmacists since 1974 when the program began," he said. "The numbers have increased drastically, and the demographics are changing. Now we're seeing younger males. That has to do with some early interventions by states with pharmacist recovery networks."

Norton pointed out that the average pharmacist the facility treats has severe problems and has been to treatment two or three times. "We see patients who have been to treatment sev-

eral times and have not done well. Most pharmacists stay 16 to 17 weeks. Now 55% of those pharmacists on initial discharge will be put on some type of psychotropic medication for depression, anxiety, or personality disorder," he said.

Norton is concerned that there may be female R.Ph.s who need treatment for drug addiction. "About 55% of the pharmacy graduates are women. We're seeing only a small percentage of those women in treatment. I see 95% men and 5% women. I think there are more women out there in need of treatment," he said.

Norton explained that women who receive treatment at Talbott have more complicated personal issues to deal with than men, including childhood traumas and being involved in abusive relationships. They may also have a strong genetic history for depression, anxiety, or addiction.

Why is the number of pharmacists needing treatment on an upward trajectory? Increased stress in the workplace is largely to blame. "A lot of them are not happy with the profession because it never met their professional expectations," said Norton. "Many had expectations of becoming doctors and did not meet that goal. Even though pharmacy can be a wonderful career, most pharmacists end up doing work a tech can do." On top of all that, he said, the average pharmacist he sees works more than 60 hours a week.

The confines of the workplace also contribute to increased stress. "The average pharmacist works in an area that's about 12 ft. by 60 ft. They are locked in there; they can't eat; they can't use the restroom as necessary—they have to cheat their employer in order to take a break," said Norton.

Another culprit is the physical strain of the job, which requires R.Ph.s to be on their feet most of the day. Many pharmacists develop hip, back, and leg problems, and, because drugs are so accessible, they begin to self-medicate their pains.

Marley provided a scenario to illustrate how increased stress and the physical demands of the job lead R.Ph.s to self-medicate and eventually develop drug dependency: "Ten years ago, a pharmacist filled 100 Rxs a day. He has a bad back and can't get relief help. All day, he dispenses Vicodin and ibuprofen. He thinks, 'I'll take a couple of these to get through the day.' He does, and the back pain goes away.

Telltale signs of drug abuse

- Changes in physical appearance, including weight loss and poor physical hygiene
- Sweatiness, irritability, forgetfulness, tardiness
- Mood swings throughout the day
- Bathroom breaks, after which mood is elevated
- Ocular changes (e.g., pinpoint-size pupils); shakiness; tremors; and, in some cases, seizures caused by drug withdrawals; speech problems (e.g., slurred speech, inability to concentrate or carry on a conversation)
- Avoidance of counseling patients because of inability to offer explanations
- Frequent absences without any notice
- Willingness to work extra shifts, weekends, and holidays and showing up on days off to seek an opportunity to steal drugs; returning after the pharmacy closes for a wallet or house keys that were intentionally left behind in case of questioning
- Giving up lunchtime so that others in the pharmacy can lunch together, leaving the abuser alone to take drugs
- Patient complaints about being shorted quantity of drug dispensed; increasing complaints from patients or co-workers as to a person's attitude
- Always volunteering to check-in orders or check controlled substances
- Adjusting perpetual inventories to reflect lost Rxs and thus cover up for stolen drugs
- Ordering items that are not needed

"Move forward 10 years," Marley continued. "That R.Ph. is filling 500 Rxs a day, with the same bad back and even more stress. A couple of Vicodins help the back pain and the stress of phones ringing, the people giving you looks, and the manager complaining about your fill rates. Tomorrow, his back might not hurt, but he remembers the stress was less when he took the pills. In 13 years of doing this work, I never met a pharmacist who set out to be a drug addict. It's just one of those things that happen."

Yet another reason pharmacists succumb to addiction is many of them believe that because they are knowledgeable about drugs, they are immune from harm. "We hear this from everybody, 'I'm a pharmacist. I know how the drugs work. I can control them.' Garbage. They are the same as everybody else. They cannot control the drugs," insisted Benedict.

Acknowledging that genetics and predisposition to addiction are strong factors in determining whether a person will develop an addiction problem, Marley said each person has his own individual addiction threshold. "A lot of people use and abuse drugs, but they don't get into compulsive use because their genetic risk or environmental stress was low enough and use of drugs was small enough that they didn't cross that line," he said.

Pharmacy schools to blame?

Many pharmacists' addiction problems can be traced back to heavy partying in school. "Some started taking narcotics during internships," said Marley. "The schools know this is going on, but no one has ever gotten serious about addressing it."

Marley believes schools should enforce alcohol laws and keep parties out of dorms, fraternities, and sororities. "We need to remind the administration there aren't any stupid people in pharmacy school. If their grades are going into the toilet, the administration needs to look at what's going on," he said.

Which drugs are being abused?

Hydrocodone and derivatives such as oxycodone top the list of impaired pharmacists' favorites, according to Norton. He has also seen abuse of Valium, Xanax, and Ativan. "Hydrocodone is a class III. It is the one that is the most abused. It's available in 25 different forms on the shelf. It would be hard for someone to come in and do an audit. Generically, you have multiples, so it can be hidden. It's ordered a lot and used a lot," he said.

"When hydrocodone was introduced, it exploded. About 70% of pharmacists I treat are abusing hydrocodone," echoed Marley.

Norton is beginning to see OxyContin (oxycodone, Purdue Pharma) being abused by pharmacists. He explained that 18 to 24 months after a drug is introduced, he usually begins to see pharmacists abusing it. "I anticipate this year I will see more abuse of OxyContin. We've had some folks come in here using 1,600 to 1,800 mg of OxyContin a day," he revealed.

Benedict agreed that oxycodone and hydrocodone are among the most commonly diverted drugs. Diazepam, alprazolam, and phentermine are also on his list. Emphasizing that addicts are looking for drugs that provide quick onset, a good high, and quick elimination from their body, he noted, "Diazepam doesn't fit that description, yet it's been abused for so long. They usually start out with the opiates and the benzodiazepines, but they move on to other things."

The average R.Ph. Benedict investigates is taking 30 pills a day and may be abusing one or more products. "That's more than 7,000 doses diverted in one year," he said. "The average pharmacist we see has been diverting drugs for two to 14 years. Many of them go for a long time just abusing the drugs, not becoming addicted—then something happens in their life, and they go crazy."

Do pharmacists realize how many pills they are abusing? "I've never seen one person in 22 years accurately estimate how much they are taking. They will downplay the quantity, and it's usually about a third of what they are taking," Benedict said.

Where can R.Ph.s go for help?

Pharmacists are not the only ones who have difficulty acknowledging they have a drug addiction problem. The industry was oblivious to the situation until the early '80s.

Ronald Williams, former leader of the pharmacy section of the University of Utah School on Alcoholism and Other Drug Dependencies and head of the American Pharmaceutical Association's pharmacy recovery network, said that in the early '80s there was no widespread recognition that there was an addiction

Where R.Ph.s can go for help

University of Utah School on Alcoholism and Other Drug Dependencies Pharmacy Section:
Sponsored by the American Pharmaceutical Association and the APhA Academy of Students of Pharmacy (APhA-ASP). For information contact Susan Langston at hsadmin1.slangsto@state.ut.us.

APhA Addiction Practitioner Interest Group:
Has as its mission to foster greater awareness and understanding of addictive disease as a public health issue and to promote treatment and recovery from addictive illnesses through education, advocacy, and peer support. For more information, visit pdelprato@aol.com.

International Pharmacists Anonymous:
Founded in 1987, IPA has 1,060 members. Services include a confidential e-mail list, e-mail updates, and a newsletter that is published three times a year. The organization holds meetings at APhA meetings, hospital pharmacy meetings, and at the Southwest Pharmacist Recovery Network meeting, which is held every fall. This year it will be held in Tucson from Sept. 13 to 15. IPA will also meet at the Heartland PRN in Nebraska, from Oct. 4 to 6, and at the Southeast PRN in Atlanta, Nov. 8 to 10. For more information, contact Mary Jo Cerny at mjc757@atcjet.net or (308) 284-8296, or Brent Clevenger at MSRBCrph@aol.com or call (601) 214-9893.

problem in pharmacy. "Back then, if a pharmacist had a problem and the board found out, he lost his license and that was the end of it. There were no facilities and no recognition of the recovery process," he said.

The pharmacy section of The University of Utah School on Alcoholism and Other Drug Dependencies has been instrumental in improving recognition of the problem as well as helping impaired R.Ph.s. Known as The Utah School, the program is held for a week every June. Attendance has grown from 20 at its inception to 250. Attendees include students, educators, and impaired pharmacists.

The Utah School began as a program for impaired pharmacists that was run by a group of students in Minnesota. Formerly called the Student American Pharmaceutical Association, it is now known as the APhA Academy of Students of Pharmacy. The group was able to influence APhA's house of delegates to pass a policy recognizing that there is an impairment problem in pharmacy and that there should be programs developed at the state level to help people with this problem.

"When the University of Utah saw APhA had adopted a policy, it asked if we wanted to sponsor the pharmacy section at the school," said Williams, who was involved with the Utah School from 1982 until 1998, when he retired. "It was a blessing. Suddenly we had a tool with which to implement this policy that had been adopted." The policy said there should be programs at the state level to identify impaired pharmacists and get them into treatment and back into practice. It also worked with state boards so they would no longer take a punitive approach, but rather recognize rehab and allow pharmacists who go into treatment back into practice at some point.

"The school has absolutely helped so many people, especially early on," continued Williams. People came and asked how they could establish a program in their states. While the number of state pharmacist recovery network programs has grown, treatment experts agree that the key to a successful program hinges on obtaining funding for full-time personnel and a full-time recovery program.

The problem is the majority of state programs operate on a strictly voluntary basis, said Marley. "They get no funding support from the pharmacy board. We've made leaps and bounds educating the profession about the problem." In 1982, he said, they had difficulty convincing people that there even was a problem in the profession. "Now the profession knows there's a problem, but we've not had enough success getting states at the regulatory level to take the next steps and create and fund these programs."

In 1995, when the North Carolina Pharmacist Recovery Network was still a volunteer program, it took six cases. From 1996 to 1997, it handled eight cases. In 1998, the first year it became a full-time funded program, the number of cases increased to 28. "That was a significant jump. We were able to make people aware the program was there and there was a staff person dedicated to running it," said Marley. How did the program get funded? Half of the program's budget comes from license fees, he said, while the other half comes from treatment fees it charges. Out of each license fee, $10 goes to partially fund this program.

The benefits of a fully funded program are evident in the way in which the North Carolina Pharmacist Recovery Network operates. Pharmacists come to the program in three ways. The smallest number of R.Ph.s (25%–30%) who come for treatment are those who were caught by their state pharmacy board or law enforcement. The program assists them through a disciplinary process and provides treatment. The client signs a five-year monitoring contract. The board takes the impaired pharmacists' licenses until the program says they're ready to return to work. "We petition for a hearing and generally get the license reinstated," said Marley.

The most referrals (60% to 65%) come from friends, coworkers, or family members. These pharmacists are not reported to the board as long as they do everything required by the program. This includes an initial assessment, referral to treatment, and a five-year monitoring program that includes drug tests. They must also stay clean for five years. "The board of pharmacy will never know who they are other than by an anonymous case number," explained Marley.

The program offers a way for friends and family to help their loved ones without getting them in trouble. "If they don't do what we tell them, then we tell the board. But many times, they can just come in, do what they're supposed to, and they do very well," said Marley.

Only 15% of the program's referrals are pharmacists who admit they have a problem. "Most people who come in are in profound denial," Marley said. "They are only there because I told them if they didn't get here within 48 hours, I'd call the board. Most come in and have a story to spin. Through training in this field, you learn how to work through that, and we also have a drug test."

The program's philosophy revolves around the 12 steps of Alcoholics Anonymous and Narcotics Anonymous. And although participants are monitored for five years only, it is expected that pharmacists' commitment to the 12-step model will be for life.

"They learn how to deal with life on life's terms, without using drugs," said Marley. "Most of our guys succeed and go back to practice. Of the 135 we've treated, 81% have stayed clean with one treatment experience and had no relapses. Of the remaining 19%, 15% were retreated a second time and went on to do just fine. Only 5% to 6% have difficulty and don't make it back to practice successfully."

Pointing out that with other societal-based drug treatment programs the success rates are generally one in 10, Marley said, "Our success rate is 80% because we do have the leverage to tell them we will notify the board of pharmacy and they'll lose their license."

The Georgia PharmASSIST program is one recovery program that is trying to become funded. In order to accomplish this goal, the Georgia Pharmacy Association and Georgia Pharmacy Foundation created the Southeastern Pharmacy Recovery Network Conference. The conference, held every year in the fall for the past six years, receives grants from pharmaceutical companies through the Georgia Pharmacy Foundation. Profits from attendance fees are used to get the program funded.

The Talbott Recovery Campus, mentioned above, is a private facility that also uses the 12-step program. Treatment consists of family and individual therapy. "Our primary roles here are as family therapists," said Norton. "You can't get the individual better without getting the family better. We have at least two weeks of family programs here."

Pharmacists also participate in physical exercise and a spiritual program. Norton said that the Talbott program has had an 85% success rate, although he said he "rarely" has heard a pharmacist voluntarily check himself in. "A wheel has to fall off, and it's usually a legal wheel," he said.

Benedict had more positive news, "Over the past decade, 80% of the R.Ph.s who went into treatment in Ohio have returned to practice without further problems."

While the issue of drug-addicted pharmacists is being addressed and recovery programs are growing, the problem isn't going to go away by itself. More recovery programs in more states are needed.

As Nan Davis, R.Ph., cofounder of International Pharmacists Anonymous, put it, "I get calls from all parts of the country. It's heartbreaking that they're out there on their own. We need more state programs that really advocate for pharmacists instead of just throwing them to the wolves."

Sandra Levy

Pharmacy Recovery Network state contact roster*

	Contact person for assistance	Contact for information
Alabama	James N. Lloyd MA, LPC (CORIP) UAB-Center for Psychiatric Medicine Phone: (205) 975-8548	Sharon Hester (CORIP) Phone: (205) 995-8043
Alaska	Clint Lillibridge Alaska Practitioner Recovery Program Phone: (907) 276-5517	Tammi Hackley E-mail: Tamhack@aol.com
Arizona	Lisa Yates Pharmacists Assisting Pharmacists of Arizona (PAPA) Phone: (480) 838-3668	
Arkansas	Kim Light - Secretary APSG Arkansas Pharmacy Support Group Phone: (501) 224-7538 E-mail: klight@aristotle.net	Arkansas State Board of Pharmacy Phone: (501) 682-0190 Paul Koesy E-mail: PKOZEE@aol.com
California	Tim Willison Phone: (415) 664-0368 E-mail: yes@sonic.net	Veronica Van Orman E-mail: vvanorman@cpha.com Phone: (800) 444-3851 (ext. 311)
Colorado	Donna Lindsey Peer Assistance Services, Inc. Phone: (303) 369-0039 E-mail: dlindsey@peerasst.org	Elizabeth Pace Phone: (303) 369-0039 E-mail: epace@peerasst.org
Connecticut	Susan G. Gaynor Connecticut Pharmacists Concerned for Pharmacists Phone: (860) 563-4619 E-mail: SusanGCPA@aol.com	
Delaware	Pat Carroll-Grant Phone: (302) 659-3088 E-mail: patsgrants@aol.com	Delaware Pharmacists Society (302) 659-3088
Florida	Raymond M. Pomm, M.D., or Jane Kalem Physicians Recovery Network Phone: (904) 277-8004 E-mail: prn@net-magic.net	
Georgia	Jim Bartling PharmAssist Phone: (404) 231-5074	Mary Meredith E-Mail: mmeredith@gpha.org
Idaho	Steve Streeper Idaho Recovery Assistance Program Phone: (208) 238-1587 E-mail: steve@poky.srv.net	

(continued on next page)

141

	Contact person for assistance	Contact for information
Illinois	Janet Pickett Illinois Professional Health Program Phone: (800) 215-4357 E-mail: Janet.Pickett@ advocatemedical.com	
Indiana	Carl Erdmann Jr. Phone: (317) 899-5915	Carol S. Dunham Phone: (317) 624-4401 E-mail:ipacarol@aol.com
Iowa	Bruce Alexander - Iowa PRN Phone: (319) 338-0581 (ext. 6118) E-mail: bruce.alexander@ med.va.gov	Jennifer Moulton Phone: 1-877-890-IPRN E-mail: jmoulton@iarx.org
Kansas	Dr. Mary Carder Heart of America Professional Network Phone: (913) 236-7575	Jenith Hoover Phone: (785) 228-2327
Kentucky	Brian E. Fingerson Phone: (502) 222-9802 E-mail: Finger@iglou.com	
Louisiana	B.Belaire Bourg Jr. Phone: (225) 752-5909 E-mail: bbourgrx@home.com	
Maryland	Tony Tommasello Phone: (410) 706-7513 E-mail: atommase@ rx.umaryland.edu	PatriciaTommasello E-mail: PEAC@ Bellatlantic.net
Massachusetts	Tim McCarthy Massachusetts Professional Recovery System Phone: (617) 727-2880 E-mail: Tim.F.McCarthy@ state.ma.us	
Michigan	Dan Smith Phone: (616) 891-1788	Michigan Pharmacists Association Phone: (517) 484-1466 E-mail: MAPI@ worldnet.att.net
Minnesota	Jim Alexander Phone: (612) 825-5533 E-mail: JimA.90mn@gateway.net	
Mississippi	Jerry M. Fortenberry Phone: (601) 936-6380	Phone: (601) 932-7117
Missouri	David Jones Phone: (417) 886-4111 E-mail: DaveJPRN@ worldnet.att.net	Phone: (573) HOT-4MPA
Montana	Jim Smith Montana State Pharmaceutical Association Phone: (877) 748-4400 (toll free)	

	Contact person for assistance	Contact for information
Nebraska	Julie Buscher, MHR,CADAC Licensee Assistance Program Phone : (800) 851-2336 or (402) 354-8055	
Nevada	Rhonda Larsen Phone: (702) 732-4638 E-mail: nvphall@lvdi.net	
New Hampshire	Paul Boisseau Phone: (603) 623-1234 E-mail: Peezu@mediaone.net	Rick Fradette Phone: (603) 623-1234 E-mail: JDRPHRICK@ aol.com
New Mexico	Suzie Clark E-mail: suziec2aol.com	Phone: (505) 271-0800 E-mail: mtp@swcp.com
New York	Kenny Balasiano Phone: (845) 897-3675 E-mail: KenB14@aol.com	
North Carolina	David Marley Phone: (336) 774-6555 E-mail: NCPRN@msn.com	
North Dakota	Tim S. Carlson Phone: (701) 838-4669 E-mail: Tcar@earthling.net	
Ohio	Mike Quigley Phone: (419) 531-5486 E-mail: QBCM@aol.com	Charlie Broussard Phone: (513) 398-1173 E-mail: BroussardC@aol.com
Oklahoma	Kevin Rich Phone: (405) 392-3595	Kim Spitz Phone: (405) 528-3338 (ext. 4 or 5) E-mail:Kspitz@opha.com
Oregon	Edwin Schneider Phone: (503) 804-1186 E-mail: ecruisers@ccwebster.net	
Pennsylvania	Robert Rossi Phone : (610) 583-9224	Michael Lenczynski Phone: (610) 583-9884, or (800) 892-4484 E-mail: mikelen@rcn.com
Rhode Island	Robert W. MacDonald Phone: (401) 732-9444	
South Carolina	C. Douglas Chavous Phone: (803) 787-1766	Recovering Professional Program Phone: (803) 737-9133
South Dakota	Mike Coley Phone: (605) 394-6688	
Tennessee	Roger L. Davis Phone: (615) 256-3023 E-mail: rld@tnpharm.org	
Texas	Robert "Bob" Hull Phone: (800) 727-5152 or (512) 836-8350 (ext 132) E-mail: bhull@txpharmacy.com	

(continued on next page)

	Contact person for assistance	Contact for information

Utah	Charles Walton M.D.
	Phone: (801) 530-6106
	E-mail:
	    brcmrc.brdopl.cwalton@
	    email.state.ut.us	

Virginia	Johnny Moore E-mail: JohnnyMoore@msn.com	

Washington	Michaelene Lippert, R.Ph.,
	    CDP
	WRAPP
	(800) 446-7220
	    or (206) 616-2729
	E-mail:
	    mlippert@u.washington.edu
		Ruth Kerschbaum CDC
		E-mail:
		    RuthK@olypen.com

Wisconsin	Scott Whitmore Phone: (608) 827-9200 E-mail: swhitmore@pswi.org	Ernest Witzke Phone: (920) 563-9351

Wyoming	Berton Toews, M.D.
	Phone: (307) 472-1222
		E-mail: WPAP@
		    wyomingrecovery.
		    com

Source: This contact information was compiled by Charlie Broussard, R.Ph. Any additions, deletions, or corrections should be brought to his attention via e-mail at BroussardC@aol.com or by phone at (513) 398-1173.

*There are no known recovery programs in Hawaii, Maine, New Jersey, Vermont, or West Virginia.

Social Science and Public Policy

DRUG ARRESTS AT THE MILLENNIUM

Erich Goode

People of conscience perforce agonize over the growing racial disparities in drug arrests and incarceration in the United States. One is forced to view with alarm the tendency of this nation to become increasingly a carceral society. That this tendency most strikingly characterizes drug offenses and more specifically the drug offenses of African Americans, should be troubling for us all. The drug war is being fought in earnest, we realize, and its enemy, it seems, is the black community.

One first confronts the racial disparities in the War on Drugs with a sense of outrage, a feeling that gross injustice is afoot in its prosecution. One concludes with no less a sense of outrage, but with the feeling that the injustices we observe begin at a much more basic and possibly more intractable level than the racial intent of the architects of the drug war. One also concludes with a sense of wonderment over how *deep*, how *ramifying*, and how *abiding* racial inequities in American society are, and how *ineluctably* they play themselves out in all corners of social life. In short, one shifts one's sense of outrage from the part to the whole.

Much of the drug policy debate centers around whether and to what extent the War on Drugs is racist. The charge can mean many things, of course, but one of its possible meanings is that African Americans are targeted for arrest specifically *because* they are black.

However, unless we find a smoking gun, it's unlikely that we will ever be able to locate direct, overt racist motives in the drug war. What we do have is a number of nearly iron-clad processes that both suggest inadvertence and are intricately intertwined with what used to be called institutional racism—that is, the structural reasons why identical factors and dynamics will produce very different outcomes for whites and blacks. In other words, it is entirely possible that, to the architects of the drug war, racial disparities represent that very ugliest of military concepts—collateral damage.

Recent Developments

In "The New Crisis of Legitimacy in Controls, Prisons, and Legal Structures," a classic of the many writings that express outrage over the racial disparities generated by the drug war, Troy Duster tracked the prison population (exclusive of inmates in jails and juvenile facilities) from 1981 to 1991, from 300,000 to 804,000 inmates—as he says, the largest absolute increase in the nation's history. What of recent developments? In the year 2000, the total number of inmates in state and federal prisons reached a total of 1,349,000—an even greater absolute jump over the past decade than was true of the previous one. Interestingly, the prison population declined one-half of one percent between the first and the second half of 2000, the first decline of any kind during the past 30 years. A ray of hope? Over the next couple of years, perhaps we shall see.

Given what everyone now knows about recent declines in the crime rate, it should come as no surprise that the increase in the prison population is *not* a result of a rise in criminal behavior. According to the Bureau of Justice Statistics, the decline in the violent crime victimization rate—which did not begin until the year *after* Duster wrote his article—continued unabated from 1994 to the year 2000, declining by nearly half, from 51.2 to 27.4 per 1,000 in the population. The decline in rates of property crime began much earlier. In fact, between 1977 and 2000, the total property crime victimization rate per 1,000 households declined by two-thirds—from 544.1 to 178.1, an astounding and unprecedented decline.

Remarkably, arrests for drug abuse violations grew almost unabated between the early 1970s and the late 1990s. Between 1970 and 1999, adult drug arrests more than quadrupled, from 322,300 to 1,337,600, and juvenile arrests doubled, from 93,300 to 194,600.

During the period of time Duster examined, that is, during the 1980s and very early 1990s, racial disparities in drug arrests prevailed. They have continued unabated throughout the decade of the 1990s and into the early 21st century. In 1970, African Americans made up 30 percent of the U.S. prison population; by 2000, it was just under half—47 percent. The 1997 rate per 100,000 adult residents of all adults held in prisons or jails was 6,838 for African American males and 990 for white males—a ratio of 6.9 to 1, up slightly from 1985, when it was 6.7 to 1.

In 1999, 54 percent of all white males incarcerated in federal prisons were convicted of a drug offense; for black males, the figure was 65 percent, and for females, the figure was 67 and 66 percent, respectively. For all inmates housed in federal penitentiaries, the percentage who had been sentenced for drug offenses increased from 16 percent of the total in 1970 to 56 percent in 2001. Interestingly, this percentage has been almost completely stable over the past decade, from 1991 to 2001.

The mean time served by federal prisoners convicted of a drug offense who were released in 1998 was 41.4 months, about the same time as that served by convicts sentenced for offenses related to arson and explosives (40.8 months), weapons charges (41.9 months), and racketeering and extortion (40.2 months). Drug offenders released from federal prisons in 1998 served only a year and a half less than violent offenders taken as a whole—41.4 versus 59.1 months.

African American federal drug offenders released in 1998 served a mean sentence of 49.2 months; whites, a mean of 38.0 months, a difference of nearly a year. The mean length of time to which drug offenders were sentenced in U.S. District courts in 1997 was 109.4 months for African Americans, and 64.1 months for whites—a disparity of just under three years. In 1998, 85 percent of persons convicted of crack cocaine offenses in U.S. District courts were black; only 6 percent were white. In contrast, 31 percent of persons convicted of powder cocaine offenses were black and 19 percent were white; the rest (49%) were classified as Hispanic.

Collateral Damage?

In *Malign Neglect*, Michael Tonry takes Duster's analysis a step further by reading intent into consequences. Tonry insists that, *in advance*, any legislator with even the dimmest perception of social and criminal processes *had to have known* that the drug war would produce racial inequities. Accelerating the War on Drugs, Tonry insists, "forseeably and unnecessarily blighted the lives of hundreds of thousands of young, disadvantaged black Americans." The forces that produced racial disparities were so widely known and firmly established in the criminological literature, Tonry insists, that these inequities provide prima facie evidence for the racist motives of the drug war. The drug war's architects "knew exactly what they were doing" and "should be held accountable for what they have done to damage young black Americans."

How are we to assess such claims? How are we to make sense of the drug war, which seems to make no sense whatsoever? What are the mechanisms and processes that produce the gross racial inequities we observe? Critics of these disparities often point to the fact that surveys indicate that racial differences in drug use are small, nonexistent, or even the opposite of what we would expect, given rates of drug arrests by race. Blacks are no more likely to use drugs than whites, they say, hence, the higher rates of arrest and imprisonment can only be attributable to racism.

It is true that racial differences among casual, recreational users are small. However, when we look at overdose statistics and drug tests, the African American edge in drug use looms large. African Americans are substantially over-represented at the upper reaches of use, among the most abusive substance users.

- According to DAWN, the Drug Abuse Warning Network's figures, 27 percent of persons who died in 1998 of a drug "overdose" were black, double their representation in the population—and double their representation among drug users as a whole. Over half of all persons whose death was caused or associated with cocaine use were African Americans. The same edge prevails with respect to DAWN's drug-related emergency room visits.
- A quarter of all admittees to public drug treatment programs are black, twice their representation in the general population.
- The Arrestee Drug Abuse Monitoring (or ADAM) data reveal that, nationwide, African American arrestees are significantly more likely to test positive for illicit drugs than whites (in 1997, 82 versus 68 percent), and strikingly more likely to test positive for cocaine—60 versus 25 percent.
- And in the state of Georgia in 1994, nine times as many African American newborns as whites—12.1 versus 1.3 per 1,000—tested positive for cocaine, indicating that their mothers used the drug.

It is not among casual, recreational, or typical users where arrest is most likely to take place but at the higher or more abusive levels of drug use. What counts here is that small but important minority that uses drugs in ways that lead to behavior associated with a high likelihood of arrest. And it is at these levels that African Americans are strikingly more likely to use illicit substances. Hence, the inevitable racial disparities we observe in arrest rates.

In addition, to the extent that the prosecution of the drug laws snares street sellers in buy and bust operations, it is more likely to arrest African Americans than if the police were to target higher-ups, who are more likely to be white. Arresting street dealers is easy and results in volume productivity. In contrast, going after major dealers is hard work, results in a low volume of arrests, and all too often comes up empty as a result of a tangle of legal and constitutional protections of suspects. Among other things, one byproduct of targeting street dealers is a major reason for racial disparities in drug arrest and incarceration.

In fact, a major reason why such disparities exist can be traced to what might be referred to as "point of contact" factors that are a product of racial and ethnic *styles* of drug dealing. As the United States Sentencing Commission observed in 1995, roughly two-thirds of crack defendants were considered by the police to be street-level dealers or couriers, only three out of 10 were regarded as mid-level dealers, and only one out of 20 was classified as a high-level dealer. Given their numbers as well as the nature of police tactics, the present distribution of African Americans and whites in arrest figures seems almost preordained.

The work of Eloise Dunlap, Bruce Johnson, and their colleagues suggests another linkage between routine police practices and racial disparities. There are two "relatively distinct" types of drug selling careers, says Dunlop—the "inner-city" and the "middle-class" career types. In both types of drug-selling careers, seller-to-user dealers are primarily youths and young adults, male, and are characteristically heavy users themselves. But these types differ radically in styles of dealing.

Middle-class dealers "almost always sell to steady customers [known to dealers] in private settings." Quantities tend to be fairly substantial, sales to each customer are intermittent, and violence tends to be rare. As the Office of National Drug Control Policy observed, powder cocaine is most likely to be bought and sold indoors—away from the open observation of the police.

Inner city dealers, in contrast, "often lack access to private settings for sales and typically sell in public [or semi-public locations—such as crack houses—which are accessible to nearly anyone walking off the street] to buyers they do not know." They sell much more often and in smaller quantities, and high customer turnover is common. Crack cocaine is most likely to be bought in transactions that are readily visible to the police. In such settings, violence is a frequent accompaniment, and hence, arrest in such venues is highly likely.

None of these "point of contact" factors addresses the very real and, for blacks, palpable fact that, in the inner city, they are subject to intense and unequal police scrutiny and, all too often, interrogation. The offense, "walking down the street while black," is a daily reality for the young, urban, African American male. But nonetheless, police tactics and the routine activities of drug use and dealing explains a major chunk of racial differences in arrests and incarceration; they cannot be ascribed to racist motives alone, and they will not disappear when and if the police no longer practice racial profiling.

In similar fashion, drawing a legal distinction between crack and powder cocaine also produces a higher volume of arrests and prosecutions of African Americans. Under federal law, the quantity of cocaine necessary to draw a five-year sentence is *one one-hundredth* for crack as that for powder cocaine—five versus 500 grams. Hence, for the same quantity, crack possession sentences are substantially longer than powder cocaine sentences.

Reformers and critics seem to be arguing that experts should explain to lawmakers that crack and powder cocaine are the same drug deserving of the same or comparable penalties. The 100-to-1-penalty ratio seems hugely excessive to me, but nothing will convince the public or any politician that the two substances are precisely "the same drug." The fact is, of course, crack and powder cocaine are "the same drug" only in the sense that wine and whiskey are the same drug: They both contain the same chemical, and both break down into the same chemical when metabolized in the body. But crack and cocaine are also ingested by different routes of administration, smoking versus intranasally, and hence, have very different effects. When smoked (or, more properly, inhaled) crack's effects are substan-

tially more pleasurable or reinforcing and therefore, a substantially higher proportion of its users become dependent.

Drug Arrest Disparities

Does the issue of racial disparities in arrests and imprisonment work as a rhetorical device? To progressives, this inequity serves as a signal or summary phenomenon—a kind of legal and judicial "horror story" so blatant as to force every sentient being to sit up, take notice, and feel that injustice is afoot. How can we not be moved to action? The figures virtually cry out for a just remedy. But does this rhetorical device work with the general public? Does it work among politicians? What about in a court of law?

So far, none of the legal challenges to drug convictions based on the injustice of prevailing racial disparities has succeeded. Randall Kennedy, a legal scholar, suggests that legally, the argument fails on the very grounds on which it is based—equal protection under the law. Kennedy points out that what Tonry fails to mention—that 11 out of the 21 African Americans who were then members of the House of Representatives voted in favor of the law that created the 100-to-1, powder-to-cocaine differential. As Kennedy says, if racism, conscious or unconscious, were behind the enactment of this bill, it is noteworthy that none of the black members of Congress made this charge at the time of the bill's debate, passage, or immediate aftermath.

In fact, he says, these politicians suggested exactly the reverse: *ignoring* crack's devastating impact would be harmful to the African American community. Declared Congressman Major Owens, a liberal Democrat from New York's Bedford-Stuyvesant: "We must make it perfectly clear that we view this drug [crack] as highly dangerous and that we will not tolerate its importation, possession, or sale." Said Alton Waldron, another liberal African American Democrat representing a predominantly black district in New York City, "For those of us who are black, this self-inflicted pain is the worst oppression we have known since slavery.... Let us crack down on crack."

I happen to think the War on Drugs is insane.

The charge that increasing the punishment for crack offenses represents an unequal burden to African American offenders and hence, to the African American community as a whole is specious, according to Kennedy, since crack dealing ravages mainly the African American community. Hence, he says, the failure to incarcerate crack dealers constitutes a failure to protect that community from harm. Does the refusal of the police to pursue a case against crack offenders in an African American community when African Americans lodge a complaint constitute a deprivation of equal protection under the law, he asks rhetorically? The fact that, in the face of the huge increases in drug arrests among African Americans and the insupportable sentences that have [been] meted out as a consequence, many black politicians have altered their position over the past dozen years is less important than the fact that *at the time*, implicit racism was simply not on the agenda of lawmakers.

The rage of the critics of racial disparities in the drug war is misplaced. It is disingenuous to argue, as some have, that rates of drug use for blacks and whites are equal, ergo, to be fair and just, rates of arrest and incarceration must also be equal. Even if overall rates of use were equal, given the very different and distinctive racial styles and patterns of drug use, rates of arrest and incarceration *cannot possibly* be equal. In fact, *even if there were no drug war*—that is, if the country were to return to pre-1970s rates of drug arrests and incarceration—these disparities would remain. Accelerating the War on Drugs intensified the racial disparities, but it did not create them.

The higher rate of arrest and incarceration among African Americans is an outrage not because the architects of the drug war may or may not have targeted blacks (I do not think they did), or because drug arrests and incarcerations do in fact result in racial disparities. The outrage should be generated because these disparities are a product of inequalities that existed before and are far more basic to drug offenses and their prosecution. The drug war inadvertently but effectively further marginalizes a segment of the population—the black underclass—very much in need of social and political inclusion.

By attributing a racial motive to the drug war, its critics have focused on an issue that has no policy purchase. There is simply nowhere to go with the issue of racial disparities because it is primarily the routine activities of use and the iron logic of the logistics of law enforcement, not racist motives, that generates them. The argument lacks both empirical grounding and rhetor-ical resonance. It is impossible to dismiss racist motives as one explanation for racial disparities in drug arrests and imprisonment, but again, we have no smoking gun. What we do have is racial differences that are firmly grounded in the dynamics of everyday life. And they are not going to disappear in a puff of speechmaking.

I happen to think the War on Drugs is insane. I am strongly committed to the reduction of harm. But any conceivable harm reduction strategy that has any hope of implementation could reduce the total number of arrests and imprisonment but cannot eliminate racial disparities. Street dealers will always be more subject to arrest than dealers who are more insulated from surveillance, and more abusive users of crack cocaine and heroin will always be more subject to arrest than recreational users of marijuana, LSD, and Ecstasy.

What would a solution to the drug war problem look like? Whose interests are served by continuing the War on Drugs? Given the dense entanglement of race with the routine activities of users and strategies of law enforcement, does the racial issue have maximum purchase for the reformer's agenda? If, in Duster's phrase, we are to "reconstruct" the drug war, we cannot afford to ignore these questions. Understanding racial disparities in drug arrests and imprisonment must be harnessed to a profound appreciation of how limited our capacity is to impose policy on the extremely rough timber of humanity.

Erich Goode, author of numerous books on deviance and drug use, teaches in the Department of Criminology and Criminal Justice at the University of Maryland.

Fetal Alcohol Syndrome Prevention Research

Alcohol consumption during pregnancy can have numerous adverse health consequences for the developing fetus, including fetal alcohol syndrome (FAS) and alcohol-related effects, and therefore is a significant public health problem. A variety of programs have been developed to prevent drinking during pregnancy and the resulting health problems. Some of these efforts, such as public service announcements and beverage warning labels, are universal and strive to increase the public's knowledge about FAS. Selective prevention approaches target women of reproductive age who drink alcohol. Such approaches may involve screening all pregnant women for alcohol consumption and counseling those women who do drink. Indicated prevention approaches target high-risk women (e.g., women who have previously abused alcohol or have had a child with FAS or other alcohol-related effects) and typically offer repeated counseling over several years. Both selective and indicated prevention efforts can reduce maternal alcohol consumption and improve the outcome of the offspring. KEY WORDS: *Fetal alcohol syndrome; prevention research; indicated prevention; selective prevention; universal prevention; targeted prevention; mass media prevention approach; public service announcement; warning label; prevention effort directed at people at risk; prevention outcome*

JANET R. HANKIN, PH.D.

Drinking during pregnancy, which can result in serious birth defects, remains a significant public health problem despite a variety of prevention efforts that have been implemented in recent years. According to national data collected in 1999 by the Behavioral Risk Factor Surveillance System (BRFSS), a telephone survey of the noninstitutionalized U.S. population, 12.8 percent of pregnant women consumed at least one alcoholic drink during the past month, a decrease from 16.3 percent reported in 1995 (Centers for Disease Control and Prevention [CDC] 2002a). The survey also assessed the prevalence of binge and frequent drinking (i.e., five or more drinks on one occasion or at least seven drinks per week) by pregnant women. Comparing data from 1995 and 1999, the investigators found that binge drinking and frequent drinking remained "substantially unchanged." A total of 3.3 percent of pregnant women inter-

viewed in 1999 reported frequent drinking and 2.7 percent reported binge drinking (CDC 2002a). These findings are subject to at least three limitations, however. First, BRFSS data are self-reported and might be subject to reporting biases, especially among pregnant women who are aware that alcohol use is not advised. Second, homeless women, women in homes without telephones, and women who were institutionalized were not surveyed. Both of these limitations could have an impact on prevalence rates. Third, because the proportion of pregnant women who were drinkers was limited in this sample, these estimated prevalence rates are subject to statistical limitations. Thus, the prevalence rates of drinking, frequent drinking, and binge drinking among pregnant women may actually be even higher than indicated in the BRFSS study.

The potential consequences of drinking during pregnancy—the

most serious of which are fetal alcohol syndrome (FAS) and other manifestations collectively called alcohol-related effects—are preventable birth defects. Nevertheless, only limited evaluation research exists on FAS prevention programs (National Institute on Alcohol Abuse and Alcoholism [NIAAA] 2002a). After briefly describing the harmful effects of alcohol on the fetus, this article reviews the spectrum of FAS prevention efforts and summarizes recent research on FAS prevention activities.

CONSEQUENCES OF DRINKING DURING PREGNANCY

Alcohol ingested during pregnancy can have a range of deleterious consequences for the developing fetus. The most severe condition caused by prenatal alcohol exposure is FAS, which is characterized by a particular pattern of facial anomalies, growth retardation, and developmental abnormalities in the central nervous system that often include, but are not limited to, mental retardation. Alcohol-related effects can be further subdivided into alcohol-related birth defects (ARBD) and alcohol-related neurodevelopmental disorder (ARND). ARBD can involve defects in several organ systems, such as the heart, kidney, vision, and hearing. ARND manifests as central nervous system developmental abnormalities and/or behavioral or cognitive abnormalities. In addition, some evidence indicates that prenatal exposure to alcohol increases the risk for internalizing disorders, including depression and negative self-cognitions (e.g., low self-esteem) in the offspring (Olson et al. 2001). Furthermore, prenatal alcohol exposure may result in long-term neurocognitive disorders, such as problems with executive functions (e.g., poor organizational skills, difficulties in impulse control, and poor decisionmaking skills). Finally, adults who had been prenatally exposed to alcohol frequently suffer from mental disorders and maladaptive behaviors that make it difficult for them to be self-sufficient and independent (Streissguth and O'Malley 2000). Unfortunately, it is not uncommon for prenatal alcohol exposure to result in such severe deficits.

Estimates of the prevalence of FAS in the U.S. population range from 0.5 to 2 cases per 1,000 live births (May and Gossage 2001; CDC 2002b). Rates of FAS surpass this prevalence in high-risk populations. For example, reported rates of FAS are 9.8/1000 live births among Southwestern Plains Indians living on reservations (May and Gossage 2001). The rate for alcohol-related effects (ARBD and ARND) may be as high as 5 cases per 1,000 live births (Stratton et al. 1996). May and Gossage (2001) estimate that the prevalence for FAS, ARBD, and ARND combined is 1 percent of all births. The range in prevalence results from differences in the populations at risk being studied and in the methods used to identify affected people. Analyses based on medical records often underestimate the rates of FAS and alcohol-related effects compared

with more aggressive case-finding approaches that include examinations of people living in the community (May and Gossage 2001; Stratton et al. 1996).

THE SPECTRUM OF FAS PREVENTION APPROACHES

FAS can be prevented if a woman abstains from alcohol consumption at conception and throughout pregnancy. The Committee to Study Fetal Alcohol Syndrome of the Institute of Medicine of the National Academy of Sciences has described an intervention spectrum for FAS that includes three major prevention strategies (Stratton et al. 1996):

- *Universal prevention of maternal alcohol abuse.* These interventions attempt to educate the broad public about the risks of drinking during pregnancy. These universal efforts might be geared toward pregnant women or women of childbearing age and often include public service announcements, billboards, pamphlets in physicians' offices, and media advertisements. The alcohol beverage warning label is an example of a universal intervention that has been extensively studied.
- *Selective prevention of maternal alcohol abuse.* These interventions target women who are at greater risk for having children with FAS or alcohol-related effects—that is, all women of childbearing age who consume alcohol. One example of selective prevention measures is the screening of all pregnant women for their alcohol use, followed by counseling of all drinkers regarding fetal risk or, if warranted, referral to specialized treatment.
- *Indicated prevention of FAS.* These measures are directed at high-risk women, including women who have previously abused alcohol while pregnant or while at risk for conception, or women who drink and have delivered an infant with FAS, ARND, or ARBD. This level of prevention includes alcoholism

treatment of pregnant women or women who are likely to become pregnant as well as measures to encourage prevention of pregnancy.

The following sections describe each of these major types of FAS prevention efforts and summarize research on their effectiveness.

UNIVERSAL EFFORTS AND THEIR IMPACT

One of the first steps in universal prevention efforts is to increase the public's knowledge of the consequences of alcohol use during pregnancy, particularly FAS. Various methods can be used to increase knowledge, including news reports, articles in the popular press, public service announcements, billboards, and the alcohol beverage warning label. With the exception of the research on the warning label, few studies have assessed the effectiveness of these efforts on knowledge of FAS, attitudes about drinking during pregnancy, and women's actual alcohol consumption during pregnancy.

Extent of Media Attention to Drinking During Pregnancy

Lemmens and colleagues (1999) reviewed the coverage of alcohol-related issues in five national newspapers (i.e., *New York Times, Los Angeles Times, Washington Post, Christian Science Monitor*, and *Wall Street Journal*) from 1985 through 1991 by randomly sampling articles dealing with beverage alcohol. Out of 1,677 articles examined, only 23 dealt with alcohol and pregnancy. Similarly, Golden (2000) reviewed national network evening news broadcasts between 1977 and 1996 for ABC, CBS, NBC and found that alcohol and pregnancy was a topic in only 36 of the newscasts. These particular newscasts often coincided with the announcement of government warnings, the discovery of scientific evidence linking alcohol to birth defects, and other incidents associated with alcohol abuse deemed newsworthy, such as the firing of a bartender and waitress who refused to serve alcohol to a pregnant woman.

Warning Posters

Warning posters to be placed where alcohol is sold have been required in some States as early as 1983. As of 1993, 18 States, 14 cities, and 2 counties required the display of such posters. Prugh (1986) examined the impact of posters warning about drinking during pregnancy in New York City. Prior to the posters, 54 percent of respondents mentioned birth defects as a result of drinking while pregnant. A year after the posters were introduced, 68 percent mentioned birth defects as a consequence of drinking.

Using a national sample of 4,000 adults in 1990–1991, Kaskutas and Graves (1994) found that 31 percent of respondents saw a sign or poster warning about health effects of alcohol. Among those seeing a sign or poster, 56 percent recalled a warning about alcohol and birth defects. The investigators also reported that the level of knowledge of the risks associated with drinking during pregnancy increased with an increasing number of different message sources (e.g., posters, warning label, and advertisements). Among the 142 women in the survey who had been pregnant in the past year, 86 percent saw 1 or more messages about drinking while pregnant. Eighty-seven percent of women who had been pregnant versus 58 percent of women of childbearing age who had not been pregnant had a discussion about alcohol and the risk of birth defects ($p<.05$). Thirty-six percent of the women who had been pregnant and were drinkers reported limiting their drinking for "health reasons" compared with 25 percent of the nonpregnant women ($p<.05$). Finally, 70 percent of the women who had been pregnant reported that they did not drink alcohol while pregnant (Kaskutas and Graves 1994).

Evidence that Knowledge of FAS Has Increased over Time

One study has tracked the level of knowledge of FAS over time using data from the National Health Interview Surveys that involved interviews with 19,000 people ages 18 to 44 in 1985 and with 23,000 people in 1990 (Dufour et al. 1994). Over the 5-year period between the two surveys, the proportion of respondents reporting that they had heard about FAS increased significantly, from 62 percent to 73 percent among women and from 49 percent to 55 percent among men.

Among women who had heard of FAS, the number of those who correctly defined the condition as a birth defect increased significantly from 25 percent to 39 percent. Among men, the percentages also increased significantly from 24 percent in 1985 to 36 percent in 1990.

Although this study did not test the effectiveness of particular universal interventions, the findings suggest that general knowledge of FAS has increased over time.

Effectiveness of the Alcohol Beverage Warning Label

In 1988, the U.S. Congress passed the Alcoholic Beverage Warning Label Act requiring that effective November 18, 1989, a warning label must be attached to all containers of alcoholic beverages. The first part of the warning reads: "Government Warning: According to the Surgeon General, women should not drink alcoholic beverages during pregnancy because of the risk of birth defects." Various researchers have examined exposure to the warning label and its impact on drinking during pregnancy. In general, the studies concluded that although awareness of the alcohol beverage warning label increased after the implementation of the law, this awareness has attenuated over time. Furthermore, the warning label's impact on drinking during pregnancy has been modest. (For a comprehensive review of the impact of the alcohol warning label on perception of risks including drunk driving, birth defects, and health problems; and drinking behavior in a variety of situations, see Mackinnon 1995.)

For example, Greenfield and Kaskutas (1998) examined exposure to the warning label among a national probability sample of adults using annual cross-sectional telephone surveys.[1] In a cross-sectional design, each participant is interviewed only once and a new sample is created for every year of the survey.)

For that study, interviews were conducted in 1989, 1990, 1991, 1993, and 1994 that included a total of approximately 8,000 respondents. In 1990, 6 months after the implementation of the label, 21 percent of respondents said they had seen the warning label during the past 12 months. By 1994 exposure to the label had reached a plateau, according to the investigators, with 51 percent of respondents reporting that they had seen the label in the past 12 months.

As part of a cross-sectional and longitudinal study of the effects of alcohol beverage warning labels, Kaskutas and colleagues (1998) conducted a phone survey of a national representative sample of 365 pregnant women from 1989 through 1994. Exposure to the warning label fluctuated over the course of the study (7 percent saw the label in 1989, 27 percent in both 1990 and 1991, 58 percent in 1993, and 42 percent in 1994 [no data was collected in 1992]). Exposure to signs or posters also varied over the study period from a high of 28 percent in 1991 to a low of 13 percent in 1993 (1989, 21 percent; 1990, 17 percent; 1994, 17 percent). Advertisements about drinking during pregnancy were seen by 81 percent of women during 1989, 1990, and 1991, but by fewer women in 1993 and 1994 (65 percent and 58 percent, respectively). Finally, 84 percent of women had conversations about drinking during pregnancy in both 1989 and 1991, and 87 percent in 1990, but only 74 percent in 1993 and 58 percent in 1994. These data suggest changes, and in some cases, decreases in the proportion of women exposed to these media messages over time.

Seventy-five percent of the women reported not drinking, whereas 21 percent had one or two drinks and 4 percent admitted drinking at least three drinks on any single day during pregnancy. However, the 1989–1994 data showed no statistically significant relation between drinking patterns during pregnancy and exposure to any of the types of messages assessed in the surveys (Kaskutas et al. 1998).

Several other studies have tracked the awareness of warning labels in various populations, as follows:

- A Detroit study using a 1995 probability sample of 1,107 women found that 39 percent of the women had seen a warning label in the past 12 months. Among abstainers, 18 percent had seen a warning label, compared with 52 percent of women who drank. Seventy-seven percent of those who had seen the label recalled that it mentioned birth defects (Hankin 1998).

- An Indiana study evaluated knowledge of the warning label among 1,211 12th grade students in the fall of 1989 (i.e., before the introduction of the label) and 2,006 students in the fall of 1990 (i.e., after the introduction of the label). The study found that in the fall of 1989, 26 percent reported having seen alcohol warning labels compared with 41 percent in the fall of 1990. In 1989, 65 percent of respondents who reported seeing the label also reported that it mentioned birth defects,[2] whereas by the fall of 1990, this proportion had increased to 83 percent (Mackinnon et al. 1993).

- Another study tracked changes in label awareness from May 1989 through June 1993 among 7,334 inner-city African American women seeking prenatal care. Over the 50-month study period, the level of label awareness continued to increase through December 1992, when it reached the maximum of about 80 percent (Hankin et al. 1996).

Using the same inner-city prenatal clinic, Hankin and colleagues (1998) examined the impact of the warning label on drinking during pregnancy. This study involved 21,127 pregnant African American women using the prenatal clinic between 1986 and 1995. Controlling for patient characteristics and the unemployment rate,[3] drinking began to decline 8 months after the implementation of the warning label (Hankin et al. 1998). However, this decline was only modest (i.e., 0.05 ounces of absolute alcohol per week or approximately 1 ounce of beer) and appeared to be short-lived. Thus, by 1992, the women's alcohol consumption rose again and by 1995, pregnant women had become accustomed to the message.

SELECTIVE EFFORTS AND THEIR IMPACT

Selective prevention targets all women in their reproductive years who drink alcohol (although most studies target heavy drinkers).

One randomized trial assessed the impact of a brief intervention on drinking during pregnancy in this population (Chang et al. 1999, 2000). Women initiating prenatal care at Brigham and Women's Hospital in Boston, MA, were screened for their alcohol use using a brief questionnaire called the T-ACE[4] (Sokol et al. 1989). The first 250 women who were identified as risk drinkers using this questionnaire and who had consumed alcohol in the previous 6 months were randomly assigned to an assessment-only group ($n = 127$) or to a brief intervention group ($n = 123$). The brief intervention consisted of a 45-minute session with a physician and included the articulation of drinking goals while pregnant, identification of risk situations for drinking and alternatives to drinking, and the recommendation of abstinence during pregnancy from the Surgeon General and the Secretary of Health and Human Services. The study investigators then interviewed women once they had given birth about their alcohol consumption since the original assessment. Women in both groups reduced their alcohol consumption during pregnancy, and no difference existed between the two groups in the decrease in average number of drinks per drinking day. Accordingly, Chang and colleagues (1999) concluded that screening alone may be related to a reduction of drinking during pregnancy.

The study also attempted to identify patient characteristics that predicted greater success of the intervention approach. For example, the brief intervention appeared most successful for women who had been drinking alcohol in the previous 6 months but who had been abstinent in the 90 days prior to their first prenatal visit. Among current drinkers at baseline in the brief intervention group, women who articulated specific drinking goals for specific reasons were more likely to reduce alcohol consumption or abstain from alcohol during pregnancy than were women without such goals (Chang et al. 2000).

An ongoing randomized clinical trial is extending these selective prevention efforts by applying them to an indicated prevention program. In this trial, recruitment focuses on a high-risk population of 300 pregnant women who are currently drinking, drank during a previous pregnancy, or drank at least one drink daily prior to current pregnancy. In this study, the investigators, led by Chang, are comparing the results of an assessment-only condition with an enhanced brief intervention that involves a support partner chosen by the pregnant woman.

Handmaker and colleagues (1999) piloted a study to evaluate the results of motivational interviewing with 42 pregnant problem drinkers. Women reporting any recent drinking were randomly assigned either to the experimental group that received a 1-hour motivational interview focused on weighing drinking against the risk of birth defects, or to a control group that received a letter explaining the risks of drinking during pregnancy and recommending the woman talk to her obstetrical provider about the risks. Women in both groups had significantly reduced their alcohol intake at followup 2 months later. Women who self-reported the highest levels of blood alcohol concentrations had the greatest decrease in alcohol consumption if they were in the experimental group compared with the control group. (Blood alcohol concentrations were estimated using computer projections that were based on self-reports of estimated number of drinks, alcohol content of drinks, length of drinking episodes, the woman's weight, and an average rate of alcohol metabolism for women.)

Another selective prevention approach that was part of the Developing Effective Educational Resources (DEER) project examined the exposure and reactions to warnings about drinking during pregnancy in samples of 321 pregnant Native Americans and African Americans living in the Northern California Bay area and Los Angeles. In this study, Kaskutas (2000) found that although the women were frequently exposed to warning messages, they were uncertain about the impact of FAS. Specifically, only about a quarter of the women could name at least one birth defect associated with FAS and only one-fifth knew that FAS was related to alcohol consumption.

Only about a quarter of the women could name at least one birth defect associated with FAS and only one-fifth knew that FAS was related to alcohol consumption.

Furthermore, the women did not understand the benefits of quitting drinking at any time during pregnancy, and they had the misconception that wine, beer, and wine coolers are safer to drink during pregnancy than liquor. Finally, most of the women underestimated their drinking. Thus, when the investigator compared alcohol intake using standard drink sizes[5] with self-defined drink sizes (assessed with the help of beverage containers and photos), consumption by risk drinkers was 2 to 3 times higher using self-defined drink sizes compared with standard size drink measurements.

Ongoing research is extending this methodology and testing a novel prevention program for pregnant women enrolled in a health maintenance organization (Kaskutas and Graves 2001). In this randomized clinical trial, the investigators use models of alcoholic beverage containers (beverage containers of various sizes, such as 12-ounce versus 40-ounce beer bottles or beer cans, or liquor bottles that range from 375 milliliters, 750 milliliters, and 1 liter) or drinking vessels (shot glasses, wine glasses, or drinking glasses with lines marked off with letters so women could tell the investigators how high they filled the glass) and a computer program to help pregnant women understand how much they actually drink.

After the women identify the bottle or glass they typically drink from, the computer program calculates the absolute ounces of alcohol consumed. These nonconfrontational approaches of using drinking vessels and beverage containers and talking about drinking in a nonthreatening way help the women discuss their drinking habits while pregnant.

INDICATED EFFORTS AND THEIR IMPACT

Indicated prevention efforts are directed toward the population at highest risk of having children with FAS or alcohol-related effects—that is, women who have a history of drinking during pregnancy or have previously delivered a child affected by alcohol. Several studies have assessed prevention approaches directed at this population to prevent the birth of further alcohol-affected children. (Handmaker and Wilbourne [2001] thoroughly review motivational interventions in prenatal clinics, describing additional approaches not mentioned here.)

One of these approaches was the Protecting the Next Pregnancy project, which targeted women who had been identified as drinking heavily during the last pregnancy (called the index pregnancy). The goal of the intervention being tested was to reduce the women's drinking during their next pregnancies (Hankin and Sokol 1995; Hankin et al. 2000). All women consuming at least four drinks per week (i.e., 0.3 ounces absolute alcohol per day) at the time they conceived during the index pregnancy were approached in the hospital's postpartum unit and asked to participate in the trial. (The women's average alcohol consumption was 1.2 ounces of absolute alcohol per day, or more than 16 drinks per week, at the time of conception for the index pregnancy.) Four weeks after giving birth, the women were randomly assigned to an experimental group that received an intensive brief intervention or a control group that received standard clinical care. The study included 300 women, who were followed up to 5 years.

The brief intervention involved a one-on-one method, which was

based on a cognitive behavioral approach, and included 5 sessions beginning at 1 month after giving birth and continuing for 12 months. In those sessions, the counselor reviewed the definition of a standard drink, helped the women set the goal of abstention or reduction of alcohol use, established limits on consumption (if not abstaining), and taught ways to reduce drinking. Additional booster sessions were conducted over the 5-year followup period. The control group was simply advised that "You can have a healthier baby if you cut back or stop drinking during pregnancy."

Of the 300 participants, 96 women delivered 1 or more infants during the followup period. The investigators found that women in the experimental group drank significantly less than did women in the control group during the subsequent pregnancies. While 25 percent of the women in the control group drank at least 0.3 ounces of absolute alcohol per day, only 11.8 percent of the women in the experimental group drank at that risk level (chi-square 2.4, $p < .06$, 1-tailed [Hankin and Sokol 1995; Hankin et al. 2000]). Furthermore, among women who drank during subsequent pregnancies, those from the experimental group drank about half as much as did women from the control group (i.e., 0.32 ounce versus 0.65 ounce absolute alcohol per day, $t = 2.08$, $p < .03$, 1-tailed). This reduced alcohol consumption resulted in improved birth outcomes among women from the experimental group, including fewer low-birth weight babies and fewer premature births. In addition, children born to women from the experimental group exhibited better neurobehavioral performance at 13 months of age compared with the children of women from the control group. These findings indicate that the brief intervention protected the next pregnancy by reducing alcohol consumption and improving infant outcomes.

In another indicated prevention effort called Project TrEAT (Trial for Early Alcohol Treatment) researchers screened almost 6,000 women ages 18 to 40 for problem drinking and then randomly assigned 205 problem drinkers to a brief intervention program or to a control group (Manwell et al. 2000). The two groups did not differ significantly with respect to various factors, such as alcohol use, age, socioeconomic status, smoking, various psychiatric disorders, lifetime drug use, or health care utilization. The brief intervention in this study consisted of two 15-minute counseling sessions conducted by physicians and including a review of the woman's current health behavior, a discussion of the adverse effects of alcohol, a drinking agreement, and cards to record alcohol intake. The control group received a booklet on general health issues. Participants were followed for 48 months. Women in the brief intervention group successfully reduced their mean alcohol intake by 48 percent, and the proportion of women reporting any binge drinking in this group decreased from 93 percent to 68 percent. The control group also exhibited modest declines in alcohol use.

During the followup period, 41 women became pregnant, including 22 in the brief intervention group and 19 in the control group. For these women, the brief intervention seemed to result in better outcomes in terms of decreased consumption because women in the brief intervention group reduced their alcohol consumption from 13.6 to 3.5 drinks per week, compared with a decrease from 13.5 drinks to 10.1 drinks per week for women in the control group.

Another example of a treatment program targeting women who have already given birth to alcohol- or drug-exposed infants was the Seattle Birth to 3 Advocacy Project (Streissguth 1997). This program was designed for women who were heavy users of alcohol or other drugs, had no prenatal care, and were not connected to service providers during their pregnancy. Specially trained paraprofessionals,[6] acting as advocates, worked on a one-on-one basis with the women and their families over a 3-year period. The 65 women in the program, most of whom were unemployed or on welfare, learned how to set goals, connect with other providers, and acquire new skills. After 2 years, 80 percent of the women had received alcohol and other drug abuse treatment, and 60 percent had remained abstinent from alcohol and

other drugs. Moreover, 62 percent of the women were using long-term birth control methods, thereby reducing the risk for another alcohol- or drug-exposed pregnancy.

ADDITIONAL EXAMPLES OF ONGOING FAS PREVENTION RESEARCH

Several other programs are studying different FAS prevention efforts in a variety of target populations and settings. For example, Project CHOICES (Changing High-Risk AlcOhol Use and Increasing Contraception Effectiveness Study), which is funded by the Centers for Disease Control and Prevention (Floyd et al. 1999), is a selective prevention effort to prevent alcohol exposure during pregnancy among women of childbearing age in special settings. These populations include women in a jail, in a substance abuse center, or in clinics as well as a group of women with concerns about problem drinking who were recruited through media announcements. The program uses a brief intervention to reduce alcohol use and/or postpone pregnancy until drinking problems are resolved.

Another recently funded study is aimed at college students, encouraging them to abstain from alcohol or to use contraception if they drink. The goal of this program is to reduce alcohol use and promote effective contraception among women who are not currently pregnant. The program uses a brief intervention that educates women about the consequences of problem drinking, the benefits and costs of changing drinking and contraception behavior, setting goals, keeping a daily diary, and followup support.

An ongoing prevention effort on Native American reservations is based on the Institute of Medicine model and incorporates universal, selective, and indicated prevention activities (May 1995). The study includes four prevention communities and two "research only" communities. The selective prevention component consists of a screening program for women in clinics and Women, Infant, and Children (WIC) sites to identify high-risk drinkers. The indicated prevention component involves

case management using motivational interviewing and community reinforcement approaches to help women who are drinking during pregnancy. The two sets of communities will be compared on a variety of outcome measures.

NIAAA is funding several other prevention studies of interventions designed to reduce drinking among pregnant women. (Information about these studies can be obtained from the Computer Retrieval Information on Scientific Projects [CRISP] database at http://crisp.cit.nih.gov.) Most of these efforts use brief interventions with motivational interviewing. Another program that is based at WIC clinics seeks to increase the detection of alcohol use during pregnancy, identify maternal characteristics contributing to the success of a brief intervention, identify characteristics of the intervention itself that contribute to its effectiveness, and evaluate the impact of the program on infant outcome. Finally, NIAAA is funding a study that is based on a more environmentally focused perspective and that examines the impact of alcohol server education in FAS prevention. All of these prevention efforts are ongoing, and researchers are still waiting for data on the results of these programs.

DISCUSSION

As noted by NIAAA, "Unfortunately, many women continue to drink during pregnancy. Furthermore, many of the women who continue to drink during pregnancy are at highest risk for having children with fetal alcohol syndrome and related problems. Thus, finding potent new ways to reach populations at risk and to influence changes in their behavior remains a challenge for alcohol research" (NIAAA 2000b, p. 3).

Researchers and clinicians already have made some progress in the efforts to prevent FAS. For example, universal prevention approaches have increased the general public's knowledge about the results of drinking during pregnancy. Studies on awareness of the alcohol beverage warning label showed an increase in awareness over time. In addition, a larger proportion of the public knows about the relationships between drinking during pregnancy and birth defects. However, knowledge is not enough to change norms and actual behavior, as indicated by recent data that almost 13 percent of pregnant women drink during pregnancy (CDC 2002a). Numerous questions remain to be answered. For example, although the alcohol beverage warning label had a modest impact on drinking during pregnancy for a short time, the public has become habituated to its message. Future analyses need to clarify why this habituation occurred and whether new labels or a system of rotating labels can prevent habituation. Additional research must identify the most effective ways to educate the public about FAS (e.g., revised alcohol beverage warning labels, warning posters, public service announcements, or news reports). Systematic studies are needed that compare various universal prevention efforts and their impacts across various social groups.

Brief interventions for pregnant women can successfully reduce alcohol intake during pregnancy.

Several researchers have examined the effects of selective and indicated prevention efforts using randomized clinical trials. The results described in this article suggest that brief interventions for pregnant women can successfully reduce alcohol intake during pregnancy. Additional studies using experimental designs (i.e., random assignment of study participants to an intervention group or to a control group that just receives standard clinical care) are necessary, however, to determine whether these findings are generalizable to pregnant women in diverse settings or whether the interventions need to be tailored to pregnant women from different ethnic and socioeconomic groups. Other unanswered questions concern the most appropriate contents for the brief intervention. Finally, it is important to understand whether the intervention results in clinically significant results across a variety of outcomes, including drinking during preg-

nancy, infant birth weight, length of gestation, and infant neurobehavioral outcomes. Although the research on the success of FAS prevention programs is still in its infancy, ongoing studies may help researchers and clinicians discover the best methods for separating alcohol from pregnancy and thus preventing FAS and alcohol-related effects.

NOTES

1. The term "probability sample" means that the sample was created to be representative of the U.S. population (e.g., included the same numbers of males, females, Blacks, Whites as the population). In a cross-sectional design, each participant is interviewed only once and a new sample is created for every year of the survey.

2. Reports of having seen warning labels before the labels actually existed are not uncommon. The explanation for such "false positives" is that subjects are likely to feel there must be a label if they are being asked about it.

3. Long-term drinking trends have been related to unemployment rates. For example, pregnant women may drink more when they have fewer resources and support. Furthermore, when unemployment is high, choices for prenatal care are limited, and more poor pregnant women may turn to the prenatal clinic where the study was conducted. Hankin and colleagues hypothesize that pregnant women may drink more when unemployment is high. They were unable to find any study that specifically examined this relationship. However, the following studies show that alcohol consumption, binge drinking, alcohol problems, and alcohol-related diseases are related to unemployment rates: Crawford, A.; Plant, M.A.; Kreitman, N.; and Latcham, R.W. Unemployment and drinking behaviour: Some data from a general population survey of alcohol use. *British Journal of Addiction* 82: 1007–1016, 1987; Brenner, M.H. Economic change, alcohol consumption, and heart disease mortality in nine industrialized

countries. *Social Science and Medicine* 25:119–132, 1987; Linksy, A.S.; Straus, M.S.; and Colby, J.P., Jr. Stressful events, stressful conditions, and alcohol problems in the United States: A partial test of Bale's Theory. *Journal of Studies on Alcohol* 46:72–80, 1985; Catalano, R.; Dooley, D.; Wilson, G.; and Hough, R. Job loss and alcohol abuse: A test using data from the Epidemiologic Catchment Area Project. *Journal of Health and Social Behavior* 34:215–225, 1993.)

4. The T-ACE consists of four questions and yields a maximum score of five points. Women who score two or more points are considered risk drinkers.

5. A standard drink frequently is defined as 12 ounces of beer, 5 ounces of wine, or 1.5 ounces of distilled spirits, each of which contains approximately 0.5 ounces (14 grams) of pure alcohol.

6. These were women with backgrounds similar to the clients' (e.g., in terms of previous obstacles in their lives, such as alcohol use, poverty, single parenthood, or family violence) who had completed 2 years of college and had been trained in alcohol and other drug treatment, child development, parenting skills, and community resources.

REFERENCES

Centers for Disease Control and Prevention (CDC). Alcohol use among women of childbearing age—United States, 1991–1999. *Morbidity and Mortality Weekly Reports, April 5,* 51(13):273–276, 2002a.

Centers for Disease Control and Prevention (CDC). Fetal alcohol syndrome—Alaska, Arizona, Colorado, and New York, 1995–1997. *Morbidity and Mortality Weekly Reports, May 24,* 51(20):433–435, 2002b.

CHANG, G.; WILKINS-HAUG, L.; BERMAN, S.; AND GOETZ, M. A brief intervention for alcohol use in pregnancy: A randomized trial. *Addiction* 94: 1499– 1508, 1999.

CHANG, G.; GOETZ, M.A.; WILKINS-HAUG, L.; AND BERMAN, S. A brief intervention for prenatal alcohol use: An in-depth look. *Journal of Substance Abuse Treatment* 18:365–369, 2000.

DUFOUR, M.C.; WILLIAMS, G.D.; CAMP-BELL, K.E.; AND AITKEN, S.S. Knowledge of FAS and the risks of heavy drinking during pregnancy, 1985 and 1990. *Alcohol Health & Research World* 18:86–92, 1994.

FLOYD, R.L.; EBRAHIM, S.; BOYLE, C.A.; AND GOULD, D.W. Preventing alcohol-exposed pregnancies among women of childbearing age: The necessity of a preconceptional approach. *Journal of Women's Health & Gender-Based Medicine* 8:733–736, 1999.

GOLDEN, J. "A tempest in a cocktail glass:" Mothers, alcohol, and television, 1977–1996. *Journal of Health Politics, Policy and Law* 25:473–498, 2000.

GREENFIELD, T.K., AND KASKUTAS, L.A. Five years' exposure to the alcohol warning label messages and their impacts: Evidence from diffusion analysis. *Applied Behavioral Science Review* 6:39–68, 1998.

HANDMAKER, N.S., AND WILBOURNE, P. Motivational interventions in prenatal clinics. *Alcohol Research & Health* 25:219–229, 2001.

HANDMAKER, N.S.; MILLER, W.R.; AND MANICKE, M. Finding of a pilot study of motivational interviewing with pregnant drinkers. *Journal of Studies on Alcohol* 60:285–287, 1999.

HANKIN, J. Label exposure and recall among Detroit Metropolitan women. *Applied Behavioral Science Review* 6:1–16, 1998.

HANKIN, J., AND SOKOL, R.J. Identification and care of problems associated with alcohol ingestion in pregnancy. *Seminars in Perinatology* 19:286–292, 1995.

HANKIN, J.R.; SLOAN, J.J.; FIRESTONE, I.J.; et al. Has awareness of the alcohol warning label reached its upper limit? *Alcoholism: Clinical and Experimental Research* 20:440–444, 1996.

HANKIN, J.R.; SLOAN, J.J.; AND SOKOL, R.J. The modest impact of the alcohol beverage warning label on drinking during pregnancy among a sample of African American women. *Journal of Public Policy and Marketing* 17:61–69, 1998.

HANKIN, J.R.; MCCAUL, M.E.; AND HEUSSNER, J. Pregnant, alcohol abusing women. *Alcoholism: Clinical and Experimental Research* 24:1276–1286, 2000.

KASKUTAS, L.A. Understanding drinking during pregnancy among urban American Indians and African Americans: Health messages, risk beliefs, and how we measure consumption. *Alcoholism: Clinical and Experimental Research* 24:1241–1250, 2000.

KASKUTAS, L.A., AND GRAVES, K. Relationship between cumulative exposure to health messages and awareness and behavior-related drinking during pregnancy. *American Journal of Health Promotion* 9:115–124, 1994.

KASKUTAS, L.A., AND GRAVES, K. Pre-pregnancy drinking: How drink size affects risk assessment. *Addiction* 96:1199–1209, 2001.

KASKUTAS, L.A.; GREENFIELD T.; LEE, M.E.; AND COTE J. Reach and effects of health messages on drinking during pregnancy. *Journal of Health Education* 28:11–17, 1998.

LEMMENS, P.H.; VAETH, P. A.; AND GREENFIELD, T. K. Coverage of beverage alcohol issues in the print media of the United States, 1985–1991. *American Journal of Public Health* 89:1555–1560, 1999.

MACKINNON, D.P. Review of the effects of the alcohol warning label. In: Watson, R.R., ed. *Alcohol, Cocaine, and Accidents: Drug and Alcohol Abuse Reviews 7.* Totowa, NJ: Humana Press, 1995. pp. 131–161.

MACKINNON, D.P.; PENTZ, M.A.; AND STACY, A.W. The alcohol warning and adolescents: The first year. *American Journal of Public Health* 83:585–587, 1993.

MANWELL, L.G.; FLEMING, M.F.; MUNDT, M.P.; et al. Treatment of problem alcohol use in women of childbearing age: Results of a brief intervention trial. *Alcoholism: Clinical and Experimental Research* 24:1517–1524, 2000.

MAY, P.A. A multiple-level comprehensive approach to the prevention of fetal alcohol syndrome (FAS) and other alcohol-related birth defects (ARBD). *International Journal of Addiction* 30:1549–1602, 1995.

MAY, P.A., AND GOSSAGE, J.P. Estimating the prevalence of Fetal Alcohol Syndrome: A summary. *Alcohol Research & Health* 25:159–167, 2001.

National Institute on Alcohol Abuse and Alcoholism. *Tenth Special Report to the U.S. Congress on Alcohol and Health.* Washington, DC: Department of Health and Human Services, 2002*a*.

National Institute on Alcohol Abuse and Alcoholism. *Alcohol Alert* No. 50: "Fetal Alcohol Exposure and the Brain." Bethesda, MD: National Institute on Alcohol Abuse and Alcoholism, 2000*b*.

OLSON, H.C.; O'CONNOR, M.J.; AND FITZGERALD, H.E. Lessons learned from study of the developmental impact of parental alcohol use. *Infant Mental Health Journal* 22:271–290, 2001.

PRUGH, T. Point-of-purchase health warning notices. *Alcohol Health & Research World* 10(4):36, 1986.

SOKOL, R.J.; MARTIER, S.S.; AND AGER, J.W. The T-ACE questions: Practical prenatal detection of risk drinking. *American Journal of Obstetrics and Gynecology* 160:863–871, 1989.

STRATTON, K.; HOWE, C.; AND BATTAGLIA, F., eds. *Fetal Alcohol Syndrome: Diagnosis, Prevention, and Treatment.* Washington, DC: National Academy Press, 1996.

STREISSGUTH, A. *Fetal Alcohol Syndrome: A Guide for Families and Communities.* Baltimore, MD: Paul H. Brookes Publishing, 1997.

STREISSGUTH, A.P., AND O'MALLEY, K. Neuropsychiatric implications and long-term consequences of fetal alcohol spectrum disorders. *Seminars in Neuropsychiatry* 5:177–190, 2000.

JANET R. HANKIN, PH.D., is a professor in the Department of Sociology, Wayne State University, Detroit, Michigan.

Campus boozing toll

Alcohol blamed for 1,400 student deaths, 70,000 sex assaults a year

By Ray Delgado
CHRONICLE STAFF WRITER

The news that 1,400 college students across the country die every year due to alcohol-related accidents comes as no surprise to Edith Heideman, a Palo Alto mother who lost her son to alcohol poisoning while he was rushing a fraternity at California State University at Chico.

"I'm surprised there haven't been more," said Heideman, an outspoken advocate of alcohol-related prevention programs since her son's death in October 2000. "I think this happens all the time, from what I've heard."

Although college drinking is seen by many as a rite of passage, there are others like Heideman who say it needs to be treated as a major health problem.

A study released today by the federally supported Task Force on College Drinking said that an estimated 1,400 college students are killed in alcohol-related accidents every year, including alcohol poisonings and traffic accidents.

Alcohol abuse also played a role in more than 500,000 injuries and 70,000 cases of sexual assault or date rape, according to the study. More than 400, 000 students between 18 and 24 years old also reported having unsafe sex due to alcohol use, researchers found.

"I think actually getting the numbers out will help the public understand that this is a very large problem, perhaps a larger problem than people might have otherwise thought," said Ralph Hingson of the Boston University School of Public Health, the chief researcher of the study.

The study does not mention whether the alcohol problem is decreasing or increasing but a Harvard School of Public Health survey released last month said that levels of binge drinking—having at least four or five drinks at a sitting—are the same as in the

early 1990s. That study also reported that more students are abstaining from alcohol.

The new report was one of 24 studies commissioned by the task force of college presidents, scientists and students convened by the National Institute on Alcohol Abuse and Alcoholism. The institute is part of the National Institutes of Health.

Most of the papers will be published in the Journal of Studies on Alcohol.

Motor vehicle fatalities were the most common form of alcohol-related deaths. The statistics included an auto fatality if the student had alcohol in his blood, even if the level was below the legal limit.

Students who died in other alcohol-related accidents, such as falls and drownings, were included. Those who died as a result of homicides or suicides were not.

> "I do think that students are finally realizing that you can die from drinking."
>
> SHAUNA QUINN
> *director of the CSU Chico Campus Alcohol and Drug Education Center*

Shauna Quinn, the director of the Campus Alcohol and Drug Education Center at CSU Chico, said she thought the statistics were accurate with what she has seen recently. Binge drinking, she said, remains a serious problem at Chico despite five alcohol-related deaths over the past five years.

Quinn said that although many students who engage in binge drinking at Chico are drinking more than ever, the university's

ongoing battle against alcohol abuse is finally getting through.

"I do think that students are finally realizing that you can die from drinking," Quinn said. "They're concerned about their friends and are taking them to the hospital" if they have been drinking excessively.

Quinn said Chico has been trying to combat its reputation as a party school, especially after the death of Heideman's son Adrian, who was found in the basement of his fraternity house with a blood-alcohol level three times the legal limit for a driver.

After Heideman's death, the university stepped up its education efforts, blanketed the campus with flyers and brought back a free ride program for students who had too much to drink.

Despite those efforts, another student who had been drinking excessively was killed the following April when he was struck by a train.

Last year, the 23-campus California State University became the first university system to institute a system-wide alcohol policy, focusing on education, restricting alcohol advertisements on campus and strict enforcement of existing drinking laws.

CSU Chancellor Charles B. Reed also offered $25,000 to each campus to do prevention work or to establish alcohol centers on campus.

"What we are trying to do is prevent alcohol abuse and also make alcohol uncool on campuses, less glamorous," said Clara Potes-Fellow, a spokesperson for the university system. "Alcohol abuse is also responsible for poor grades, date rape, property damage and fights at the schools. It is important to make the students understand what is safe and what is abuse and what is reasonable."

Chronicle news service contributed to this report

E-mail Ray Delgado at rdelgado@sfchronicle.com.

Colombia

Drug Treatment Programs

BY ROB HANSER

Colombia is a country with a drug culture that can be traced back to the earliest inhabitants of the region (Kusinitz, 1988; Perez-Gomez, 1998). Some researchers argue that social acceptance of the moderate use of the coca leaf may contribute to the diminished awareness of the impact of cocaine dependence among citizens of Colombia (Kusinitz, 1988; Perez-Gomez, 1998). Further, priorities for rectifying poverty and alleviating depressed living conditions have undermined any chance for improvement in mental health and addiction services in most Latin American countries (Boulez & Vaughn, 1995; Francisco, 1995; Kusinitz, 1988; Perez-Gomez, 1998). This is an extremely difficult area to explore because of the social censoring and disorder that exists within Colombia. Further, Colombia has no national comprehensive system of statistics for monitoring characteristics of those who obtain drug treatment within its borders (Perez-Gomez, 1998). Institutions are not obligated to report data, and families pay "out of pocket" for treatment since it is not covered by any form of government assistance; demonstrating a low priority for treatment within the Colombian government (Perez-Gomez, 1998). Thus, underdiagnosing and a lack of reporting systems go hand-in-hand with understaffed substance abuse programs in this nation's public health sector (Perez-Gomez, 1998).

Historical and Cultural Considerations

The mountains and rain forests of South America have numerous species of plants known to alter consciousness (Kusinitz, 1988). The use of the coca plant, from which cocaine is derived, has been dated from as early as 2500 B.C. (Kusinitz, 1988). In the past, Colombian cocaine traffickers obtained their coca paste from Peru and Bolivia and then processed it into cocaine to be distributed abroad (Kusinitz, 1988). But during the 1970s, Colombian drug dealers tried to grow their own coca plants in the mountains of northern and western Colombia (Francisco, 1995; Kusinitz, 1988). These crops were inferior to the imported coca and were not suitable for processing into the white powder drug popular in the United States and Europe. Further, wholesale prices took a drastic drop during the 1980s (Kusinitz, 1988).

Faced with this threat to their profits, Colombian dealers turned their own people into addicts by supplying them with this inferior brand of cocaine. The dealers mixed their surplus with tobacco to produce "bazuco," a cigarette that provides a quick, intense high, followed by an intense craving for more of the drug (Kusinitz, 1988; Perez-Gomez, 1998). Bazuco traffickers targeted Colombia's marijuana smokers, essentially providing the drug for free to build a customer base (Kusinitz, 1988; Perez-Gomez, 1998). The paste contains high amounts of the active ingredient as well as toxic chemicals such as ether, gasoline, kerosene, etc. used in the refining process (Kusinitz, 1988; Montoya & Chilcoat, 1996). Thus, in addition to its high addiction rate, bazuco also poses a serious toxic hazard to those who use it (Montoya & Chilcoat, 1996). The introduction of bazuco has created an enormous growth in the population of drug addicts in Colombia (Kusinitz, 1988; Montoya & Chilcoat, 1996; Perez-Gomez, 1998). The vast majority of drug abusers use alcohol, marijuana, cocaine, bazuco, or any combination of these drugs (Montoya & Chilcoat, 1996). It is cocaine and bazuco, however, that are largely singled out as the culprits behind the majority of Colombia's major domestic drug problem (Kusinitz, 1988; Perez-Gomez, 1998).

Profile of the Typical Colombian Drug Abuser

The typical client in most Colombian drug treatment programs is male, single, unemployed, and anywhere from 18 to 30 years of age (Kusinitz, 1988; Perez-Gomez, 1998; Torres de Galvis, 1993). Over three-fourths of these drug abusers are polydrug users who have progressed from alcohol, to bazuco, and ultimately coca paste (Torres de Galvis, 1993). In fact, alcohol, cannabis, and varieties of cocaine are the chief drugs of choice in Colombia (Torres de Galvis, 1993). Throughout the 1990s and into the 2000s, the profile of drug abusers in Colombia has begun to change. Increasingly, there are more young adolescents who are 14 to 16 years of age and more abusers are female. Although cocaine and bazuco abuse are still the most prevalent drug problem in Colombia, other substances such as Rohypnol and other benzodiazepines are being used more frequently as well (Perez-Gomez, 1998; Torres de Galvis, 1993). Heroin is likewise gaining slow but increased popularity among the Colombian drug subculture (Perez-Gomez, 1998; Torres de Galvis, 1993).

Overview of Treatment Programs

It is important to note that the World Health Organization has held numerous regional workshops to promote uniformity on the standards of service in drug treatment programs in a variety of Latin American nations (Kusinitz, 1988; Perez-Gomez, 1998). Other Latin American countries such as Chile, Venezuela, Panama, and Costa Rica have developed adjusted standards of care and monitoring programs, including accreditation requirements (Perez-Gomez, 1998). Still, in countries like Colombia, very few institutions publish detailed accounts of their procedures which can vary significantly. This lack of information is likewise indicative of governmental ambivalence toward the drug problem (Perez-Gomez, 1998). In Colombia, there is no reliable and publicly available information on the evaluation of drug treatment (Perez-Gomez, 1998).

From the available information, despite its poor quality, it can be seen that some of the local intervention programs hold some promise of success. In principle, all drug treatment institutions in Colombia are members of the Colombian Health Network, which is under the Ministry of Health (Perez-Gomez, 1998). But it has not functioned well because there is an acknowledged lack of expertise; with most governmental resources going toward prevention of drug traf-

ficking rather than treatment of drug abuse. Regardless, treatment institutions within Colombia still struggle to address the addiction difficulties that are ingrained in Colombian culture (Kusinitz, 1988; Perez-Gomez, 1998). These programs come in a variety of approaches and are presented to give a general overview of basic types of programs utilized.

Day Clinics and Nonresidential Hospital Wards

Day Clinics and Nonresidential Hospital Wards have played an increasingly important role in drug treatment programs during the 1990s. Some are funded by the government while others are operated as charities. Typically, these clinics focus on physical recuperation and the adoption of new lifestyles (Perez-Gomez, 1998). Most of these programs have good reputations, at least according to drug addicts who have participated in this regime. Some of the staff in these programs are licensed professionals (psychologists, psychiatrists, social workers), and others are former addicts who have received moderate training to qualify as paraprofessionals (Perez-Gomez, 1998).

Therapeutic Communities and Short-Term Residential Clinics

Therapeutic communities came into vogue during the 1980s in Colombia. Most Colombians do not prefer these types of interventions; their ideology and repressive style, coupled with the extended seclusion (from 6 months to 3 years) that is imposed, creates great difficulty in resocializing these patients back into the community (Perez-Gomez, 1998). Still, these programs are well suited for clients with extensive drug abusing histories or those who have histories of criminal or delinquent behavior (Perez-Gomez, 1998). These programs were implemented as an alternative to psychiatric and mental hospitals. Such hospitals overused various psychotropic medications ignoring cognitive and life-skills interventions (Perez-Gomez, 1998). Because of this ineffective treatment modality, most patients of these hospitals experienced relapse within a month or so of discharge. Interestingly,

therapeutic communities have had high drop-out rates that make it questionable if these interventions are, in fact, an improvement over previous hospitalization (Perez-Gomez, 1998).

Short-term residential clinics, on the other hand, utilize some similar characteristics but are only 30 to 90 days in length (Perez-Gomez, 1998). Treatment is residential, but is highly confrontational, attempting to implement quick and directly applied interventions in a condensed period of time (Perez-Gomez, 1998). These programs are highly cognitive in nature, being reminiscent of a rational emotive therapeutic orientation (Perez-Gomez, 1998). These programs are also very expensive for most Colombians and have not necessarily been shown to be effective. However, it is generally thought that methods of confronting ineffective beliefs revolving around addiction, coupled with teaching cognitive techniques of coping, hold the most hope in producing long-term rather than temporary recoveries.

Outpatient Centers

In outpatient programs, clients attend voluntarily for this intensive form of treatment. Some clients may receive up to 24 hours of face-to-face therapy per week. La Casa, in Bogota, exemplifies this treatment modality. Patients of these programs are often very young (with over 90 percent being between the ages of 13 and 25) and desire to become completely abstinent (Perez-Gomez, 1998). Outpatient centers like La Casa in Bogota do not make the commitment to abstinence a prerequisite for treatment (Perez-Gomez, 1998).

Clients in these programs receive individual, family, and group therapy, and their parents are expected to take part in the process by attendance at special weekly meetings. These programs include motivational interventions and extensive relapse prevention strategies that are routinely implemented within the structure of the treatment schedule (Perez-Gomez, 1998). These programs also network effectively with other agencies to provide for total reintegration, such as with job placement and housing programs (Perez-Gomez, 1998). Lastly, fees for these programs are kept affordable, in part, due to the low overhead of outpatient treatment. Outpatient treatment programs have emerged as the primary and favored form of intervention with Colombia (Perez-Gomez, 1998).

Treatment Strategies in Outpatient Centers

Most treatment centers in Colombia employ a combination of individual, family, and group strategies as well as psycho-educational programs (Perez-Gomez, 1998). During the past decade, there has been an increased combination of treatment methods in a multimodal pattern. Thus, individual therapy is augmented by several other forms of group therapy, community support and outreach services, family involvement, and faith-based interventions. Fundamental to this approach is the involvement of family members, and unless the person is homeless and socially cut-off from family, this approach is given primary emphasis (Perez-Gomez, 1998).

Most all of these treatment centers emphasize self-responsibility and a sense of internal locus of control. The therapy administered is in many ways similar to a Reality Therapy scheme such as that originally touted by William Glasser. While pointing to self-responsibility as a key ingredient to overcoming addictions, these treatment programs make efforts to avoid stigmatization of guilt (Kusinitz, 1988; Perez-Gomez, 1998). Instead, the object of intervention is to instill both self-awareness and self-control, including techniques to avoid situations and circumstances that may trigger relapse. The choice to abuse licit or illicit substances, then, is up to the individual, and this is the premise for accepting only voluntary clients to this type of treatment program (Perez-Gomez, 1998).

Conclusion

Given the current cultural attitudes toward drug use and the amount of social and economic instability in Colombia, treatment programs for substance abuse are likely to experience numerous setbacks and challenges (Madrigal, 1998). Out of those programs available day clinics and outpatient intensive treatment centers seem to hold the most promise for drug abuse treatment. It is hard to be overly optimistic about the future of substance abuse treatment programs in Colombia (Madrigal, 1998). Indeed, the social, political, and economic dimensions of Colombia are very unstable, and this may stimulate drug use that continues to increase among the population that sees little hope for the future (Boulez & Vaughn, 1995; Madrigal, 1998). Further, drug abuse programs do not seem to rank very high on the list of governmental priorities, potentially leading to an ever further deterioration of prevention and treatment for drugs within Colombia's borders.

References

Boulez, E. E., & Vaughn, M. S. (1995). Violent crime and modernization in Colombia. *Crime, Law & Social Change, 23,* 17–40.

Francisco, T. E. (1995). *Political economy and illegal drugs in Colombia.* Boulder, CO: L. Rienner.

Kusinitz, M. (1988). *Drug use around the world.* New York: Chelsea House Publishers.

Madrigal, E. (1998). Drug policies and tradition: Implications for the care of addictive disorders in two Andean countries. In H. Klingemann & G. Hunt (Eds.). *Drug treatment systems in an international perspective* (pp. 195–197). Thousand Oaks, CA: Sage Publications.

Montoya, I. D., & Chilcoat, H. D. (1996). Epidemiology of coca derivatives use in the Andean region: A tale of five countries. *Substance Use & Misuse, 31,* 1227–1240.

Perez-Gomez, A. (1998). Drug consumption and drug treatment in a drug-producing country: Colombia between myth and reality—a view from the inside. In H. Klingemann & G. Hunt (Eds.). *Drug treatment systems in an international perspective* (pp. 173–181). Thousand Oaks, CA: Sage Publications.

Torres de Galvis (1993). Epidemiologic surveillance system of drug use and abuse (VESPA) in Medellin, Colombia. In National Institute on Drug Abuse (Ed.). *Epidemiologic trends in drug abuse* (pp. 418–432). Rockville, MD: National Institute on Drug Abuse.

Rob Hanser is a Ph.D. candidate at Sam Houston State University.

UNIT 7

Creating and Sustaining Effective Drug Control Policy

Unit Selections

Key Points to Consider

- As you read the following articles, attempt to identify additional questions and issues that mold public opinion and shape public policy on drugs. Some examples worthy of discussion are: How serious is the drug problem perceived to be? Is it getting worse?

- What are the impacts of drugs on children and schools? How do drugs drive crime? What are the impacts of drugs on policing, the courts, and corrections?

- How are public opinion and public policy affected by public events, drug education campaigns, announced government policies, and media coverage?

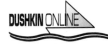 **Links: www.dushkin.com/online/**
These sites are annotated in the World Wide Web pages.

The Drug Reform Coordination Network (DRC)
http://www.drcnet.org

Drug Watch International
http://www.drugwatch.org

United Nations International Drug Control Program (UNDCP)
http://www.undcp.org

Marijuana Policy Project
http://www.mpp.org

Office of National Drug Control Policy (ONDCP)
http://www.whitehousedrugpolicy.gov

The drug problem consistently competes with all major public policy issues, including the economy, education, and foreign policy. Formulating and implementing effective drug control policy is a troublesome task. Some would argue that the consequences of policy failures have been worse than the problems they were attempting to address. Others would argue that although the world of shaping drug policy is an imperfect one, the process has worked generally as well as could be expected. Although the majority of Americans believe that failures and breakdowns in the fight against drug abuse have occurred in spite of various drug policies, not because of them, there is ever-increasing public pressure to rethink the get-tough, stay-tough, enforcement-oriented ideas of the last two decades.

Policy formulation is not a process of aimless wandering. Various levels of government have responsibility for responding to problems of drug abuse. At the center of most policy debate is the premise that the manufacture, possession, use, and distribution of psychoactive drugs without government authorization is illegal. The federal posture of prohibition is an important emphasis on state and local policy making. Currently, federal drug policy emphasizes President Bush's goal of reducing drug use by 10 percent over 2 years and 25 percent over 5 years. Core priorities of the overall plan are to stop drug use before it starts, heal America's drug users, and disrupt the illegal market. These three core goals are reinforced by specific objectives outlined in a policy statement produced by the White House Office of Drug Control Policy.

One exception to prevailing public views that generally support drug prohibition is the softening of attitudes regarding the medical use of marijuana. Another surrounds the controversy of whether to prosecute and incarcerate first-time users or those found in possession of drugs. There is much public consensus that criminalizing addiction that is not related to other criminal misconduct is unjustified. Prison is the nursery for human pathologies that simply wait to infect all who enter. Prison and punishment cause anger and focus—something that is often returned to society in terms of tragedy. Society struggles at determining the levels at which drug users and addicts become criminals and felons.

Still, surveys typically report that the majority of Americans think that legalizing, and in some cases even decriminalizing, dangerous drugs is a bad idea. The fear of increased crime, increased drug use, and the potential threat to children are the most often stated reasons. Citing the devastating consequences of alcohol and tobacco use, most Americans question society's ability to use any addictive, mind-altering drug responsibly. Currently, the public favors both supply reduction and demand reduction as effective strategies in combating the drug problem. Concomitantly, policy analysts struggle with objectives. Shaping public policy is a critical function that greatly relies upon public input. Policy-making apparatus is influenced by public opinion, and public opinion is in turn influenced by public policy. When the president refers to drugs as threats to national security, the impact on public opinion is tremendous.

The prevailing characteristic of today's drug policy still reflects a punitive, "get tough" approach to control. The leveling off of both adult as well as youth drug use over the past years serves to sustain this policy. The prison experience thus remains primarily one of retribution, not rehabilitation. There is typically little opportunity for treatment afforded to the vast majority of prisoners suffering from drug problems. A drug-abusing prisoner, initially committed to the prison system for drug offenses, who receives no drug treatment while in custody, is a virtual guarantee to reoffend. Correctional settings that are offering drug treatment to qualified offenders are reducing recidivism significantly. Court-directed coercion of drug offenders, as a mechanism to force offenders into treatment, is generally meeting with positive results. And in some cases, successful treatment and rehabilitation accompany the incentive to have arrests ultimately expunged and be rewarded with reentering society as a citizen, not a felon. A state of California study found that every dollar spent on treatment saved $7 in hospital admissions and law-enforcement costs. Nevertheless, the degree to which Americans are willing to support and sustain a less enforcement-oriented response to drug policy questions remains to be seen. There is concern that even with a shift in policy toward education, prevention, and treatment, an intense, enforcement-oriented perspective will remain on the nation's poor, inner-urban, largely minority subpopulations.

Another complicated aspect of creating national as well as local drug policy is consideration of the growing body of research on the subject. The past 20 years have produced numerous public and private investigations, surveys, and conclusions relative to the dynamic of drug use in American society. Most literature reflects, however, an indirect influence of research on large-scale policy decisions. There is a saying that "policy makers use research like a drunk uses a lamppost—for support, rather than illumination." One exception, however, to the continued enforcement-oriented nature of federal policy is the consistently increasing commitment to treatment. This commitment comes as a direct result of research related to progress achieved in treating and rehabilitating users. Treatment, in terms of dollars spent, can compete with all other components of drug control policy.

Further complicating the research/policy-making relationship is that the policy-making community is largely composed of persons of diverse backgrounds, professional capacities, and political interests. Some are elected officials, others are civil servants, and many are private citizens from the medical and educational communities. In some cases, such as with alcohol and tobacco, powerful industry players assert a tremendous influence on policy. As you read on, consider the new research-related implications for drug policy, such as those addressing the incarceration of drug offenders.

Higher Learning

The court also backs schools' right to randomly screen students for drugs

By RON STODGHILL

ONE MIGHT SAY THAT LOCKNEY, A SMALL FARMING COMMUNITY in the Texas panhandle, was ahead of its time. A couple of years ago, with local drug trafficking and addiction on the rise, the local school district adopted one of the strongest drug-testing policies in the country: all kids in Grades 6 through 12 were subject to mandatory drug tests, with spot checks throughout the semester. "Our purpose was to provide a deterrent for the students, not to catch them," says superintendent Raymond Lusk. "If they were caught, there'd be consequences, certainly, but that's not why we did it."

At $18 a student per test, the price was manageable, and the district's administrators believed that random testing of even 10% of the student body each month was worth it. That is, until a parent, backed by the American Civil Liberties Union (A.C.L.U.), sued to have the testing stopped, claiming a violation of the Fourth Amendment protection against unreasonable search and seizure. The district settled the suit and discontinued testing after just one year.

The Lockney officials are vindicated by last week's Supreme Court ruling that random drug testing of students involved in extracurricular activities is constitutional. Still, Lusk is reluctant to give testing another try for fear of rekindling local opposition. "It's opened the door," he says of the ruling. "We just don't know how wide or even if we want to walk through it again or not."

The court's 5-to-4 decision came in a case brought by an Oklahoma girl who objected to her town's policy of randomly testing students who participated in any school-sponsored group. It expanded a 1995 ruling that sanctioned drug tests for members of school athletic teams. Civil libertarians have argued that such policies violate young people's privacy. But in his majority opinion, Justice Clarence Thomas wrote, "Securing order in the school environment sometimes requires that students be subjected to greater controls than those appropriate for adults."

Even those administrators who have the will to test may not have a way to do it. Many of them say testing is simply too expensive for their cash-starved districts. The cost of testing a student for drugs ranges from $10 to $20, while the more complicated drug-testing kits for athletes can be double that price because of the need to monitor for performance-enhancing steroids. Even after the court upheld drug testing of student athletes, only a fraction of school districts followed through. Many holdouts cite budget constraints; others cite privacy issues. A.C.L.U. attorney Graham Boyd warns, "If drug testing now becomes a rite of passage... the door will be cracked open wider to government demands for DNA, medical records, financial information and other personal data."

Fairness is another concern. Edwin Darden, senior staff attorney for the National School Boards Association, agrees that the ruling "captures the imagination that some nice kid who blows the trumpet, is in the chess club or is in the Future Farmers of America will be subjected to all these drug tests." But in practice Darden expects "a nonreaction" similar to what followed the 1995 ruling on athlete testing.

But for schools that are willing and able to pay the price, the court's ruling provides one more weapon in the war against drugs. Oklahoma school officials say that after everything from surveillance cameras to canine patrols failed to reduce drug use, random testing was a desperate last resort—and proved the most effective deterrent of all. "Without testing for drugs, we just weren't effectively eliminating the problem," says Linda Meoli, attorney for the Oklahoma school district. "We really needed another, better tool."

—With reporting by Joe Pappalardo/New York

U.S., Canada clash on pot laws

Parliament's plan to decriminalize possession creates rift

By Donna Leinwand
USA TODAY

The Bush administration is hinting that it could make it more difficult for Canadian goods to get into this country if Canada's Parliament moves ahead with a proposal to drop criminal penalties for possession of small amounts of marijuana.

The proposal, part of an effort to overhaul Canada's anti-drug policies, essentially would treat most marijuana smokers there the same as people who get misdemeanor traffic tickets. Violators would be ticketed and would have to pay a small fine, but they no longer would face jail time.

Canada's plan isn't that unusual: 12 U.S. states and most of the 15 nations in the European Union have eased penalties on first-time offenders in recent years. That's a reflection of how many governments have grown weary of pursuing individual marijuana users.

But U.S. officials, while stressing that they aren't trying to interfere in Canada's affairs, are urging Canadians to resist decriminalizing marijuana.

In a lobbying campaign that has seemed heavy-handed to some Canadians, U.S. officials have said that such a change in Canada's laws would undermine tougher anti-drug statutes in the USA, lead to more smuggling and create opportunities for organized crime. Bush administration aides note that marijuana is an increasing problem along the Canadian border, where U.S. inspectors seized more than 19,000 pounds of the leaf in 2002, compared with less than 2,000 pounds four years earlier.

In December, U.S. anti-drug czar John Walters stumped across Canada, criticizing the decriminalization plan. He told business groups in Vancouver, where police allow public pot-smoking in some areas, that they would face tighter security at the U.S. border if Canada eased its marijuana laws.

The backlash was immediate across Canada, where surveys have shown that nearly 70% of the country believes that possessing a small amount of marijuana should be punishable only by a small fine. Canadian newspapers accused the USA of being arrogant and called Walters paranoid.

For years, the USA and Canada have squabbled over border issues like longtime friends with a few habits that annoy each other. U.S. officials dislike Canada's looser immigration laws and limited regulation of prescription drugs, particularly pseudoephedrine, used to make methamphetamine.

Canadian officials complain that Colombian cocaine and Mexican heroin often enter Canada via the USA. Canadians argue that the USA should do more to curb Americans' demand for illegal drugs, because restricting the supply only increases prices.

Canada's full Parliament is likely to consider a decriminalization proposal soon.

Committees in the House of Commons and the Senate have issued reports that say police should not arrest people for smoking marijuana, adding momentum to the decriminalization effort. Early versions of the proposal say those caught with no more than 30 grams—about an ounce—of marijuana for personal use would be ticketed and fined an undetermined amount.

'Drug tourist' penalties

Marijuana possession in Canada now is a criminal offense that can carry jail time. Although people convicted of such an offense rarely are sent to jail, they do end up with a criminal record. In the USA, states generally prosecute marijuana-possession offenses, and sentences vary from mandatory jail time to fines. Under federal sentencing guidelines, a person convicted of possession could be sentenced to a year in jail.

Canada would keep criminal penalties for marijuana offenses that pose a significant danger to others, such as illegal trafficking, selling to minors or driving while under the influence of the drug. To prevent "drug tourists," Canadian officials say they would consider special penalties for sales to non-Canadians.

Walters and other U.S. officials said they are worried that such a policy change would make marijuana more available in Canada, leading to more smuggling. They say drug gangs, sensing a more tolerant climate, probably would move their operations near the Canadian-U.S. border, and more Ameri-

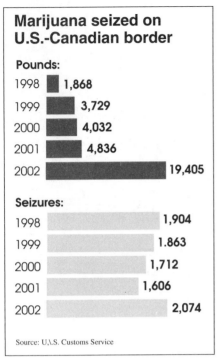

Marijuana seized on U.S.-Canadian border

Pounds:

1998 — 1,868
1999 — 3,729
2000 — 4,032
2001 — 4,836
2002 — 19,405

Seizures:

1998 — 1,904
1999 — 1.863
2000 — 1,712
2001 — 1,606
2002 — 2,074

Source: U,\.S. Customs Service

By Julie Snider, USA TODAY

can teens would cross the border to smoke pot.

Looser marijuana laws in Canada would make it "probable we will have to do more restrictive things at the border," Walters said.

For Canadians who have been slowed by security checks imposed by the USA since the Sept. 11, 2001, terrorists attacks, that would mean more delays in crossing the border, he said. That could damage Canadian business; trade with the USA accounts for 70% of Canada's exports.

Canadian Sen. Pierre-Claude Nolin, head of the panel that released the Senate report and a supporter of eased penalties, doubts that a new marijuana policy in Canada would lead U.S. officials to hinder trade.

Walters "should have respect for our courts and our public," Nolin says. "He cannot stop 8,000 semitrailers at the Windsor (Detroit) border every day. He's saying that, but he will not do that."

Marijuana use in the USA has risen during the past decade. A 2001 study by U.S. government and university researchers indicated that 49% of high school seniors had smoked pot, up from 32.6% in 1992.

In Canada, authorities say their studies indicate that about 30% of Canadians ages 12 to 64 have used marijuana at least once. Although drug use generally is presumed to be rising, Canadian officials say they do not have accurate data they could use to plot a trend.

Canadians say America's rising demand for marijuana makes smuggling appealing to criminal organizations. They also cite the dozen U.S. states that have cut penalties for marijuana possession in recent years—Alaska, California, Colorado, Maine, Minnesota, Mississippi, Nebraska, Nevada, New York, North Carolina, Ohio and Oregon—and say the U.S. government should focus more attention on them.

"It is up to each country to get its own house in order before criticizing its neighbor," a Canadian Senate report said. In the USA, state and local prosecutors handle most marijuana cases. Federal prosecutors usually handle cases that involve large amounts of the leaf or that involve suspects who cross state or national borders.

Asa Hutchinson, a former head of the U.S. Drug Enforcement Administration who now is a top official at the Department of Homeland Security, said last year that "we have to accept responsibility, and we're trying to reduce demand. But without being critical of Canada, we're simply stating a reality: The decision of the Canadian government will have a consequence in this country."

More from Mexico

U.S. Customs agents say the amount of marijuana entering the USA for Canada is dwarfed by that from Mexico. The Royal Canadian Mounted police says 800 tons of marijuana circulates in Canada each year. It's grown mostly in British Columbia, Ontario and Quebec—all of which border the USA. Canadian and U.S. officials say they do not know how much Canadian pot reaches the USA.

"B.C. Bud," the potent, hydroponically grown marijuana from British Columbia, and its eastern counterpart, "Quebec Gold," sell for as much as $4,500 a pound, the DEA says.

If Canada decriminalizes marijuana, U.S. Customs officials expect to see more marijuana coming over the northern border, Customs spokesman Dean Boyd says. "It doesn't take a rocket scientist to come to that conclusion."

Canadian Justice Minister Martin Cauchon, who soon will present the government's plan for decriminalization, says he wants to bring Canadian law in line with public opinion and with judicial rulings favoring lighter penalties for marijuana possession. "We're not talking about being weak. We want to have tougher law enforcement. Our policy toward trafficking will remain the same.

WASHINGTON'S UNSAVORY ANTIDRUG PARTNERS

"The willingness of U.S. administrations to collaborate with the most-odious dictatorships in the war on drugs is long-standing and continuing."

BY TED GALEN CARPENTER

AMERICAN OFFICIALS have frequently cooperated with unsavory regimes in an attempt to stem drug trafficking, even when Washington has treated those regimes as pariahs on all other issues. A graphic example of that dual approach occurred in May, 2002, when a senior member of the military junta ruling Burma, Col. Kyaw Thein, came to Washington for discussions with Bush Administration officials on ways to improve his government's efforts to eradicate illicit opium production. Kyaw met with Assistant Secretary of State Rand Beers, as well as officials of the Drug Enforcement Administration (DEA), the Justice and Treasury departments, and the White House Office of National Drug Control Policy.

Kyaw's visit was curious on multiple levels. He was a prominent figure in the junta that had strangled Burma's aspirations for democracy and harassed the leader of the democratic forces, Nobel laureate Aung San Suu Kyi, for years. That mistreatment has included placing her under house arrest for nine months—an episode that had just ended in early May. Kyaw's trip was a departure from the ban imposed in 1996 on visits to the U.S. by high-ranking members of the junta. Indeed, Kyaw had been specifically named as being ineligible to receive a visa. Yet, to discuss drug policy, he was now welcome

in Washington. His visit could not even be interpreted as a reward to Burma's military leaders for freeing Suu Kyi. Administration officials conceded that the visit had been planned for weeks—long before her release. Yet, the Administration emphasized that the extensive talks with Kyaw did not herald a loosening of the economic sanctions that had been imposed on Burma. Cooperation was to take place on the drug issue alone.

That was not the first time U.S. officials had sought to make an exception to general policy toward Burma in the name of waging the war on drugs. In 1995, Lee P. Brown, director of the White House Office of National Drug Control Policy under Pres. Bill Clinton, led a push for expanded cooperation with the Burmese military to eradicate poppy fields and arrest traffickers. Thomas A. Constantine, director of the DEA; Assistant Secretary of State Robert Gelbard; and Under Secretary of State for Global Affairs Timothy E. Wirth supported Brown's effort. They waged their campaign even though the State Department's most-recent human rights report had concluded that Burma had a highly authoritarian regime that had killed or jailed its political opponents, squelched free speech and demonstrations, and impressed thousands of people into forced labor to assist the military.

Brown summarized his attitude and that of his colleagues on that uncomfortable issue: "I'm very concerned about human rights violations in Burma. But I'm equally concerned about human rights in America and the poison being exported from Burma that ends up on the streets of our cities." In other words, fighting drug trafficking took precedence over any qualms Americans might have about the brutally repressive nature of the Burmese junta. Although Brown did not get his wish entirely, some American cooperation with Burma continued throughout the remainder of the 1990s, despite Washington's overall policy of trying to isolate the military regime.

Throughout the decades since Pres. Richard Nixon first proclaimed a war on drugs in 1971, the U.S. has repeatedly made a "drug war exception" in its foreign policy toward repugnant and repressive regimes. Policy toward Burma has been no means an aberration. The U.S. adopted a similar approach to Panama's dictator, Manuel Noriega; Peru's authoritarian president, Alberto Fujimori; and even Cuban dictator Fidel Castro. Incredibly, Washington even sought to cooperate with the infamous Taliban regime in Afghanistan and praised its effort to eradicate the cultivation of opium poppies.

When the Taliban announced a ban on opium cultivation in early 2001, U.S. officials were most complimentary. James P. Callahan, director of Asian affairs for the State Department's Bureau of International Narcotics and Law Enforcement Affairs, uncritically relayed the alleged accounts of Afghan farmers that "the Taliban used a system of consensus-building" to develop and implement the edict. That characterization was more than a little dubious, since the Taliban was not known for pursuing consensus in other aspects of its rule. *Los Angeles Times* columnist Robert Scheer was scathing in his criticism of the U.S. response. "That a totalitarian country can effectively crack down on farmers is not surprising," he noted, but Sheer contended that "it is grotesque" for a U.S. official to describe the drug-crop crackdown in such benign terms.

The Bush Administration did more than praise the Taliban's announced ban on opium cultivation. In mid May, 2001, Secretary of State Colin Powell announced a $43,000,000 grant to Afghanistan in addition to the humanitarian aid the U.S. had long been providing to agencies assisting Afghan refugees. Given Callahan's comment, there was little doubt that the new stipend was a reward for Kabul's anti-drug efforts. That $43,000,000 grant needs to be placed in context. Afghanistan's estimated gross domestic product at the time was a mere $2,000,000,000. The equivalent financial impact on the U.S. economy would have required an infusion of $215,000,000,000. In other words, the $43,000,000 was very serious money to Afghanistan's theocratic masters.

To make matters worse, U.S. officials were naive to take the Taliban edict at face value. The much-touted crackdown on opium poppy cultivation appears to have been little more than an illusion. Despite U.S. and United Nations reports that the Taliban had virtually wiped out the poppy crop in 2000–01, authorities in neighboring Tajikistan reported that the amounts coming across the border were actually increasing. In reality, the Taliban gave its order to halt cultivation to drive up the price of the opium the regime had already stockpiled.

Even if the Taliban had tried to stem cultivation for honest reasons, U.S. cooperation with that regime should have been morally repugnant. Among other outrages, the Taliban government prohibited the education of girls, tortured and executed political critics, and required non-Muslims to wear distinctive clothing—a practice reminiscent of Nazi Germany's edict that Jews must display the Star of David on their clothes. Yet, U.S. officials deemed none of that to be a bar to cooperation with the Taliban on drug policy.

Even if the Bush Administration had not been dissuaded by moral considerations, it should have been by purely pragmatic concerns. In an eerily prescient passage, Sheer noted in May, 2001, "Never mind that Osama bin Laden still operates the leading anti-American terror operation from his base in Afghanistan, from which, among other crimes, he launched two bloody attacks on American embassies in Africa in 1998." Sheer was on the mark when he concluded, "The war on drugs has become our own fanatics' obsession and easily trumps all other concerns."

Washington's approach came to an especially calamitous end in September, 2001, when the Taliban regime was linked to bin Laden's terrorist attacks on the World Trade Center and the Pentagon that killed more than 3,000 people. Moreover, evidence quickly emerged that the Taliban all along had been collecting millions of dollars in profits from the illicit drug trade, with much of that money going into the coffers of the terrorists. Rarely is there such graphic evidence of the bankruptcy of American drug policy.

When it comes to waging the war on drugs, no moral or ideological impediment has seemed sufficient to keep the U.S. government from cooperating with any regime. In recent years, the U.S. has even worked with Fidel Castro on drug matters. As early as 1996, Cuban and U.S. authorities collaborated in the interception and search of a Colombian freighter carrying six tons of cocaine. Cuban officials acted as prosecution witnesses in the trial of the crew in a U.S. court.

In May, 1999, Barry McCaffrey, director of the White House Office of National Drug Control Policy, praised the Cuban government for its cooperation on the drug issue and urged a broader dialogue. He rejected allegations that the Cuban government itself was involved in drug trafficking, even though previous U.S. administrations had cited evidence of such activity. (McCaffrey's exoneration of the Castro regime drew a stinging rebuke from Alberto Hernandez, chairman of the Cuban American National Foundation. "Cooperating with Castro on drugs is like asking Don Corleone to help you fight organized crime in New York," he stated.)

What was striking about Washington's willingness to collaborate with Castro's regime on antidrug activities was that it stood in such sharp contrast to overall American policy toward Cuba. The U.S.

had severed diplomatic relations with Castro's communist regime at the beginning of the 1960s and had maintained a far-reaching economic embargo against the island since that time. Indeed, sanctions had actually been tightened during the Clinton years. Although there were scattered voices of dissent, leaders of both the Republican and Democratic parties strongly endorsed the hard-line policy. Yet, on one issue—drugs—U.S. officials were willing to deviate from the strategy of making the communist autocrat a pariah. Castro's American critics routinely excoriated him for jailing political opponents, suppressing a wide range of freedoms, and turning his country into an economic disaster. His record, in their view, precluded U.S. trade with Cuba and even made it necessary to prevent American tourists from visiting the island. However, none of that apparently was an impediment to collaborating with his security forces in the war on drugs.

The policy of cooperating with the Castro regime on the drug war has drawn praise in two Council on Foreign Relations Task Force reports on policy toward Cuba. In the second, issued in 2001, the Task Force recommended that the U.S. develop "an active program of counternarcotics contacts with Cuban counterparts," and stated that such cooperation should involve "limited exchanges of personnel" with Cuba's security agencies.

On another occasion, McCaffrey reiterated that he thought cooperation with the Castro regime was a splendid idea and urged the Bush Administration to intensify mutual counterdrug activities. Although there is no evidence of an intensification of cooperation under Bush, there is likewise no indication that the existing level has been scaled back.

When most people think of Manuel Noriega, they recall the U.S. invasion of Panama and the capture of the odious dictator. One declared purpose of the December, 1989, U.S. military operation in Panama was to apprehend Noriega and bring him to Florida for trial on narcotics trafficking charges.

That was hardly the beginning of the relationship between the U.S. and Noriega, though. In the years before the 1989 invasion, Washington's relationship with him had been of a very different nature. For years, there had been close cooperation as the Panamanian strongman assisted Washington in its drive to undermine the leftist Sandinista regime in Nicaragua and prop up the right-wing government of El Salvador against Marxist rebels. Noriega had also received praise from the DEA for his cooperation in helping to stanch the flow of narcotics through his country. The latter was no small consideration, since Panama was a major transit point in the illegal drug trade.

Washington's enthusiasm for Noriega's apparent dedication to the drug war began as early as 1978 when DEA administrator Peter Bensinger thanked him for his support in the fight against drugs. Eight years later, one of Bensinger's successors, John Lawn, sent Noriega an effusive thank you letter. "I would like to take this opportunity to reiterate my deep appreciation for the vigorous anti-drug trafficking policy that you have adopted, which is reflected in the numerous expulsions from Panama of accused traffickers," Lawn wrote. In May, 1987, Lawn praised the Panamanian leader for his "personal commitment" to one important drug investigation: "I look forward to our continued efforts together. Drug traffickers around the world are now on notice that the proceeds and profits of their illegal ventures are not welcome in Panama." The following year, DEA spokesman Cornelius Dougherty conceded that there had been many such letters of praise over the years. "The bottom line is that he was helpful and cooperative," Dougherty maintained.

Yet, throughout the 1980s, Noriega systematically undermined democratic rule—typically by rigging elections to ensure the victory of compliant civilian front men while he held the real reins of power as the head of Panama's armed forces. Noriega was also not above harassing, jailing, and torturing political opponents. Indeed, he was apparently not above murdering them.

Noriega's domestic political troubles first became acute in late 1987 when Roberto Diaz, a retired high-ranking Panamanian military officer and former Noriega confidant, made a series of explosive accusations. Most notably, Diaz presented evidence that the general had set up the 1984 murder of a leading opposition politician who had spoken out against Noriega's alleged involvement in drug trafficking.

Until these high-profile allegations, Washington seemed impervious to evidence that Noriega was perverting Panama's political system and brutalizing political opponents. In that respect, the actions of American officials were consistent with an increasingly familiar pattern. As long as the ruler in question seemed cooperative on the drug war, U.S. leaders were willing to look the other way regarding his conduct, however repugnant. What is per-

haps more surprising is that U.S. officials seemed impervious to evidence that Noriega himself was involved in the drug trade.

Ironically, throughout the period when Noriega was winning praise for his anti-drug measures, there were mounting indications of his corruption. He had been cited by at least one source as the person at the center of Panama's drug trafficking network a decade before his indictment and the subsequent U.S. invasion. As *Wall Street Journal* correspondent Frederick Kempe noted, "Noriega had been arresting many drug traffickers and extraditing some of them to the United States, but just as often he extorted traffickers before they could gain their release." In essence, while appearing to help the Americans fight the drug trade, "he was only turning in his competition, as he skimmed off the profits from a multibillion-dollar industry," Kempe pointed out.

Noriega was engaged in a delicate balancing act, protecting the interests of the Colombian cartels while retaining the support of U.S. officials. "It was a tricky game," Kempe indicates, "but American agents in Panama were particularly easy to con," and it worked for many years. "With each major drug bust that Noriega assisted, and with each fugitive that he helped to extradite, Noriega grew in the DEA's esteem, at the same time that he was expanding business with the cartel. It was a remarkable balancing act that can only be explained one way: Noriega was using the DEA as his own private enforcer." The invasion of Panama and the arrest of Noriega were a dramatic admission of just how misguided previous U.S. policy had been.

Anyone who might have assumed that the Noriega experience had taught U.S. officials a sobering lesson about cooperating with corrupt dictators in the name of waging the war on drugs soon received evidence to the contrary. The most-graphic example was the increasingly cozy relationship between Washington and the government of Peru's autocratic president, Alberto Fujimori, in the 1990s.

The trend toward democracy in Latin America experienced a major blow in April, 1992, when Fujimori declared to the nation that he had assumed exclusive control of the government in an *autogolpe* ("self-coup") with the support of the military. His revamped regime moved quickly to shut down all independent branches of the government. He dissolved the Peruvian congress and eviscerated the judicial system by summarily dismissing 13 supreme

court justices as well as all the judges on the Tribunal of Constitutional Guarantees. During the early years of his authoritarian rule, the U.S. State and Justice departments frequently condemned the regime's human rights abuses. As the Fujimori government pressed its campaign against the Maoist Sendero Luminoso (Shining Path) guerrillas, there was an abundance of such abuses.

Fujimori's offensive against the Shining Path affected many of the peasants in the Upper Huallaga Valley and other remote locales, who grew much of the coca crop and at least countenanced, if not actively supported, the guerrillas. As the effort to stamp out the Shining Path gained momentum in the mid and late 1990s, Washington began to look on the autocratic regime in Lima with greater tolerance. Indeed, from the standpoint of U.S. officials, Fujimori's decision to unleash the military offered the promise of a dual benefit. Not only did it promise to weaken a dangerous radical-left political force, it seemed to be disrupting the source of the bulk of the cocaine flowing from the Andrean region.

Between 1995 and 1998, the acreage under coca cultivation in Peru dropped 40%. By 1999, the decline reached 56%. U.S. officials used terms such as "amazing" and "astonishing" and were quick to credit the Peruvian government. In truth, however, the principal reason for the decline was a fungus that swept through the Peruvian coca crop during those years.

During the 1990s, the U.S. military assisted the Peruvian government in interdicting planes carrying drugs out of Peru to processing facilities in Colombia. American radar monitoring of suspect flights was crucial to that operation. By 1998, Washington was significantly expanding its drug war financial aid to the Peruvian government in other ways. Under one program, a five-year, $60,000,000 effort, the U.S. sought to expand Peru's force of river patrol boats greatly to combat the drug trade in the Amazon basin. At that time, the Peruvian military had just 16 such boats. The U.S. aid would provide another 54, as well as funds to train the additional military personnel needed to man them.

The Fujimori government's prosecution of the drug war was more apparent than real, though. As far as the Peruvian military was concerned, the principal offense of the peasants engaged in growing coca was not that they were involved in the drug trade, but that they helped fund the Shining Path. A cynic might even argue that the military's real complaint was that too many peasants paid off the Shining Path instead of the military.

Throughout the 1990s, allegations surfaced repeatedly that Vladimiro Montesinos, the head of the National Intelligence Service, used his office to shield friendly drug traffickers, even as the military used force against drug-crop peasants who were deemed enemies of the regime. After Fujimori fell from power and fled the country in late 2000, those allegations soared in number. Evidence surfaced that Montesinos may have received as much as $1,000,000 from a leading Mexican drug cartel. At the same time, he and his intelligence apparatus were apparently receiving up to $1,000,000 a year from the CIA.

Despite the unsavory nature of the Fujimori-Montesinos regime, U.S. praise for Peru's antidrug efforts increased steadily during the 1990s. Between 1995 and 1998, coca production in Peru supposedly declined by 40% and the price of coca leaves fell by half. That result drew praise from U.S. Ambassador Dennis Jett. Peru had "demonstrated that the battle can be won against an enemy that doesn't respect frontiers or laws," he stated. It didn't seem to bother Washington unduly that it was cooperating with a regime that had used the military to undermine democracy in Peru.

Learning from the past

The willingness of U.S. administrations to collaborate with the most-odious dictatorships in the war on drugs is long-standing and continuing. It is more than a little distressing to see the U.S. government betray America's values in that fashion. Moreover, it has been a myopic, utterly futile policy. In case after case, Washington's ostensible partners in the antidrug crusade have themselves been extensively involved in trafficking. The fiascos with Noriega and Afghanistan's Taliban government were just the most-notorious examples.

One might well speculate about why a succession of administrations, Republican and Democrat, conservative and liberal, would engage in such conduct. The core reason is probably continued frustration at the lack of lasting, meaningful results in the international phase of the war on drugs. Over the last three decades, the U.S. has made a concerted effort to cut off, or at least significantly reduce, the flow of drugs into the country from Latin America, Central Asia, and Southeast Asia. Despite that effort, more illegal drugs enter the U.S. from those sources today than did when the "supply-side" campaign began.

Instead of facing the reality that a prohibitionist strategy is doomed to fail, that it merely creates a lucrative black-market premium that attracts new producers, U.S. officials are willing to make common cause with any regime that promises to combat the scourge of narcotics, even when the regime in question is thoroughly repressive.

The folly of collaborating with unsavory partners in the international war on drugs may be of more than historical interest. Bush Administration officials and Congressional drug warriors alike are fairly gushing with enthusiasm over the election of Alvaro Uribe as Colombia's new president. Uribe campaigned on a platform advocating vigorous resistance to Colombia's leftist insurgents and an intensified effort to eradicate the country's lucrative drug trade. Perhaps Uribe is a sincere and honorable man who is merely mistaken in his belief that pursuing a prohibitionist strategy toward drugs can ever be effective.

Nevertheless, there are troubling signs that he may be from the same mold as some of Washington's repugnant partners in the drug war. One disturbing indicator was that members of the principal right-wing paramilitary organization, the United Self-Defense Forces of Colombia (AUC), openly backed Uribe's candidacy. The AUC is on the State Department's list of terrorist organizations, and Colombia's outgoing president, Andres Pastrana, has accused it of being responsible for at least 70% of the atrocities committed in his country's complex civil war.

In addition to the unsettling reality of the AUC's enthusiasm for Uribe, one of the new president's closest associates has been accused of involvement in the drug trade. Perhaps these factors will prove to be nothing more than ephemeral dark clouds, but it is also possible that Washington is acquiring another unsavory associate in the war on drugs.

Ted Galen Carpenter, vice president for defense and foreign policy studies, Cato Institute, Washington, D.C., is the author of Bad Neighbor Policy: Washington's Futile War on Drugs in Latin America.

Illegal Drug Use and Public Policy

One can support the war on drugs' goal of reducing
consumption without supporting the war itself.

Michael Grossman, Frank J. Chaloupka, and Kyumin Shim

ABSTRACT

The period from the 1980s to the present has witnessed a
lively and unsettled debate concerning the legalization of
marijuana, cocaine, heroin, and other illicit substances in
the United States. Proponents of legalization argue that
the demand for these harmful and potentially addictive
substances is not responsive to price. Opponents argue
that prices will fall tremendously in a regime characterized by legalization and that the option of legalization
and taxation is not feasible. In this paper we summarize
theoretical and empirical evidence suggesting that none
of these propositions is correct.

From the 1980s to the present a lively debate has taken
place concerning the legalization of marijuana, cocaine,
heroin, and other illegal drugs in the United States. Opponents argue that legalization of these potentially addictive goods would reduce their prices. By the law of the
downward-sloping demand function, their consumption
would rise, as would the harmful effects associated with
increased use. Foes of legalization assert that these effects
may be substantial. Some proponents of legalization
adopt the conventional wisdom that the consumption of
illegal addictive substances is not very responsive to
price. Others are willing to trade off an increase in consumption for reductions in the violence, crime, and other
costs of the current regime.

The present situation is especially grim. The United
States spends approximately $26 billion a year on its war
on drugs, whose aim is to apprehend and punish drug
dealers and users. Ten percent of all arrests are for nonviolent drug offenses. Forty percent of drug arrests are for
possession of marijuana. Twenty percent of those arrested are juveniles, and the actual number of youths arrested rose more than 80 percent between 1993 and 1997.
Drug offenders account for 25 percent of the U.S. prison
population. Largely because of the war on drugs, the per
capita number of prisoners more than doubled between
1985 and 1997. The U.S. imprisonment rate for drug offenses (149 per 100,000 population in 1995) exceeds the
rates of most Western European nations for all crimes (for
example, 95 per 100,000 population for France in 1995).
Almost all drug offenders in U.S. prisons committed non-
violent crimes. Although racial patterns in drug use do
not differ markedly, nonwhites account for almost 75 percent of drug offenders in prison.[1] These costs of the war
on drugs have been compounded by the spread of HIV
and AIDS among intravenous drug users.

In this paper we address three of the most contentious
issues in the legalization debate. First, we summarize recent evidence that casts doubt on the contention made by
proponents of legalization that the demand for illegal
drugs is not responsive to price. Second, we question the
assertion made by opponents of legalization that prices
will fall tremendously if drug consumption is legalized.
Finally, we question the argument of opponents that the
option of legalization and taxation is not feasible. We
raise the possibility that the market price of drugs with an
excise tax could be greater than the price induced by a
war on drugs, even when producers could ignore the tax
and produce substances illegally underground.

As the reader may already have gathered, our aim is to
debunk myths concerning the price-sensitivity of drug
consumption, the effect of legalization on price, and a regime in which drugs are legal but taxed in much the same
way that cigarettes and alcohol are taxed. Thus, our aim
is to provide "grist for the policy mill" rather than to conduct a full cost-benefit analysis of legalization and taxation. In raising alternatives to the current regime, we
realize that the consumption of the addictive substances
at issue generates external costs (harm to others), and we
ignore internal costs (harm to self).

One can support the drug war's goal of reducing consumption without supporting the war itself. Moreover,
changes in perceptions concerning drug consumption
and in the political climate suggest that there are alternatives worth considering. Increasingly, drug abuse is
viewed as a disease to be addressed by treatment and pre-

vention rather than as illegal behavior to be addressed by the criminal justice system. State initiatives to decriminalize the possession of small amounts of marijuana in the 1970s were followed by initiatives to legalize the use of marijuana for medical purposes in the 1990s. According to Gallup polls, the percentage of Americans who favored legalization of marijuana use rose from 18 percent in 1973 to 31 percent in 1999.[2] These developments highlight the timeliness of a discussion of the "sacred cows" adopted by proponents and opponents of drug legalization.

Trends

To put studies of the effects of drug prices on consumption in perspective, we examine trends in cocaine, marijuana, and heroin prices in the United States from 1981 to 2000. While these are not the only three substances used illicitly, they are the three for which data are available for long periods of time …. Moreover, marijuana has been the most widely used illicit substance since the early 1970s, and cocaine was the second most widely used substance during much of the period considered here.

These real prices (the money price of each substance divided by the Consumer Price Index for all goods) are based on purchases made by drug enforcement agents to apprehend drug dealers as recorded in the System to Retrieve Information from Drug Evidence (STRIDE) maintained by the Drug Enforcement Administration (DEA) of the U.S. Department of Justice. Despite large allocations of resources to interdiction and criminal justice as part of the federal war on drugs, the real price of one pure gram of cocaine fell by 50 percent, and heroin, 37 percent, between 1981 and 2000. Most of the cocaine price decline took place in the 1980s; the price of heroin was fairly stable until 1987 and fell thereafter.

The real price of marijuana shows a different trend. It increased by almost 20 percent during the period as a whole. This overall upward trend can be decomposed into an expansion from 1981 to 1991, followed by a decline. The price more than tripled in the earlier period but declined by more than 60 percent in the later period.

- **Decline in real price of cocaine.** The decline in the real price of cocaine has attracted the most attention in the popular press. Researchers have pointed to a number of causal factors.[3] One was the development of the production sector and the results of learning by doing that followed the reintroduction of cocaine into the U.S. market in the early 1970s after a long period of absence. Much of the learning-by-doing phenomenon may have taken the form of technological progress in evading law enforcement. A second factor was vertical integration, which reduced the number of levels in the chain of distribution and the cost of wholesaling and retail-

ing. In addition, there was a shift to low-cost labor as the professionals who dealt cocaine in the 1970s were replaced by unemployed inner-city residents in the 1980s. Finally, the degree of competition in the illegal cocaine industry may have increased over time. While there is little "hard" empirical evidence to support these explanations, Suren Basov and colleagues have found that the 25 percent decline in the relative wage of low-skilled labor since 1979 can account for approximately 20 percent of the decline in the real price of cocaine since that year.[4]

- **Implications for the war on drugs.** The downward trend in the real price of cocaine that has accompanied the upward trend in resources allocated to enforcement does not mean that the war on drugs has been a failure. Using data for cities during 1985–1996, Ilyana Kuziemko and Steven Levitt have found that cocaine prices are positively related to the certainty of punishment, as measured by per capita drug-offense arrests, and the severity of punishment, as measured by the fraction of drug arrests that result in the criminal's being sentenced to prison.[5] On balance, however, the rise in enforcement has been swamped by other factors.

- **Connection between price and use.** Elsewhere, we have examined trends in the use of cocaine, heroin, and marijuana since 1981.[6] Space limitations prevent us from including that material. Here we note that several trends suggest that the number of persons who use illegal drugs rises as the real prices of these substances fall. More definitive evidence on this issue is contained in the studies discussed below.

Demand Studies

Economists use price elasticity of demand to summarize the magnitude of the response in consumption to a change in price. This is defined as the percentage change in consumption caused by a 1 percent change in price. For example, a price elasticity of demand of -0.5 means that a 10 percent reduction in price causes a 5 percent increase in consumption.

"Own-price" effects or elasticities are concerned with changes in the consumption of a certain good as the price of that good changes; "cross-price" effects or elasticities are concerned with changes in the consumption of a good as the prices of other goods vary. If the cross-price elasticity of cocaine, for example, with respect to the price of marijuana is positive, marijuana and cocaine are substitutes in that consumption of cocaine falls and consumption of marijuana rises when the price of marijuana falls. If the cross-price elasticity is negative, the two goods are complements in that a reduction in the price of marijuana causes the consumption of both to rise. Cross-price effects or elasticities are relevant in evaluating a policy to legalize marijuana but not cocaine or heroin. They also are relevant because legalization may have impacts on the consumption of cigarettes and alcohol.

Some theoretical and empirical analyses of the demand for harmful substances such as cigarettes, alcohol, cocaine, heroin, marijuana, and opium employ a conventional framework that ignores the addictive properties of these substances. Others explicitly incorporate addiction, forward-looking behavior, and linkages between past and future consumption.[7] For our purposes, all of these approaches predict that illegal drugs should exhibit downward-sloping demand functions.

Most of the studies reviewed here use city- and year-specific illegal drug prices from STRIDE and self-reported drug use from the National Household Survey on Drug Abuse or the Monitoring the Future national survey. Typically, the outcomes are past-year or past-month participation and frequency of use, given positive participation. At the individual level, the elasticity of participation with respect to price can be interpreted as the percentage increase in the probability of use caused by a 1 percent reduction in price. In a fixed population, this elasticity also shows the percentage of increase in the number of users caused by a 1 percent reduction in price.

Own-price effects.   Cocaine. Estimates in several studies of the price elasticity demand for cocaine participation in the past year range between -0.41 and -1.00.[8] These estimates imply that a 10 percent reduction in price would cause the number of people who use cocaine to rise by between 4 percent and 10 percent. The price elasticity of the frequency of annual use conditional on positive use falls between -0.35 and -0.44. That is, a 10 percent reduction in price would cause the number of occasions on which a participant uses cocaine to rise by approximately 4 percent.

The largest price elasticities emerge from studies that are limited to teenagers and young adults, which implies that this group is more sensitive to price than are adults or the general population. This finding has important policy implications because the prevalence of illegal drug use is highest among persons ages 17–29. Since few people initiate drug use after age twenty-nine, the most effective way to curtail consumption in all segments of the population may be to prevent initiation and consumption among youths and young adults.

The studies just cited do not consider consumption by the homeless and by prison inmates, who may behave very differently from the population at large. Jonathan Caulkins, however, reports an even larger price elasticity of demand for cocaine (-2.50) using data on the percentage of persons arrested and brought to booking facilities in various U.S. cities who tested positive for cocaine based on urine specimens.[9] Caulkins also finds an elasticity of the number of hospital emergency department mentions for cocaine with regard to price of -1.30 in an annual U.S. time series for 1978–1996.[10] These two studies suggest that heavy users may be more, rather than less, price-sensitive than the general population.

Marijuana. Marijuana has been the most widely used illicit substance in the United States since data first became available in the early 1970s. Marijuana price-elasticity estimates are particularly important in light of the reduction in participation between 1978 or 1979 and 1992 and the increase since then.

Rosalie Pacula and colleagues present a fairly wide range of estimates of marijuana participation price elasticities for high school seniors but indicate that a conservative lower-bound figure is -0.30.[11] Their upper-bound figure of -0.69 may be too small given the measurement error in price discussed in the study. They also show that the upward trend in price between 1982 and 1992 and the downward trend between 1992 and 1998 can explain at least part of the "1980s' marijuana recession" and the "1990s' expansion."

Cross-price effects and the "gateway hypothesis." Unlike the studies that contain estimates of own-price effects or elasticities, many fewer definitive conclusions can be drawn from the recent literature on cross-price effects or elasticities. In light of the popularity of the "gateway hypothesis," which postulates that marijuana is a stepping stone to harder drugs, researchers have focused on the impacts of marijuana price changes on the consumption of other addictive substances. Cigarettes and alcohol have been included in the set of substances whose consumption may be affected by changes in illegal drug prices in light of the negative consequences associated with the consumption of these legal addictive goods.

Some of the research in this area capitalizes on the decriminalization of the possession of small amounts of marijuana by eleven U.S. states between 1973 and 1978. Presumably, this reduced the full price of marijuana (the sum of the money price and the expected penalty for conviction of use).

John DiNardo and Thomas Lemieux have found that decriminalization had a negative effect on the relevance of alcohol use by high school seniors, which suggests that alcohol and marijuana are substitutes for one another.[12] Their study provides supporting evidence that increases in state minimum legal drinking ages in the 1980s raised the prevalence of marijuana use. But decriminalization had no impact on the prevalence of marijuana. Clifford Thies and Charles Register have obtained results suggesting complementarity between marijuana and alcohol and between marijuana and cocaine; the use of both substances was higher among persons who resided in decriminalized states.[13] As in the DiNardo-Lemieux study, no firm conclusions can be drawn because marijuana prevalence was not affected by decriminalization.

Studies that use money prices tend to find complementarity. Henry Saffer and Frank Chaloupka have conducted the most comprehensive investigation of money cross-price effects because they estimate demand functions for alcohol, marijuana, cocaine, and heroin that contain the money price of each substance except marijuana.[14] Their results are consistent with complementary relationships among these substances in the sense that a reduction in the price of one of these substances increases the use of all of them. But the absence of a marijuana price from the demand functions limits to some extent the generalizability of their estimates.

Proponents of the gateway hypothesis argue that youth and young adult substance users progress from the legal (at least for adults) substances of cigarettes and alcohol to marijuana and then to cocaine and other hard drugs. Positive cross-sectional correlations among these substances or findings of correlations between early cigarette and alcohol use and later marijuana use or between early marijuana use and later hard-drug use shed little light on this hypothesis. Temporal precedence and statistical correlation are only necessary conditions for establishing causality because these correlations may reflect unobserved individual factors such as the propensity to engage in risky behavior.

Jeffrey DeSimone studies the effect of past marijuana use on current cocaine use using a technique that is meant to eliminate the correlation between unobserved factors and marijuana use.[15] He has found that prior use of marijuana increases the probability of using cocaine by more than 29 percent, even after one controls for unobserved individual characteristics. This is the strongest evidence to date in support of the gateway hypothesis.

Expected penalty effects. The expected penalty for possessing an illegal drug, defined as the probability of apprehension and conviction multiplied by the fine or monetary value of the prison sentence for conviction, raises the full price of the substance confronted by the user. We already have referred to the impacts of the decriminalization of the possession of small amounts of marijuana by eleven states between 1973 and 1978 in our discussion of cross-price effects. DiNardo and Lemieux and Thies and Register have found no effects of this development on marijuana participation, while Chaloupka and colleagues and Saffer and Chaloupka have reported positive effects of decriminalization on participation.[16] The mixed results may arise because nearly every state liberalized its treatment of marijuana possession in the 1970s.

Chaloupka and colleagues and Matthew Farrelly and colleagues have shown that marijuana and cocaine use are negatively related to state fines for conviction of possession.[17] These effects are weak, most likely because the probability of apprehension and conviction is low. For example, according to the former study, doubling the fines for marijuana possession would reduce the probability of marijuana use by high school seniors by less than 1 percent.

Policy Implications

It appears that we have added fuel to the fire of the advocates against legalization. After all, the weight of the empirical evidence is that demand functions for illegal drugs, like demand functions for other goods, slope downward. Youths and young adults appear to be more responsive to price than older adults are. This is troubling, because the former group may discount the future most heavily and may be most susceptible to the type of time-inconsistent behavior described by Jonathan Gruber and Botond K? szegi.[18] Moreover, price elasticities for heavy users are larger than those for the general population, although these results must be interpreted with caution because they are based on small samples and sometimes inferred from outcomes related to consumption.

The magnitudes of the effects or elasticities often are substantial, especially for teenagers and young adults. For example, according to the cited study by Grossman and Chaloupka, a 10 percent reduction in the price of cocaine would cause the number of youths and young adults who use cocaine to grow by approximately 10 percent and would increase the frequency of use among users by a little more than 3 percent.[19] According to the study by Pacula and colleagues, the same 10 percent reduction in the price of marijuana would raise the number of high school seniors who use marijuana by 3 percent.[20] This is smaller than the cocaine price response but may be a lower-bound estimate because the price of marijuana is subject to more measurement error than is the price of cocaine. Even if the price elasticity of marijuana participation were as low as -0.3, legalization might provoke a large increase in the number of users if there were as much as a fifteenfold decline in price, as predicted by Mark Moore.[21]

There is some evidence that illegal drugs, cigarettes, and alcohol are complements, which implies that the use of all of these substances would increase if marijuana were legalized. Finally, reductions or eliminations in expected penalties imposed on users also would stimulate demand.

Impact of legalization on prices. Two factors add fuel to the fire of the advocates for legalization. The increase in consumption that accompanies legalization depends on the price elasticity of demand and on the magnitude of the price reduction caused by the removal of penalties for production and distribution. Published studies suggest extremely large price reductions: seventyfold in the case of heroin, twentyfold in the case of cocaine, and fifteenfold in the case of marijuana.[22]

Jeffrey Miron's extremely careful and detailed empirical analysis indicates, however, that these estimates are overstated.[23] He compares the markup from raw material (which he terms "farmgate") to retail for cocaine and heroin to such legal products as chocolate, coffee, tea, beer, spices, tobacco, and potatoes. While retail cocaine and heroin prices are many times the costs of the raw materials requried to produce them, markups also are large for these legal goods, although smaller than those for cocaine and heroin. These data suggest that the black-market price of cocaine is 2.5–5 times larger than the price that would prevail if it were legalized, while the black-market price of heroin is 8–19 times larger than the price in a legal market. Miron reaches similar conclusions based on prices of cocaine, morphine, and heroin used for legal purposes. He attributes these results to evasion of costs by black-market suppliers. These costs include taxes on labor and capital; costs associated with environmental, safety, health, and labor-market regulation; and advertising costs. The avoidance of these costs by black-market suppliers offsets some but not all of the expected penalties imposed by the government on these suppliers. While the impact on price is smaller than suggested by previous analysts, Miron's estimates still imply that legalization would result in significant reductions in drug prices and, consequently, large increases in drug use.

Legalization and taxation.   A second factor that throws even more fuel onto the pro-legalization fire is that a regime in which drug production and consumption are fully legal, but drug use is discouraged by excise taxes on production or consumption, has not been and should be evaluated. Monetary taxes have been considered a poor substitute for a drug war because excise taxes have been assumed to be unable to reduce drug use as much as a war on drugs can. The argument is that producers could always choose to go "underground" and sell illegally if a monetary tax made legal prices higher than underground prices.

In preliminary research, Gary Becker and colleagues have shown that the market price of drugs with a monetary excise tax could be greater than the price induced by a war on drugs, even when producers could ignore the monetary tax and produce substances illegally underground.[24] This is because the government could allocate resources to preventing production in the illegal market. In effect, it imposes a nonmonetary tax in this market whose expected value exceeds the tax in the legal market. Becker and colleagues conclude that in certain circumstances the threat of imposing a cost on illegal producers that is above the excise tax if they produced legally is sufficient to discourage illegal production. Hence, the threat does not have to be carried out on a large scale and is much less costly to implement than is a war on drugs when drugs are illegal.

Excise taxes imposed on producers or consumers of drugs play the same role when drugs are legal as do expected penalties imposed on producers and consumers when drugs are illegal. Both raise the full price of consumption and reduce the quantity demanded. But excise taxes are simply transfers, while penalties and efforts to enforce and evade them use real resources. Hence, social welfare potentially is greater in a regime in which drugs are legal and taxed. Tax revenue could be redistributed to the population in a lump-sum fashion or used to fund drug treatment and prevention programs. In the long run, legalization might lead to a lower level of consumption than the present situation.

Deterring youth consumption.   To address the problem of consumption by youths, legalization and taxation could be combined with minimum-purchase-age laws already in place for alcohol and cigarettes. Even if these laws are partially evaded, the higher money price of drugs that might characterize the legalization regime might be a powerful deterrent to youth consumption. Legalization eliminates the current expected penalty costs imposed on users. The latter costs are much higher for adults than for youths because adults place a higher value on their time and youths are much more likely to heavily discount the future effects of their current decisions. Hence, an increase in money price accompanied by the elimination of prison terms, community service, and the acquisition of a police record for possession would raise the full or effective price of drugs faced by youths even if this price fell for adults.

We have not provided enough evidence to conclude definitively that the use of cocaine, marijuana, and other illicit substances should be legalized. We have, however, highlighted three factors that have been ignored or not emphasized in the debate concerning legalization. The first is that legalization of all drugs or legalization of marijuana is likely to increase consumption greatly if prices fall by as much as that suggested by many contributors to the debate. The second is that these price reductions, while almost certainly sizable, may have been greatly overestimated. The third is that legalization and tax-ation "the combined approach that characterizes the regulation of cigarettes and alcohol" may be better than the current approach.

Clearly, more research on the characteristics of the taxation and legalization regime is required before it can be recommended. We hope, however, that we have convinced the reader to treat with great skepticism the propositions that the demand for illegal drugs is not sensitive to price; that tremendous price reductions will occur if drugs are legalized; and that legalization and taxation is not a feasible policy option.

The authors thank the editorial staff at Health Affairs; Rosalie Liccardo Pacula; and the participants in the 4 October 2001 conference, "Non-Medical Determinants of Health Status," sponsored by Princeton University's Center for Health and Wellbeing, for helpful comments. They also thank Patrick Johnston and Ryan Kling for providing data on cocaine, heroin, and marijuana prices and Inas Rashad for research assistance. This paper has not undergone the review accorded official National Bureau of Economic Research (NBER) publications; in particular, it has not been submitted for approval by the Board of Directors. Any opinions expressed are those of the authors and not those of the NBER.

NOTES

1. Bureau of Justice Statistics, U.S. Department of Justice, Sourcebook of Criminal Justice Statistics 2000 (Washington: U.S. Government Printing Office, 2001); and R. MacCoun and P. Reuter, Drug War Heresies: Learning from Other Vices, Times, and Places (Cambridge: Cambridge University Press, 2001).

2. Bureau of Justice Statistics, Sourcebook of Criminal Justice Statistics 2000.

3. Jonathan P. Caulkins, Carnegie Mellon University, personal communication with Michael Grossman, 15 May 1995; and S. Basov et al., "Prohibition and the Market for Illegal Drugs: An Overview of Recent History" (Working Paper, Boston University, 2001).

4. Basov et al., "Prohibition and the Market for Illegal Drugs."

5. I. Kuziemko and S. Levitt, "An Empirical Analysis of Imprisoning Drug Offenders" (Working Paper, University of Chicago, 2001).

6. M. Grossman et al., "Illegal Drug Use and Public Policy" (Working Paper, City University of New York Graduate Center, 2001).

7. For approaches that assume forward-looking behavior, see G. S. Becker and K. M. Murphy, "A Theory of Rational Addiction," Journal of Political Economy 96, no. 4 (1988): 675–700; and J. Gruber and B. K?szegi, "Is Addiction Rational'? Theory and Evidence," Quarterly Journal of Economics (November 2001): 1261–1303.

8. M. Grossman and F. J. Chaloupka, "The Demand for Cocaine by Young Adults: A Rational Addiction Approach," Journal of Health Economics 17, no. 4 (1998): 427–474; F. J. Chaloupka et al., "The Demand for Cocaine and Marijuana by Youth," in The Economic Analysis of Substance Use and Abuse: An Integration of Econometric and Behavioral Economic Research, ed. F. J. Chaloupka et al. (Chicago: University of Chicago Press, 1999), 133–155; H. Saffer and F. J. Chaloupka, "The Demand for Illicit Drugs," Economic Inquiry 37, no. 3 (1999): 401–411; and M. C. Farrelly et al., "The Joint Demand for Cigarettes and Marijuana: Evidence from the National Household Surveys on Drug Abuse," Journal of Health Economics 20, no. 1 (2001): 51–68.

9. J. P. Caulkins, "Estimating Elasticities of Demand for Cocaine and Heroin with DUF Data" (Working Paper, Heinz School of Public Policy, Carnegie Mellon University, 1996).

10. J. P. Caulkins, "Drug Prices and Emergency Department Mentions for Cocaine and Heroin," American Journal of Public Health 91, no. 9 (2001): 1446–1448.

11. R. L. Pacula et al., "Marijuana and Youth," in Risky Behavior among Youths: An Economic Analysis, ed. J. Gruber (Chicago: University of Chicago Press, 2000), 271–326.

12. J. DiNardo and T. Lemieux, "Alcohol, Marijuana, and American Youth: The Unintended Effects of Government Regulation," Journal of Health Economics 20, no. 6 (2001): 991–1010.

13. C. F. Thies and C. A. Register, "Decriminalization of Marijuana and the Demand for Alcohol, Marijuana, and Cocaine," Social Science Journal 30, no. 4 (1993): 385–399.

14. Saffer and Chaloupka, "The Demand for Illicit Drugs."

15. J. DeSimone, "Is Marijuana a Gateway Drug?" Eastern Economics Journal 24, no. 2 (1998): 149–164.

16. DiNardo and Lemieux, "Alcohol, Marijuana, and American Youth"; Thies and Register, "Decriminalization of Marijuana"; Chaloupka et al., "The Demand for Cocaine and Marijuana by Youth"; and Saffer and Chaloupka, "The Demand for Illicit Drugs."

17. Chaloupka et al., "The Demand for Cocaine and Marijuana by Youth"; and Farrelly et al., "The Joint Demand for Cigarettes and Marijuana."

18. Gruber and K?szegi, "Is Addiction Rational'?"

19. Grossman and Chaloupka, "The Demand for Cocaine by Young Adults."

20. Pacula et al., "Marijuana and Youth."

21. M. H. Moore, "Supply Reduction and Drug Enforcement," in Drugs and Crime, ed. M. Tonry and J. W. Wilson (Chicago: University of Chicago Press, 1990), 109–157.

22. For a summary of these studies, see J. Miron, "The Effect of Drug Prohibition on Drug Prices" (Working Paper, Boston University and Bastiat Institute, 2001).

23. Ibid.

24. G. S. Becker, M. Grossman, and K. M. Murphy, "The Simple Economics of the War on Drugs" (Working Paper, University of Chicago, 2001).

How to Win the Drug War

The drug war has trampled our liberties, broken up families, and done nothing to stop the flow of illegal drugs. So how can people of good will end this pernicious war?

by James Gray

For more than two decades I was a soldier in the War on Drugs. In the course of my career, I have helped put drug users and dealers in jail; I have presided over the breakup of families; I have followed the laws of my state and have seen their results.

At one point, I held the record for the largest drug prosecution in the Los Angeles area: 75 kilos of heroin, which was and is a lot of narcotics. But today the record is 18 tons. I have prosecuted some people, and later sentenced others, to long terms in prison for drug offenses, and would do so again. But it has not done any good. I have concluded that we would be in much better shape if we could somehow take the profit out of the drug trade. Truly, the drugs are dangerous, but it is the drug money that is turning a disease into a plague.

I saw the heartbreaking results of drug prohibition too many times in my own courtroom. I saw children tempted by adults to become involved in drug trafficking for $50 in cash, a lot of money to a youngster in the inner city, or almost anywhere else. Once the child's reliability has been established in his roles as a lookout or gofer, he is trusted to sell small amounts of drugs. Of course, that results in greater profits both for the adult dealer and his protégé. The children sell these drugs, not to adults, but to their peers, thus recruiting more children into a life of taking and selling drugs. I saw this repeated again and again. Like others in the court system, I didn't talk about it.

More than once, I saw a single mother who made a big mistake: she chose the wrong boyfriend, a drug dealer. One day, he offered her $400 to carry a particular package across town and give it to a fellow dealer. She strongly suspected that it contained drugs, but she needed the money to pay her rent. So she did it. And she was arrested, convicted, and sentenced to five years in prison for the transportation of cocaine. Since the mother legally abandoned her children because she could not take care of them, they all came to me, in juvenile court, to be dealt with as abused and neglected children.

I tell these mothers that unless they are really lucky and have a close personal friend or family member that is both willing and able to take care of their children until they are released from custody, their children will probably be adopted by somebody else. That is usually enough to make a mother hysterical.

Taxpayers shouldn't be very happy, either. Not only does it cost about $25,000 to keep the mother in prison for the next year; it also costs about $5,000 per month to keep a child in a group home until adoption. For a family of three, that means that our local government has to spend about $145,000 of taxpayer money for the first year simply to separate a mother from her children. And it falls upon me to enforce this result. I do it, because I am required by my oath of office to follow the law.

But there came a time when I could be quiet about this terrible situation no longer.

I concluded that helping to repeal drug prohibition was the best and most lasting gift I could make to my country. On April 8, 1992, I held a press conference outside the Courthouse in Santa Ana and recommended that we as a country investigate the possibility of change.

Since that time, I have spoken on this subject as often as possible, consistent with getting my cases tried. Most people listen; some agree, and others still want to punish me for my attempts to have an open and honest discussion of drug policy. I remember a short introduction I received before one of my talks, which was along the lines of: "I know you all want to hear the latest dope from the courthouse, so here's Judge Gray."

The major parties will never begin the process of ending the War on Drugs. It takes another party to do that—one that holds dear the principles of liberty.

During the next few years, I worked on a book to expose the evil anti-drug crusade. In 2001, my book, *Why Our Drug Laws Have Failed and What We Can Do About It—A Judicial Indictment of the War on Drugs*, was published by Temple University Press. It was the culmination of my experience as a former federal prosecutor with the United States Attorney's Office in Los Angeles, criminal defense attorney in the United States Navy JAG Corps, and a trial judge in Orange County, California since 1983, experience which had long before convinced me that our nation's program of drug prohibition is not simply a failure, but a hopeless failure.

In February, I took another step to end the War on Drugs. After being a Republican for all of my adult life, I registered as a member of the Libertarian Party. I realized that the major parties will never begin the process of ending the War on Drugs. It takes another party to do that—one that holds dear the principles of liberty. I had taken the "World's Smallest Political Quiz," and discovered that I was already a libertarian. I was frustrated and concerned about our country's lack of principled leadership, the direction of our economy, and the continued subversion of the protections of our Bill of Rights. The Libertarian Party is my natural home. And it is the Libertarian Party's historic mission to begin the peace process in the War on Drugs.

Drug prohibition has resulted in a greater loss of civil liberties than anything else in the history of our country. The United States of America leads the world in the incarceration of its people, mostly for non-violent drug offenses. Statistics show that all racial groups use and abuse drugs at basically the same rate, but most of those incarcerated are people of color. The War on Drugs has contributed substantially to the increasing power, bureaucracy, and intrusiveness of government. And, of course, the sale of illicit drugs is by far the largest source of funding for terrorists around the world. If we were truly serious about fighting terrorism, we would kill the "Golden Goose" of terrorism, which is drug prohibition.

It is important to understand that the failure of these laws is not the fault of law enforcement. It makes as much sense to blame the police and the criminal justice system for the failure of drug prohibition as it would be to blame Elliot Ness for the failure of alcohol Prohibition. The tragic results are the fault of the drug laws themselves, and not those who have been assigned the impossible task of enforcing them.

"We the People" are facing radicals at the controls of government who are impervious to the harm they are causing. When the head of the Drug Enforcement Administration expressly flouts the will of the people as expressed, for example, by California's medical marijuana Proposition 215, that is one thing. He is a policeman, enforcing the law as ordered. But what about when the head of the Department of Justice subverts that will? When John Ashcroft, as the United States Attorney General, directly acts against the expressed will of the people in this area, simply because he disagrees with it, he is not being conservative. We should call this action what it is: extremist. And when various officials of the federal government use our tax money actively to oppose state ballot initiatives all around the country, we should call that what it is: illegal.

The Republican and Democratic parties are invested in the drug war, committed to it. If we wait for them to act against drug prohibition, we will be waiting a very long time. However, we Libertarians are singularly in a position to help. I suggest that the Libertarian Party make the issue of the repeal of drug prohibition the centerpiece issue of all state and federal political campaigns for 2004. R. W. Bradford has made a similar argument in speeches over the past several years, and in an article in the December 1999 *Liberty*, and so possibly have others. The idea is not original with me, but it is a good idea.

I understand that, historically, the Libertarian Party has been largely unsuccessful in putting its candidates into office. But that can change, and in many ways the voters are ahead of the politicians on this issue. If we can make it clear that every vote for a state or federal Libertarian candidate represents a vote to end the War on Drugs and we capture only a third of the votes of people who want drug reform, we will get ten percent of the vote. That would be enough to make us a political force to be reckoned with and to put the drug war into the nation's political debate.

I want to make this very clear. If we focus our campaign on the drug issue, people who agree with us will not worry about "throwing away their vote" on a third-party candidate. For a change, *every* vote will be seen to matter.

Many Americans have seen and suffered through the unnecessary harms perpetrated by our failed drug policy. And many of these people are organized. By the time this article is published, I will have contacted all the drug policy reform groups I know, such as the Drug Policy Alliance, Families Against Mandatory Minimums, Common Sense for Drug Policy, Families Against Three Strikes, the National Organization for the Reform of Marijuana Laws, the Marijuana Policy Project, the Drug Policy Foundations of Texas, Hawaii, and New Mexico. I will call their members to join me and become dues-paying members of the Libertarian Party, and request their friends and family members to do the same.

The people in these groups are frustrated by the absence of a tangible national movement that they can support. In addition, in many ways they have learned through their experiences to share libertarian principles and values. The more people who register Libertarian, the more public attention will be paid to the issue of drug policy reform. This, in turn, will attract additional members, and additional attention. I think this plan will be successful, because most of the people in these groups are active; they are committed; they vote, and they have friends who vote.

Today, most Americans realize that our country is not in better shape with regard to the use and abuse of drugs and all the harm and misery that accompany them than we were five years ago. They also are beginning to understand that since that is the case, we can have no legitimate expectation of being in better shape next year than we are today unless we change our approach. Accordingly, many of our fellow citizens are beginning to realize that it is okay to discuss this subject.

Whether they know it or not, Americans are looking to the Party of Principle for guidance and leadership. Our slogan in 2004 should be "This Time It Matters."

From *Liberty*, May 2003, pp. 33-34, 40. © 2003 by Liberty Magazine.

UNIT 8

Prevention, Treatment, and Education

Unit Selections

Key Points to Consider

- How effective are drug education and prevention programs? Are they too generic? How are they assessed and evaluated?

- Does the responsibility for drug education and prevention programs lie with the family, the schools, the police, or the federal government? Explain. Who is willing or unwilling to get involved?

- How effective is drug treatment? Do you agree or disagree that providing free, publicly sponsored drug programs would be one way to greatly reduce America's drug problem?

- What must treatment programs and treatment philosophy consider when providing services to a diverse population of clients? If an addicted friend or loved one asked your advice on finding treatment, how would you respond? What are your options?

- How does the prevailing American attitude toward drug addiction reflect an uncomfortable resistance toward becoming involved?

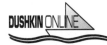 **Links: www.dushkin.com/online/**
These sites are annotated in the World Wide Web pages.

Creative Partnerships for Prevention
http://arts.endow.gov/partner/Creative.html
D.A.R.E.
http://www.dare-america.com
Hazelden
http://www.hazelden.org
Indiana Prevention Resource Center
http://www.drugs.indiana.edu/home.html

There are no magic bullets for preventing drug abuse and treating drug-dependent persons. As one commentator stated, "Drug addicts can be cured, but we're not very good at it!" History is replete with accounts of the diverse attempts of frustrated societies to reclaim or reject their fallen members. Addicts have been executed, imprisoned, and treated with ambivalent indifference. In some circles, the debate still rages as to whether addicts suffer from a pernicious disease or simply a weak character. The evolution of processes used to rehabilitate addicted persons and prevent future abuse has been slow and filled with paradox. Yet the case is not lost. On the contrary, great new strides have been made in not only understanding the various genetic, physiological, psychological, and environmental frameworks that combine to serve as a basis for addiction but in using these frameworks successfully to treat and prevent dependency. Research continues to establish and strengthen the role of treatment as a critical component in the fight against drug abuse. Some drug treatment programs have been shown to reduce dramatically the costs associated with high-risk populations of users. For example, recidivism associated with drug abuse has been shown to decrease by 50 percent after treatment. Treatment is a critical component in the fight against drug abuse, but it is not a panacea. Society cannot "treat" drug abuse away just as it cannot "arrest" it away.

Drug prevention and treatment philosophies subscribe to a multitude of modalities. Everything seems to work a little and nothing seems to work completely. The articles in this unit illustrate the diversity of methods utilized in prevention and treatment programs. Also illustrated is the struggle in which prevention and treatment programs compete for local, state, and federal resources.

Prevention/Education: A primary strategy of drug prevention programs is to prevent and/or delay initial drug use. A secondary strategy is to discourage use by persons minimally involved with drugs. Both strategies include (1) educating users and potential users, (2) teaching adolescents how to resist peer pressure, (3) addressing problems associated with drug abuse such as teen pregnancy, failure in school, and lawbreaking, and (4) creating community support and involvement for prevention activities.

Prevention and education programs are administered through a variety of mechanisms. Schools are an important delivery apparatus, as are local law enforcement agencies. The latest federal drug budget provides for a $10 million increase to the Drug Free Communities Support program and $5 million for a new Parents Drug Core. A total of $8 million was made available to local communities for schools, to implement drug testing in situations where educators and parents deem it necessary. Other prevention programs are community-based and sponsored by civic organizations, church groups, and private corporations. All programs pursue funding through public grants and private endowments. Federal grants to local, state, and private programs are critical components to program solvency.

The multifaceted nature of prevention programs makes them difficult to assess categorically. School programs that emphasize the development of skills to resist social and peer pressure

produce generally varying degrees of positive results. Research continues to make more evident the need to focus prevention programs with specific populations in mind.

Treatment: Like prevention programs, drug treatment programs enlist a variety of methods to treat persons dependent upon legal and illegal drugs. There is no single-pronged approach to treatment for drug abuse. Treatment modality may differ radically from one user to the next. The user's background, physical and mental health, personal motivation, and support structure all have serious implications for treatment type. Lumping together the diverse needs of chemically dependent persons for purposes of applying a generic treatment process provides confounding results at best. In addition, most persons needing and seeking treatment have problems with more than one drug—polydrug use. Current research also correlates drug use with serious mental illness (SMI). Among adults who used an illegal drug in the past year, over 17 percent had an SMI as compared with 6.9 percent of adults who did not use an illegal drug. Among adults with SMI, 29 percent had used an illegal drug in the past year. When binge drinking and SMI are examined, similar correlations emerge. The implications of dual diagnosis are serious, as it is estimated that there are 30 to 40 million chemically dependent persons in this country. The existing harmful drug use and mental health nexus is exacerbated by the fact that using certain powerful drugs, such as methamphetamine, push functioning persons into the dysfunctional realm of mental illness. Providing treatment services to dually diagnosed persons is one of the most difficult and troubling aspects of the treatment equation. Historically, drug treatment programs have avoided or denied services to addicts suffering from psychological disorders such as schizophrenia. Mental health service providers have responded similarly owing to their inability to treat drug addiction.

Although treatment programs differ in methods, most provide a combination of key services. These include drug counseling, drug education, pharmacological therapy, psychotherapy, relapse prevention, and assistance with support structures. Treatment programs may be outpatient-oriented or residential in nature. Residential programs require patients to live at the facility for a prescribed period of time. These residential programs, often described as therapeutic communities, emphasize the development of social, vocational, and educational skills.

The number of available treatment programs is a continual political controversy with respect to federal and state drug budget expenditures. The current trend is to increase the availability of treatment programs. Despite drug prevention efforts, 16 million Americans use drugs on a monthly basis, and roughly 6 million meet the clinical criteria for needing drug treatment. One key component of federal drug strategy was to fund a new treatment initiative in 2004 that would provide drug treatment to individuals otherwise unable to obtain it. More than $600 million was committed over 3 years whereby local governments, through a voucher system, could be reimbursed for providing services at a multitude of levels. Even though most agree that drug treatment is costly, not providing it is more costly.

MICHAEL DARBY'S JOURNEY

A new weapon in the war on drugs: family

A New York program that focuses on drug treatment through family
support is a revolutionary new model.

By Alexandra Marks
Staff writer of The Christian Science Monitor

NEW YORK—Michael Darby has five new reasons to stay off drugs and out of jail: His girlfriend, Denise Ruiz, and her four daughters.

It's the family the 24-year-old parolee has always wanted. And despite the challenges and frustrations that come with such close relationships, he's determined to work to keep them.

"It's crazy because she and the girls got here right on time," says Mr. Darby, who was paroled in September and moved in with Ms. Ruiz shortly thereafter. "I always prayed for a family and someone who could love me a much as I loved her."

The new Darby/Ruiz family is part of what's being touted as a "revolutionary" approach to drug treatment and probation. Called La Bodega de la Familia, it's proven to have significant success in reducing substance abuse and a return to crime among parolees such as Darby. The reason: It looks at the parolee not as an individual but part of a whole family that has its own set of separate issues that need to be addressed for real healing and recovery to take place.

It sounds like simple common sense. And in fact, many of the private treatment centers for middle-class addicts that have insurance make working with the whole family a priority. But because most poor people get their drug treatment through the criminal-justice system, families are usually an afterthought at best.

WE ARE FAMILY: Denise Ruiz and two of her four children helped parolee Michael Darby stay off drugs by particpating in a program started by Carol Shapiro.

"It is one of those things that is so intuitive, but its never really been used," says Carol Shapiro, the founder of La Bodega de la Familia.

"Government in poor people's lives tends to discount the power and influence of family; it tends to think they have all the answers."

A study by the Vera Institute for Justice released in Washington on Tuesday found that illegal drug use by participants in La Bodega declined from 80 percent to 42 percent, significantly more than in the comparison group. La Bodega participants were also less likely to be arrested again and they, along with their families, reported an "enhanced sense of well-being" as a result of the increased access to—and use of—support services.

Principles with policy implications

The findings have caught the attention of policymakers in a wide range of fields from drug treatment to public housing. The reason: using La Bodega's systematic approach to family healing can be taught to social workers and case managers in any field. And with an estimated 600,000 people being released from prison each year and the worst budget crisis in generations—the hope is that any government agency can tap and leverage the power of the family to help in recovery.

An expanded program

In 2001, Miss Shapiro started a new nonprofit called Family Justice which is designed to teach La Bodega's principles to thousands of people in the criminal justice system around the country.

"Considering that we have limited resources, we're always looking for what works," says Rick Levy, New York City's first deputy commissioner of probation. There are currently about 60 probationers in the program and he would like to expand that number.

When La Bodega was started in 1996 as an experimental project in an old bodega on New York's predominantly Hispanic Lower East Side, Shapiro and the other founders thought that family involvement would help participants stay in drug treatment longer. So researchers were stunned to see the significant drop in drug use with no correlating increase in the use of treatment. They went back to try understand why.

"It wasn't the formal treatment," says Chris Stone, the director of the Vera Institute of Justice. "But it appears people were adjusting their behavior because of their changed and stronger relationships with their families."

One of things that distinguishes La Bodega's approach is the program's definition of "family."

The family case managers make it a point of going beyond just the immediate family to provide support by asking their participants about other figures in their lives. As a result the "family" grows to include girlfriends and even close neighbors from childhood.

In Michael Darby's case, it included Ms. Ruiz and her children. They'd met while he was in prison. Ruiz was a born-again Christian. She'd gone to visit Darby as a favor to his grandmother. The two eventually became romantically involved.

Building a support network

When Darby first arrived home after spending most of the past six years in prison primarily for drug dealing, he had a difficult time adjusting to his new freedom and responsibilities. Ms. Ruiz had expected that he'd immediately get back to work. The two clashed, and the relationship almost ended.

"I had my downs and I went real down, but I didn't know how to stop," says Darby. "I almost lost her."

He easily could have been sent back to prison for violating his parole. Instead, his case manager Amy Alverez worked closely with Darby and also helped Ruiz gain a new understanding of the challenges her boyfriend was facing.

"It helped me understand that I have to be patient," she says.

"I expected a lot from him quick, but jail is all he's ever really known, he hasn't really been in a healthy, structured environment."

The two are committed to building a life together. And Darby is ready now, because his life no longer feels like a "black hole" filled with pain, but something that's blessed and is his own.

Harm Reduction: A Promising Approach for College Health

Ralph J. Castro, MS; Betsy D. Foy, MHS, CHES

In college health, we struggle to find effective and salient prevention and early intervention strategies in the realm of alcohol and other drug use. Efforts that stress pure abstinence and prohibition have fallen short in achieving our goal of creating a sustained, healthy campus environment, as is shown by the uprisings and riots on various college campuses over the past few years and the lack of consistent improvement with high-risk, heavy episodic drinkers.[1] As members of institutions of higher learning, we must be the forerunners who test and create novel and innovative forms of prevention and early intervention models that show promising results, just as faculty are charged to do so in their specific areas of scholarship. Hence, we must be willing to look at all approaches, whether controversial or not, to find the most effective methods. One such approach is termed *harm reduction.*

A single definition for harm reduction cannot be found; each harm-reduction program defines its goals and purpose differently. Nevertheless, the guiding public-health principal is the same—reducing the harm associated with a specific high-risk behavior.[2] Harm is synonymous with consequence and risk; however, risk has more complex underpinnings in empirical public health studies. Harm is not seen as a dichotomous variable, but rather as a fluid entity on a continuum; thus, an individual can be in grievous harm on one end and in slight harm on the other end. Therefore, harm-reduction programs must fit the nature of the perceived harm.

In harm reduction, the following 6 community-focused features are present:

- Pragmatism, or working in the parameters of what exists,
- A humanistic approach in which acceptance and the value of others are stressed,
- Focus on the nature of the harm and not the criminal element of the behavior,
- A cost-and-benefit balance to best meet the needs of all involved,
- A peer-based model, and
- Prioritization of immediate goals that lead to quick successes.[3–4]

These features are developed to meet the target populations in their environments where they are most comfortable and are most likely to seek services. For example, much outreach is done on the streets, in shelters, or, in the case of college health, in residence halls.

Examples of community-based harm-reduction initiatives include needle-exchange programs, condom distribution in schools, HIV outreach with prostitutes, methadone programs, designated-driver programs, and onsite ecstasy drug testing. Many programs have the potential to be labeled as harm reduction if their intention is to reduce harm. For a program to be true harm reduction, however, it must actually reduce harm and not merely intend to reduce the harm associated with a high-risk behavior.[5]

One approach to encourage individuals to curb or extinguish drug use is to distribute information on how harmful drugs are and to impose strict penalties. Another approach is to "meet them where they are." In other words, to realize that individuals may currently be using alcohol or drugs or both and provide objective and accurate information on safe and unsafe use while focusing on the problem behaviors and the immediate consequences of the person's actions. This approach allows individuals to make informed choices about their health behaviors—not simply be told what to do. In both of these cases, the goal is for the individual ultimately to stop using risky substances, but the approach is different.

Challenges exist to the harm-reduction model, which is seen as controversial and provocative. Most of these challenges come from our society's moralistic and legalistic nature, which emphasizes temperance when it comes to drugs. Also, many harm-reduction programs work with oppressed and marginalized groups who do not have a strong political voice. Furthermore, the legal issues associated with many harm-reduction programs lead to a polarization of good and bad and the mentality of "because it is the law, it is automatically right." Finally, many harm-reduction programs that show promising results do not receive the attention they deserve because other socially entrenched prevention programs or traditional abstinence-based treatment programs are still the mainstay in the United States. Many of these older prevention and treatment models produce more income for the field than a harm-reduction program, simply because of program requirements such as hospitalization and various psychopharmacological treatments. In some cases, vast amounts of money are spent on outdated programs with little concern for their effectiveness. Providers and institutions that could lose substantial funds are reluctant to look closely at harm-reduction approaches for good reasons. However, we are now witnessing more emphasis on harm-reduction principles in the development of public health messages and strategies with alcohol and tobacco.

Nevertheless, certain myths regarding harm-reduction practices will not go away. Opponents state that harm-reduction methods encourage illegal activity and focus only on moderate and safe use. On the contrary, many harm-reduction programs see abstinence as the ultimate goal in their work.[6] Often, the only real difference between traditional approaches and harm-reduction approaches is that harm-reduction techniques allow individuals to have control in choosing the methods that will best suit their immediate needs.

Harm Reduction and Ecstasy: A Case Example

Ecstasy or MDMA (3, 4-methylenedioxymethamphetamine) is an illegal and controlled drug that has stimulant and mood-elevating properties. Recent studies indicate a rise in the recreational use of this drug among U.S. college-age students, as well as a growing concern in the scientific community about the possible long-term cognitive effects of even onetime use of the substance.[7]

Much of the harm-reduction work with ecstasy and other club drugs has focused on the venues, such as raves and underground parties, where these substances are used. Raves are large parties where music and dancing are the primary event. At raves, some participants, hoping to enhance feelings of closeness and bonding with others while dancing, use substances such as ecstasy.

Harm-reduction programs at raves focus on drug testing and education about making safe decisions. Organizations such as Dancesafe (a nonprofit, harm-reduction organization with groups across the nation) set up testing booths at raves to test ecstasy tablets. The testing is offered because many other highly dangerous substances such as DXM (dextromethorphan) and PMA (para-methoxyamphetamine) have caused deaths to unsuspecting partygoers who are sold the pills as MDMA.[8] The goal of harm-reduction drug testing is to provide accurate and clear information about what is being ingested so that the users can make informed choices about whether to take the drug. Most of the testing methods screen for the presence of MDMA or MDA in the tablet. The outreach worker places a small amount scraped from the pill on a plate and gives the pill back to the user. The tester then dabs a small amount of a chemical on top of the scraping. The chemical reaction and subsequent color changes indicate the presence of different chemical properties in the tablet (eg, MDMA properties). The participant is given a color chart indicating what was detected in the drug test. The testers remain neutral and neither encourage nor discourage the use of the substance. No drugs are seized at the booths, and the tester offers information about the substance and its effects and consequences to the individual whose drug is being tested.[9] The tester offers general information about keeping hydrated and describes overdose reactions as well as interactions from mixing drugs.

In addition to testing pills and providing educational materials, some harm reduction groups distribute water. A number of rave-related deaths have resulted from heat exhaustion and dehydration. Ecstasy is known to increase body temperatures to dangerous levels. Raves commonly take place in crowded and hot environments; and some rave organizers, to increase profits, have been known to sell water at very high prices, as much as $20 per bottle. The outrageous cost can be a contributing factor to heat exhaustion and dehydration if attenders are unwilling or unable to pay such prices.

Harm-reduction groups also distribute educational information about negative behavioral outcomes (eg. heatstroke, legal consequences) from the use of ecstasy. One of the characteristic effects of ecstasy is that it is known to diminish serotonin levels in the brain. Using ecstasy can cause an acceleration of a major depressive episode or a phenomenon users call *blue Tuesday*, in which a person can become sad, tired, and dysphoric for as long as a week after using the drug.[9] The depressed episode lasts until the body can replenish serotonin levels in the brain and achieve homeostasis. The literature the tester gives to the individual explains this common reaction in detail for potential users of ecstasy, highlighting the risks and dangers associated with this outcome. As we progress in the "human ecstasy experiment" over the next several years, we will learn more about the effects of long-term use on memory, cognitive functioning, and other physiological processes and will provide this important information to at-risk populations as well.

Harm Reduction and College Students

At this time, we can and should provide students with accurate information about alcohol and drug use and empower them to think critically and make healthy decisions about their high-risk behaviors. Harm-reduction approaches can be successful with college students because students are a perfect target population: intelligent and open-to-new experiences, with the ability to think abstractly and willingness to help others. We know that we will never be able to eliminate drug use completely among college students, but we can work to lessen the harm associated with high-risk behaviors and can strongly encourage abstinence. Most adolescents who use drugs in high school or college stop using them at some point in their lives and do not go on to become substance dependent. By offering assistance to them in the interim, we may help create an environment that leads to healthy (and less deadly) choices when students are confronted with high-risk and dangerous situations.

Furthermore, harm-reduction stresses a peer-based model that complements the existing peer health model we offer in college health. In addition to the basic health information we currently provide to peer educators, we could easily teach them harm-reduction strategies. By training peer health educators in harm-reduction principles and strategies, we strengthen the messages that we give and also increase the credibility of the medium. For example, at Stanford University, peer health educators are trained in a harm-reduction framework in alcohol and drug issues. From various in-house evaluations, we learned that peer health educators were viewed by their fellow students as credible leaders and resources. Students are not apprehensive when they are speaking with peer health educators because they know they will not be judged and will receive accurate and objective information about any health-related topic. In addition, the cornerstone for a new 3-year alcohol-prevention grant to Washington University in St. Louis targets peer education based on harm-reduction principles. Thirty-six student leaders will receive intensive training in harm-reduction methods specific to high-risk drinking situations and will provide outreach to high-risk peer groups.

Many college and university alcohol and other drug abuse prevention programs already use harm-reduction methods. For example, the social-norm model provides students with accurate and objective information on their peers' use patterns in the hope that fellow students will make informed and responsible choices about their own behavior and, in turn, create a safe and healthy campus culture.

We in college health are in a prime position to implement and evaluate harm-reduction strategies. In a sense, we are already doing much of that work. It is our charge to further the scope of prevention efforts and to push the envelope to discover the methods that we can best use to produce and encourage positive change with our students. Harm-reduction strategies stress the values and ideas that are basic to our university charters and mission statements. Therefore, we must be bold in the work we do and in the methods we choose. Incorporating harm-reduction strategies is a solid beginning.

NOTE

For further information, please address communications to Ralph J. Castro, manager, Stanford University Alcohol and Other Drug Prevention Programs, Room 222, Vaden Health Center, 866 Campus Drive, Stanford, CA 94305–8580 (e-mail: rjcastro@stanford.edu).

REFERENCES

1. Wechsler H, Lee JE, Kuo M, Seibring M, Nelson TF, Lee H. Trends in college binge drinking during a period of increased prevention efforts: Findings from 4 Harvard School of Public Health College Alcohol Study Surveys: 1993–2001. *J Am Coll Health.* 2002;50(5):203–217.

2. Drucker E. Harm reduction: A public health strategy. *Current Issues in Public Health.* 1995;1:64–70.

3. Conley P, Hewitt D, Mitic W, et al. Harm reduction: Concepts and practice. Paper presented at the Canadian Centre on Substance Abuse National Working Group on Policy. Toronto, 1996; 1–15.

4. Des Jarlais DC. Harm reduction: A framework for incorporating science into drug policy. *Am J Public Health.* 1995;85: 10–12.

5. Single E. The concept of harm reduction and its application to alcohol. 6th Dorothy Black Lecture. Presented at the Canadian Centre on Substance Abuse conference. Toronto: 1996.

6. Marlatt GA. Harm reduction: Come as you are. *Addict Behav.* 1996;21(6):779–788.

7. Strote J, Lee JE, Wechsler H. Increased MDMA use among college students. Results of a national survey. *J Adolesc Health.* 2002;30:64–72.

8. Felgate HE, Felgate PD, James RA, Sims DN, Vozzo DC. Recent paramethoxyamphetamine deaths. *J Anal Toxicol.* 1998;2(2):169–172.

9. *The Truth About Club Drugs.* The Harm Reduction Training Institute; Oakland, CA: July 17, 2000.

Ralph J. Castro *is manager of the Alcohol and Other Drug Abuse Prevention Program, which is part of Health Promotion Services at the Vaden Health Center, Stanford University, Stanford, California, and* ***Betsy D. Foy*** *is assistant director of the Student Health and Counseling Center and the Substance Abuse Specialist at Washington University, St. Louis, Missouri.*

From *The Journal of American College Health*, September 2002, pp. 89-91. Reprinted with permission of the Helen Dwight Reid Foundation. Published by Heldref Publications, 1319 Eighteenth St. NW, Washington, DC 20036-1802. © 2002.

Smoking Cessation

Smoking is a risk factor for the four leading causes of death in the United States, yet 48 million Americans—24% of the U.S. adult population—continue to smoke. Approximately 70% of people who smoke visit a physician each year, yet only half report ever being advised to quit smoking by their physician. Smoking cessation is difficult due to nicotine addiction and withdrawal symptoms. Expert groups such as the National Cancer Institute and the Agency for Health Care Policy and Research offer protocols for smoking cessation that primary care physicians can use in their office practice. Recent developments in the pharmacotherapy of smoking cessation has led the U.S. Public Health Service to update the practice guidelines for treating tobacco use and dependence. Pharmacotherapy, which includes nicotine replacement therapy, offers assistance to patients who want to stop smoking. However, the cost of pharmacotherapy may be a barrier for some. Other nonpharmacologic therapies, such as counseling, are also effective. **Am J Med. 2002; 112:399–405.** © 2002 by Excerpta Medica, Inc.

Bernard Karnath, MD

Cigarette smoking is the most important modifiable risk factor for premature mortality [1]. Smoking accounts for over 400,000 deaths in the United States each year [2], and is a risk factor for the four leading causes of death: heart disease, cancer, stroke, and chronic obstructive pulmonary disease [3]. Smoking prevalence peaked in 1966 when 43% of the adult U.S. population smoked [4]. In 1998, an estimated 48 million men and women (24% of the U.S. population) smoked [5]. Approximately one third to half of those who smoke will die from smoking [6].

Fewer than half of all patients who smoked reported that they had never been advised by their physician to quit smoking.

Addiction can be defined as the compulsive use of a drug that may be associated with tolerance and withdrawal symptoms after cessation of the drug [7]. Nicotine dependence disorder is a form of substance abuse that leads to clinically important impairment or distress [8]. Fagerstrom proposed a questionnaire to determine the degree of nicotine dependence [9,10]. However, only the number of cigarettes smoked per day has been shown to correlate with the degree of dependence [11].

In 1989, the National Cancer Institute developed recommendations for physicians who treat patients who smoke [12]. This recommended approach is often referred to as "the four As." In 1996, the Agency for Health Care Policy and Research recommended a 5-step approach (Table 1)[13]. This approach, known as the 5As, is similar to the original approach by the National Cancer Institute, except for the additional step of assessing the patient's willingness to stop. The 5 steps are:

Table 1. The 5 Steps (5As) for Smoking Cessation*

Step 1	*Ask*—systematically identify all patients who smoke ("Vital sign" stamp that includes smoking status.)
Step 2	*Advise*—strongly advise all who smoke to quit. (Tailor the advice towards the patients' clinical situation.)
Step 3	*Assess*—assess the patient's willingness to quit. (Ask every patient if he or she is willing to attempt to quit. If the patient is not ready, then provide motivational intervention to promote future attempts.)
Step 4	*Assist*—assist patients in their efforts to quit. (Pharmacotherapy and counseling.)
Step 5	*Arrange*—schedule a close follow-up. (Follow-ups should occur around the date that the patient ceases smoking.)

*Adapted from the Agency for Health Care Policy and Research[13], with permission from *JAMA*. 1996; 275: 1270-1280. Copyright 1996, American Medical Association.

Vital Sign Stamp

Blood pressure _____

Pulse _____

Temperature _____

Respiratory rate _____

Smoking Status <u>Current Former Never</u>
(Circle)

Figure 1. "Vital signs" stamp that includes smoking status. Adapted from Fiore[16], with permission from *JAMA*. 1991; 266: 3183–3184. Copyright 1991, American Medical Association.

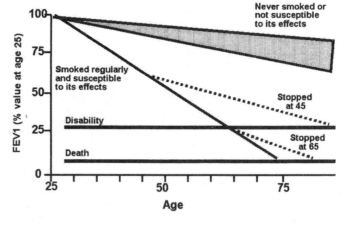

Figure 2. Change in forced expiratory volume in 1 second with smoking cessation. FEV_1 = forced expiratory volume in 1 second. Adapted from Fletcher and Peto[24], with permission from *BMJ*. 1977; 1: 1645–1648.

Ask about smoking. Physicians should ask every patient on every visit about their smoking status.

Advise about smoking cessation. Personalizing the advice can also help.

Assess the patient's willingness to stop smoking. Ask every patient if he or she is willing to attempt to quit.

Assist patients who are willing to stop. Assess the need for nicotine replacement.

Arrange a close follow-up. A follow-up visit around the date of smoking cessation will assure the patient that assistance and counseling are available.

Recent developments in the pharmacotherapy of smoking cessation has led the U.S. Public Health Service to update the practice guidelines for treating tobacco use and dependence[14,15]. The U.S. Public Health Service endorses the use of the "5 As."

Some have suggested including smoking status as a fifth "vital sign." Adding smoking status to routine assessment will ensure that those who smoke are identified (Figure 1)[16,17]. In a study by Frank and colleagues, fewer than half of all patients who smoked reported that they had ever been advised by their physician to quit smoking[18]. A study by Fiore and colleagues evaluate the effectiveness of a vital sign stamp, which included smoking status (current, former, or never), along with the traditional vital signs on the progress note paper[19]. The results of the study showed that there was a significant increase in the percentage of patients who smoked who reported that their clinician had advised them to quit smoking.

Benefits of Smoking Cessation

In a prospective study of 7178 people aged 65 years of older, total mortality among those who smoked was twice that of those who had never smoked[20], whereas subjects who smoked previously had cardiovascular mortality rates similar to those who had never smoked. The risk of developing coronary artery disease can be reduced by half after 1 year of smoking cessation, and after 2 years the risk equals that of people who never smoked[21]. Another study found that among men who had quit smoking, mortality from coronary heart disease decreased to almost the level of subjects who had never smoked after 5 years or more of smoking abstinence[22]. In the Nurses' Health Study, subjects who used to smoke had a 24% reduction in cardiovascular disease mortality after 2 years of smoking cessation[23]. Furthermore, after 10 to 14 years of smoking cessation, the adverse effects on total mortality resolved completely.

Cessation rates at 6 months of follow-up were 33% in the counseled group, compared with 21% in the controlled group.

Forced expiratory volume in 1 second (FEV1) decreases gradually with age[24], but smoking accelerates the rate of decline in FEV1. This can return to a normal rate of decline with smoking cessation (Figure 2)[25]. The risk of lung cancer in patients who used to smoke decreases progressively with the number of years of abstinence, but always remains higher than that of those who had never smoked[26].

Nonpharmacologic Methods of Smoking Cessation

Counseling. A MEDLINE search was performed to find articles that addressed the efficacy of counseling in smoking cessation. Key words used included smoking, cessation, and counseling in combination. Articles published since 1990 were considered for review. Articles were selected based on the presence of statistical data ad-

Table 2. Pharmacotherapy of Smoking Cessation*

Pharmacotherapy	Adverse Effects	Dose	Pharmacokinetics (Peak Plasma Concentration)	Duration
Nicotine gum	Dyspepsia, jaw ache	2 mg gum if < 25 cigarettes daily; 4 mg gum if ≥ 25 cigarettes daily (up to 24 pieces daily)	30 minutes	Up to 12 weeks
Nicotine inhaler	Throat irritation, coughing	6-16 cartridges daily	30 minutes	Up to 6 months
Nicotine nasal spray	Nasal irritation, rhinorrhea, coughing	8-40 doses daily	10 minutes	3-6 months
Nicotine patch	Local skin reaction	21 mg/24 hours 14 mg/24 hours 7 mg/24 hours 15 mg/16 hours	6 hours	4 weeks then 2 weeks then 2 weeks 8 weeks
Sustained-release bupropion hydrochloride	Dry mouth, insomnia, contraindicated in seizure disorder	150 mg daily for 3 days, then 150 mg twice daily	***	7-12 weeks

*From references 15,31,35-37.

dressing the efficacy of counseling intervention in smoking cessation.

Physician communication about the benefits of smoking cessation and encouragement to quit has proven to be successful. A study by Slama and colleagues showed that brief advice on smoking cessation given by physicians resulted in higher cessation rates compared with no advice[27]. Another study evaluating the effect of brief (3 to 5 minutes) counseling by a physician found higher rates of smoking cessation at 6 and 12 months of follow-up for patients who received brief counseling[28]. Similarly, Pederson et al.[29] found that among hospitalized patients with chronic obstructive pulmonary disease, the counseled group had higher cessation rates at 6 months of follow-up. All patients were advised to quit smoking, and half of the patients were provided with a self-help manual and brief 15- to 20-minute counseling sessions. Cessation rates at 6 months of follow-up were 33% (10 of 30) in the counseled group, compared with 21% (6 of 28) in the control group. A study by Wadland and colleagues[30] found that six sessions of telephone counseling improved smoking cessation rates—21% (23 of 110) for the group that underwent telephone counseling versus 8% (10 of 123) for those who received usual care.

Tobacco withdrawal. The development of nicotine replacement therapy offers assistance in the reduction of nicotine withdrawal symptoms during smoking cessation. The Fagerstrom Test for Nicotine Dependence emphasizes the "time to the first cigarette of the day"[9,10]. Nicotine has a relatively short half-life, and smokers may experience discomfort upon waking unless they smoke a cigarette[31]. A study of 554 patients who were attempting to quit smoking without assistance observed that 87%

(482 of 554) of the subjects reported withdrawal symptoms during the first week of follow-up[32]. Restlessness and an increased appetite were the most common symptoms. The signs and symptoms of tobacco withdrawal include craving for tobacco, irritability, anxiety, difficulty concentrating, restlessness, insomnia, and increased hunger[33]. Anxiety, poor concentration, irritability, restlessness, and nocturnal awakening returned to precessation levels by 30 days, but hunger symptoms remained increased at 30 days postcessation[34].

Pharmacologic Methods of Smoking Cessation

Types of nicotine replacement therapy include nicotine polacrilex gum, the transdermal patch, the nicotine nasal spray, and the nicotine inhaler[31,35-37] (Table 2). The U.S. Public Health Service recommends that all persons who are trying to quit smoking should receive pharmacotherapy for smoking cessation[14,15]. However, special consideration should be given before using pharmacotherapy in certain patients, including those with medical contraindications, who are pregnant or breast feeding, and who are adolescents. Medical contraindications include severe reactive airway disease among patients desiring nicotine nasal spray[15]. Pregnant women who smoke should be encouraged to quit first without pharmacologic aid[15]. A MEDLINE search was performed to find articles addressing the efficacy of pharmacotherapy in smoking cessation. Key words included smoking cessation, nicotine replacement, and bupropion. Articles published since 1990 were considered. Articles were selected based on the presence of statistical data addressing the efficacy of nicotine replacement, bupropion, or combination therapy in smoking cessation.

The overall continuous abstinence rates at 15 weeks of follow-up were 23% for nicotine gum, 23% for the patch, 23% for the spray, and 28% for the inhaler.

A comparative trial by Hajek and colleagues that evaluated the efficacy of the four types of nicotine replacement products found no significant difference in the rates of abstinence at 12 weeks of follow-up[38]. The continuous abstinence rates were 20% (25 of 127) for nicotine gum, 21% (26 of 124) for the patch, 24% (30 of 126) for the spray, and 24% (31 of 127) for the inhaler. A study on whether preference for a nicotine replacement product correlated with abstinence rates reported no difference at 15 weeks of follow-up[39]. Subjects were allowed to rank their preference for a nicotine replacement product (gum, patch, nasal spray, or inhaler). Those who smoked heavily preferred the spray or inhaler, but the patch was the most preferred product overall. The overall continuous abstinence rates at 15 weeks of follow-up were 23% (29 of 127) for nicotine gum, 23% (29 of 124) for the patch, 23% (29 of 126) for the spray, and 28% (36 of 127) for the inhaler. There was no difference in cessation rates for subjects who received their preferred products.

Nicotine gum. The U.S. Food and Drug Administration (FDA) approved nicotine polacrilex gum in 1984[31] and its nonprescription sale in 1995[35]. Approximately 50% of the nicotine in the gum is released in the mouth and absorbed through the mucosa. The gum comes in 2-mg and 4-mg doses and can be chewed every 1 to 2 hours for a maximum daily dose of 60 mg[35]. The typical daily dose is 10 pieces, and the recommended duration of therapy is 1 to 3 months[15]. The gum should be chewed slowly and then "parked" between the cheek and gum to facilitate nicotine absorption. The gum should be "chewed and parked" for about 30 minutes[15]. Common adverse effects include jaw ache and dyspepsia[35].

A survey of 25 insurance plans found that only 7 covered some form of treatment for smoking cessation.

A study conducted of the 2-mg and 4-mg doses of nicotine gum found a slightly (but not significantly) increased cessation rate with the 4-mg dose among subjects who had high nicotine dependence[40]. Subjects in this study were classified as having high or low nicotine dependence based on the Fagerstrom test. Subjects were randomly assigned to receive placebo, or the 2-mg or 4-mg dose of nicotine gum. Of the 608 subjects, 92 were ab-

stinent at 1 year. One-year cessation rates for those with low nicotine dependence were 11% (10 of 92) for the placebo group, 18% (17 of 92) for those who received the 4-mg dose. In contrast, 1-year cessation rates for subjects with high nicotine dependence were 8% (7 of 92) for the placebo group, 20% (18 of 92) for those assigned to the 2-mg dose of gum, and 26% (24 of 92) for those who received the 4-mg dose.

Nicotine patch. The nicotine patch was introduced in 1992[35]. There are three major brands: Habitrol (Novartis Consumer, East Hanover, New Jersey), Nicoderm CQ (SmithKline Beecham, Philadelphia, Pennsylvania), and Nicotrol (McNeil Consumer, Fort Washington, Pennsylvania). The first two formulations are intended for 24-hour use; these patches are available in 21-mg, 14-mg, and 7-mg doses. The dose can be progressively weaned over 2 to 4 months[15]. The recommended taper is 21 mg for 4 weeks, then 14 mg for 2 weeks, followed by 7 mg for 2 weeks. The Nicotrol patch is intended for 16-hour daytime use and should be removed before bedtime. The patch is available as a 15-mg dose. The recommended duration of treatment is 6 weeks[35]. Generic nicotine patches are also available. Skin irritation, a common adverse effect of nicotine patches, can be reduced by rotating the patch site[36].

A meta-analysis of 17 studies involving various nicotine patches reported abstinence rates of 22% (319 of 1466) at 6 months for the treatment group as compared with 9% (118 of 1261) for the group receiving the placebo patch[41]. A randomized placebo-controlled trial reported 1-year cessation rates of 19% (163 of 842) for the nicotine patch versus 12% (100 of 844) for the placebo patch[42]. A study of the efficacy of varying doses of the nicotine patch found that patients assigned to the 21-mg patch had higher abstinence rates at long-term follow-up[43]. The self-reported continuous cessation rates at 48 to 62 months of follow-up were 20% (39 of 193) for the patients assigned to the 21-mg patch, 10% (21 of 202) for those assigned to the 14-mg patch, 12% (15 of 127) for those assigned to the 7-mg patch, and 7% (15 of 202) for patients assigned to the placebo patch.

Another study evaluated varying doses of nicotine patches combined with different counseling treatments[44]. One group received 8 weeks of 22-mg transdermal nicotine therapy with group counseling, and another received 4 weeks of 22-mg transdermal nicotine therapy followed by 2 weeks of 11-mg transdermal nicotine therapy with brief individual counseling. Each group was placebo controlled. Six months after initiation of therapy, smoking cessation rates were 34% (15 of 44) for the group that received 8 weeks of the patch plus group counseling versus 21% (9 of 43) for the placebo group, compared with 18% (10 of 57) for the group that received 6 weeks of the patch plus individual counseling versus 7% (4 of 55) for the placebo group.

Table 3. Approximate Number Needed to Treat* Per Patient Who Quits Successfully, At 1-Year Follow-up

Type of Treatment (Reference)	Quit Rate		Difference	Number Needed to Treat
	Placebo	Treatment		
	Percentage			
Nicotine gum, 2 mg (40)	20	38	18	6
Nicotine gum, 4 mg (40)	20	43	23	4
Nicotine inhaler (49)	8	13	5	20
Nicotine nasal spray (47)	10	26	16	6
Nicotine patch (42)	12	19	7	14
Sustained-release bupropion hydrochloride (52)	12	23	11	9

*From de Craen et al (59).

One study found that the 21 mg per 24-hour patch yielded better control of morning craving symptoms than did the 15 mg per 24-hour patch, and also had longer abstinence rates[45].

Nicotine nasal spray. The nicotine nasal spray, which was introduced in 1996[35], delivers nicotine more rapidly than does gum or the patch[46]. The results of a randomized double-blind trial showed that 32% (37 of 116) of patients who used the active formulation were abstinent at 6 months, compared with 12% (13 of 111) who received the placebo[47]. One-year abstinence rates were 26% (30 of 116) for the group that received the active formulation and 10% (11 of 111) for the group that received the placebo spray. The spray is available by prescription in a quantity of 10 mL. Each 0.05-mL spray delivers 0.5 mg of nicotine[35]. The daily dose may be titrated to a maximum of 40 mg. The recommended dosage is 1 to 2 sprays every hour for 6 to 8 weeks. The minimum recommended treatment is 8 doses per day for 3 to 6 months[15]. Tapering of doses in the subsequent 4- to 6-week period is optimal to prevent withdrawal symptoms[35]. Common adverse effects include nasal irritation, rhinorrhea, sneezing, throat irritation, and coughing[36].

Nicotine inhaler. The nicotine inhaler was introduced in 1998[35]. It is available by prescription and consists of a mouthpiece and a plastic cartridge that contains 4 mg of nicotine. Approximately 80 inhalations are needed to equal the amount of nicotine obtained from 1 cigarette[35]. Common adverse effects include throat irritation and coughing[36]. The recommended dose is 6 to 16 cartridges per day for 6 to 12 weeks, with tapering over the subsequent 3 months[15]. A randomized double-blind trial found 1-year abstinence rates of 28% (35 of 123) for the nicotine inhaler group as compared with 18% (22 of 124) for the placebo group[48].

Another double-blind placebo-controlled trial found that the inhaler was useful for short-term smoking cessation with some potential for long-term cessation[49]. Cessation rates were 46% (52 of 112) in the group assigned to the nicotine inhaler compared with 28% (31 of 111) in the placebo group at 1 week, 24% (n = 27) versus 10% (n = 11) at 3 months, and 13% (n = 15) versus 8% (n = 9) at 1 year of follow-up.

Nicotine replacement in patients with coronary artery disease. Although there has been concern about the safety of nicotine replacement in patients with cardiovascular disease, two studies suggest that it is safe. One study randomly assigned 584 patients who had cardiovascular disease to a 10-week course of transdermal nicotine or placebo[50]. Primary endpoints after 14 weeks of follow-up included death, myocardial infarction, cardiac arrest, and admission to the hospital for angina, arrhythmia, or heart failure. The study showed no significant increase in cardiovascular events for patients receiving nicotine replacement therapy. In a similar study[51], 156 patients with coronary artery disease who smoked at least 1 pack of cigarettes per day were randomly assigned to receive transdermal nicotine or placebo. After 5 weeks of follow-up, the study showed no significant difference in the rate of cardiac events.

Bupropion hydrochloride. Bupropion hydrochloride was introduced in 1997 as an aid for smoking cessation[35]. The recommended dose is 150 mg once daily for 3 days, then 150 mg twice daily for up to 12 weeks[35]. A cessation date should be set 1 to 2 weeks after initiating therapy. A double-blind placebo-controlled trial of sustained-release bupropion found that cessation rates increased with the dose of the medication[52]. The 7-week cessation rates were 19% (29 of 153) for the placebo group, 29% (44 of 153) for the 100-mg group, 39% (59 of 153) for the 150-mg group, and 44% (69 of 156) for the 300-mg group. The 1-year abstinence rates were 12% (19 of 153) for the placebo group, 20% (30 of 153) for the 100-mg group, 23% (35 of 153) for the 150-mg group, and 23% (36 of 156) for the 300-mg group.

Bupropion became available as an immediate-release formulation in 1988, however, seizures were a concern

Table 4. Cost of Pharmacotherapy for Smoking Cessation*

Pharmacotherapy	Availability	Cost Per Day (Typical Daily Dose)	Cost Per Recommended Course of Therapy ($)	Estimated Cost Per Successful Quitter Based on Number Needed to Treat[†] ($)
Nicotine gum	Over the counter	$6.25 for 10 pieces (2 mg)	563 for 3 months	3400
		$6.87 for 10 pieces (4 mg)	618 for 3 months	2500
Nicotine inhaler	Prescription	$10.94 for 10 cartridges	985 for 3 months	19 700
Nicotine nasal spray	Prescription	$5.40 for 12 doses	486 for 3 months	2900
Nicotine patch	Prescription and over the counter (includes generic)	$3.50-$4.50 per patch	240 for 2 months	3400
Sustained-release bupropion hydrochloride	Prescription	$3.33 for 2 doses (150 mg)	300 for 3 months	2700

*From references 15,31,35-37

[†]From de Craen et al (59).

with the high-dose immediate-release formulation[53]. The FDA approved the sustained-release formulation in late 1996. Compared with the immediate-release formulation, the sustained-release formulation is associated with fewer adverse effects, including seizures. Common adverse effects include dry mouth, agitation, insomnia, headaches, and dizziness[54].

Combination therapy. A double-blind trial comparing placebo with sustained-release bupropion, the nicotine patch, and combined sustained-release bupropion and nicotine patch reported that combination therapy was superior to either therapy alone[55]. One-year cessation rates were 16% (26 of 160) for placebo, 16% (40 of 244) for sustained-release bupropion, 30% (74 of 244) for the nicotine patch, and 36% (87 of 245) for combination therapy. The difference in abstinence rates between the combination treatment and bupropion alone was not statistically significant, but the difference in abstinence rates between combination treatment and the nicotine patch was statistically significant.

Another double-blind study found higher abstinence rates for subjects who received a nicotine patch and nicotine gum when compared with subjects who received a nicotine patch and placebo gum[56].

Cost of Pharmacotherapy

A survey of 25 insurance plans found that only 7 (28%) covered some form of treatment for smoking cessation[57]. The average cost for each person who stopped smoking successfully ranged from $797 for patients with standard coverage, which covered 50% of behavioral services and all of the costs of nicotine replacement therapy, to $1171 for patients with full coverage[58].

The estimated numbers of people who smoke who need to be treated per person who quits successfully varies from 6 to 20 for pharmacologic therapies

(Table 3) [40-42,47,49,52,59]. The cost per person who quits based on the number needed to treat, varies from about $2500 to almost $20 000 (Table 4) [15,31,35-37]. The broader availability of over-the-counter nicotine replacement products has resulted in a higher utilization rate of pharmacotherapy[60].

Conclusion

Smoking prevalence in the United States has decreased since the 1960s, probably because of the recognition that smoking is a major modifiable risk factor for the leading causes of death. However, nearly one fourth of men and women in the United States continues to smoke. Recent advances in pharmacotherapy offer help for patients who are attempting to quit smoking.

REFERENCES

1. Smoking-attributable mortality and years of potential life lost—United States, 1984. *MMWR Morb Mortal Wkly Rep.* 1987; 36: 693–697.
2. Smoking-attributable mortality and years of potential life lost—United States, 1988. *MMWR Morb Mortal Wkly Rep.* 1991; 40: 62–71.
3. McGinnis MK, Foege WH. Actual causes of death in the United States. *JAMA.* 1993; 270: 2207–2212.
4. Achievements in public health, 1900–1999: tobacco use—United States, 1900–1999. *MMWR Morb Mortal Wkly Rep.* 1999; 48: 986–993.
5. Cigarette smoking among adults—United States, 1998. *MMWR Morb Mortal Wkly Rep.* 2000; 49: 881–884.
6. Doll R, Peto R. Mortality in relation to smoking: 20 years' observation of male British doctors. *BMJ.* 1976; 2: 1525–1536.
7. Benowitz NL, Henningfield JE. Establishing a nicotine threshold for addiction. The implications for tobacco regulation. *N Engl J Med.* 1994; 331: 123–125.
8. American Psychiatric Association. Diagnostic and Statistical Manual of Mental Disorders. 4th ed. Washington, DC: American Psychiatric Association; 1994: 195.

9. Fagerstrom KO. Measuring degree of physical dependence to tobacco smoking with reference to individualization of treatment. *Addict Behav.* 1978; 3: 235–241.

10. Heatherton TF, Kozlowski LT, Frecker RC, Fagerstrom KO. The Fagerstrom Test for Nicotine Dependence: a revision of the Fagerstrom Tolerance Questionnaire. *Br J Addict.* 1991; 86: 1119–1127.

11. Etter JF, Duc TV, Perneger TV. Validity of the Fagerstrom test for nicotine dependence and of the heaviness of smoking index among relatively light smokers. *Addiction.* 1999; 94: 269–281.

12. Manley M, Epps RP, Husten C., et al. Clinical interventions in tobacco control: a National Cancer Institute training program for physicians. *JAMA.* 1991; 266: 3172–3173.

13. The Smoking Cessation Clinical Practice Panel and Staff. The Agency for Health Care Policy and Research Smoking Cessation Clinical Practice Guideline. *JAMA.* 1996; 275: 1270–1280.

14. The Tobacco Use and Dependence Clinical Practice Guideline Panel, Staff, and Consortium Representatives. A clinical practice guideline for treating tobacco use and dependence: a US Public Health Service Report. *JAMA.* 2000; 283: 3244–3254.

15. Fiore MC. US Public Health Service clinical practice guideline: treating tobacco use and dependence. *Respir Care.* 2000; 45: 1200–1262.

16. Fiore MC. The new vital sign: assessing and documenting smoking status. *JAMA.* 1991; 266: 3183–3184.

17. Fiore MC, Pierce JP, Remington PL, Fiore BJ. Cigarette smoking: the clinician's role in cessation, prevention, and public health. *Dis Mon.* 1990; 36: 186–241.

18. Frank E, Winkleby MA, Altman DG, et al. Predictors of physician's smoking cessation advice. *JAMA.* 1991; 266: 3139–3134.

19. Fiore MC, Jorenby DE, Schensky AE, et al. Smoking status as the new vital sign: effect on assessment and intervention in patients who smoke. *Mayo Clin Proc.* 1995; 70: 209–213.

20. LaCroix AZ, Lang J, Scherr P, et al. Smoking and mortality among older men and women in three communities. *N Engl J Med.* 1991; 324: 1619–1625.

21. Rosenberg L, Kaufman DW, Helmrich SP, Shapiro S. The risk of myocardial infarction after quitting smoking in men under 55 years of age. *N Engl J Med.* 1985; 313: 1511–1514.

22. Tverdal A, Thelle D, Stensvold I, et al. Mortality in relation to smoking history; 13 years' follow-up of 68,000 Norwegian men and women 35–49 years. *J Clin Epidemiol.* 1993; 46: 475–487.

23. Kawachi I, Colditz GA, Stampfer MJ. Smoking cessation in relation to total mortality rates in women. A prospective cohort study. *Ann Intern Med.* 1993; 119: 992–1000.

24. Fletcher C, Peto R. The natural history of chronic airflow obstruction. *BMJ.* 1977; 1: 1645–1648.

25. Anthonisen NR, Connett JF, Kiley JP, et al. Effects of smoking intervention and the use of an inhaled anticholinergic bronchodilator on the rate of decline of FEV1. *JAMA.* 1994; 272: 1497–1505.

26. Samet JM. The health benefits of smoking cessation. *Med Clin North Am.* 1992; 76: 399–414.

27. Slama K, Redman S, Perkins J, et al. The effectiveness of two smoking cessation programs for use in general practice. A randomized clinical trial. *BMJ.* 1990; 300: 1707–1709.

28. Demers RY, Neale AV, Adams R, et al. The impact of physicians' brief smoking cessation counseling: A MIRNET study. *J Fam Pract.* 1990; 31: 625–629.

29. Pederson LL, Wanklin JM, Lefcoe NM. The effects of counseling on smoking cessation among patients hospitalized with chronic obstructive pulmonary disease: a randomized clinical trial. *Int J Addict.* 1991; 26: 107–119.

30. Wadland WC, Soffelmayr B, Ives K. Enhancing smoking cessation of low-income smokers in managed care. *J Fam Pract.* 2001; 50: 138–144.

31. Henningfield JE. Nicotine medications for smoking cessation. *N Engl J Med.* 1995; 333: 1196–1203.

32. Gritz ER, Carr CR, Marcus AC. The tobacco withdrawal syndrome in unaided quitters. *Br J Addict.* 1991; 86: 57–59.

33. Hughes JR, Hatsukami D. Signs and symptoms of tobacco withdrawal. *Arch Gen Psych.* 1986; 43: 289–294.

34. Hughes JR. Tobacco withdrawal in self-quitters. *J Consult Clin Psychol.* 1992; 60: 689–697.

35. Okuyemi KS, Ahluwalia JS, Harris KJ, et al. Pharmacotherapy of smoking cessation. *Arch Fam Med.* 2000; 9: 270–281.

36. Helge TD, Denelsky GY. Pharmacologic aids to smoking cessation. *Cleve Clin J Med.* 2000; 67: 818, 821–824.

37. Ellsworth AJ, Witt DM, Dugdale DC, Oliver LM. *2001–2002 Medical Drug Reference.* Philadelphia, PA: Mosby; 2001.

38. Hajek P, West R, Foulds J, et al. Randomized comparative trial of nicotine polacrilex, a transdermal patch, nasal spray, and an inhaler. *Arch Intern Med.* 1999; 159: 2033–2038.

39. West R, Hajek P, Nilsson F, et al. Individual difference in preferences for and responses to four nicotine replacement products. *Psychopharmacology.* 2001; 153: 225–230.

40. Garvey AJ, Kinnunen T, Nordstrom BL, et al. Effects of nicotine gum dose by level of nicotine dependence. *Nicotine Tob Res.* 2000; 2: 52–63.

41. Fiore MC, Smith SI, Jorenby AE, Baker TB. The effectiveness of the nicotine patch for smoking cessation. A meta-analysis. *JAMA.* 1994; 271: 1940–1947.

42. ICRF General Practice Research Group. Randomized trial of nicotine patches in general practice: results at one year. *BMJ.* 1994; 308: 1476–1477.

43. Daughton DM, Fortmann SP, Glover ED, et al. The smoking cessation efficacy of varying doses of nicotine patch delivery systems: 4 to 5 years post-quit day. *Prev Med.* 1999; 28: 113–118.

44. Fiore MC, Kenford SL, Jorenby DE, et al. Two studies of the clinical effectiveness of the nicotine patch with different counseling treatments. *Chest.* 1994; 105: 524–533.

45. Shiffman S, Elash CA, Paton SM, et al. Comparative efficacy of 24-hour and 16-hour transdermal nicotine patches for relief of morning craving. *Addiction.* 2000; 95: 1185–1195.

46. Schneider NG, Lunell E, Olmstead RE, Fagerstrom KO. Clinical pharmacokinetics of nasal nicotine delivery. A review and comparison to other nicotine systems. *Clin Pharmacokinet.* 1996; 31: 65–80.

47. Sutherland G, Stapleton JA, Russell MA, et al. Randomised controlled trial of nasal nicotine spray in smoking cessation. *Lancet.* 1992; 340: 324–329.

48. Hjalmarson A, Nilsson F, Sjostrom L, Wiklund O. The nicotine inhaler in smoking cessation. *Arch Intern Med.* 1997; 157: 1721–1728.

49. Schneider NG, Olmstead R, Nilsson F, et al. Efficacy of a nicotine inhaler in smoking cessation: a double-blind, placebo-controlled trial. *Addiction.* 1996; 91: 1293–1306.

50. Joseph AM, Norman SM, Ferry LH, et al. The safety of transdermal nicotine as an aid to smoking cessation in patients with cardiac disease. *N Engl J Med.* 1996; 335: 1792–1798.

51. Working Group for the Study of Transdermal Nicotine in Patients with Coronary Artery Disease. Nicotine replacement therapy for patients with coronary artery disease. *Arch. Intern Med.* 1994; 154: 989–995.

52. Hurt RD, Sachs DP, Glover ED, et al. A comparison of sustained-release bupropion and placebo for smoking cessation. *N Engl J Med.* 1997; 337: 1195–1202.

53. Davidson J. Seizures and bupropion: a review. *J Clin Psychiatry.* 1989; 50: 256–266.

54. Settle EC Jr. Bupropion sustained release: side effect profile. *J Clin Psychiatry.* 1998; 59 (suppl 4); 532–536.

55. Jorenby DE, Leischow SJ, Nides MA, et al. A controlled trial of sustained-release bupropion, a nicotine patch, or both for smoking cessation. *N Engl J Med.* 1999; 340: 685–691.

56. Kornitzer M, Boutsen M, Dramaix M, et al. Combined use of nicotine patch and gum in smoking cessation: a placebo-controlled clinical trial. *Prev Med.* 1995; 24: 41–47.

57. Aakko E, Piasecki TM, Remington P, Fiore MC. Smoking cessation services offered by health insurance plans for Wisconsin state employees. *WMJ.* 1999; 98: 14–18.

58. Curry SJ, Grothaus LC, McAfee T, Pabiniak C. Use and cost effectiveness of smoking-cessation services under four insurance plans in a health maintenance organization. *J Engl J Med.* 1998; 339: 673–679.

59. de Craen AJ, Vickers AJ, Tijssen JG, Kleijnen J. Number needed to treat and placebo-controlled trials. *Lancet.* 1998; 351: 310.

60. Shiffman S, Gitchell J, Pinney JM, et al. Public health benefit of over-the-counter nicotine medications. *Tob Control.* 1997; 6: 306–310.

From the University of Texas Medical Branch at Galveston, Galveston, Texas.

Requests for reprints should be addressed to Bernard Karnath, MD, Department of Internal Medicine, University of Texas Medical Branch, 301 University Boulevard, Galveston, Texas 77555-0566.

PERINATAL CARE FOR WOMEN WHO ARE ADDICTED:

Implications for Empowerment

This article explores societal responses to perinatal drug abuse, including stigmatic attitudes and behaviors of health care workers that are directed toward women who abuse drugs during pregnancy. Health care providers' stigmatic responses can deter women from receiving perinatal care and place women and their unborn children at risk. Because poor women and women of color face a greater probability of being prosecuted or losing custody of their children for using drugs while they are pregnant, the article emphasizes societal responses to these client populations. Empowering strategies are suggested by which social workers and clients can potentially redefine perinatal drug abuse as a health problem rather than a legal issue and improve the environment in which perinatal care is provided.

Key words
empowerment
health care
maternal drug abuse

Carolyn S. Carter

Perinatal drug abuse is the use of alcohol and other drugs among women who are pregnant. The National Institute on Drug Abuse estimates that 5.5 percent of the women in the United States have used illicit drugs while pregnant, including cocaine, marijuana, heroin, and psychotherapeutic drugs that were not prescribed by a physician. More than 18 percent used alcohol during their pregnancy, and 20.4 percent smoked cigarettes (Marwick, 1998).

Literature reports the increased use of drugs during pregnancy (Lieb & Sterk-Elifson, 1995), using therapeutic communities (Stevens & Arbiter, 1995) and neighborhood context (Perloff & Jaffee, 1999) for addressing perinatal drug abuse; access barriers for low-income ethnic minority women who are addicted and pregnant (Cook, Selig, Wedge, & Gohn-Baube, 1999); the importance of effective policy making (Harrison, 1991); referrals to child protection services (Azzi-Lessing & Olsen, 1996); and other responses to perinatal drug abuse (Azzi-Lessing & Olsen; Irwin, 1995; Lieb & Sterk-Elifson; Marwick, 1998).

Women who abuse drugs while pregnant face severe consequences, which include becoming stigmatized as immoral and deficient caregivers (Carter, 1997; Kearny, Murphy, & Rosenbaum, 1994; Lieb & Sterk-Elifson, 1995). A behavioral outcome of societal attitudes toward perinatal drug abuse is the degree to which the drug-taking behavior of pregnant women is criminalized (Lieb & Sterk-Elifson). Criminalization refers to using legal approaches, such as incarceration, for medical problems of clients rather than referring them for treatment (Keigher, 1999). Community response to the increasing number of women who give birth to infants addicted to crack cocaine, for example, has been to prosecute women for perinatal drug abuse (Lieb & Sterk-Elifson). Similarly, the number of mentally ill inmates in jails and prisons is estimated as being twice that in state hospitals (Keigher).

Individuals in helping professions also display stigmatic attitudes toward perinatal drug abuse. Disparaging interactions with women in some perinatal care facilities (Irwin, 1995), for example, include rude and judgmental comments to clients and violation of their confidentiality. Uncomfortable relationships with health care providers and fear of reprisal on the part of pregnant women who are addicted make women four times less likely to receive adequate care (Carten, 1996; Cook et al., 1999), thereby creating health risks for women who are addicted, their unborn fetuses, and their other children.

In this article I discuss contemporary responses to perinatal drug abuse, including ways in which the behavior of women who abuse drugs is criminalized or subjected to legal interventions. Vignettes from an ethnographic study of 120 women who used heroin, crack cocaine, and methamphetamine while pregnant (Irwin, 1995) depict the attitudes and behaviors of health care providers, society at large, and women themselves toward maternal drug abuse. This article demonstrates how poor women and women of color encounter legal interventions—such as prosecution or reports to city or state child protective services (CPS)—more frequently for using drugs during pregnancy than their more affluent, white counterparts. Because criminalizing perinatal drug abuse presents substantial risks to the health of women and children, empowering (Gutierrez, De-Lois, & GlenMaye, 1995) strategies are suggested for redefining perinatal drug abuse less as a legal issue and more as a health concern. The strategies are consistent with elements of the national health plan of the U.S. Department of Health and Human Services (DHHS), such as creating access to health care and minimizing risks to maternal, infant, and child health (DHHS, 2000).

SOCIETAL ATTITUDES TOWARD PERINATAL DRUG ABUSE

Over the past 100 years, there has been an overall shift in obstetric medicine to a focus on fetal protection (Harrison, 1991). In cases involving material drug abuse, the shift has sometimes resulted in adversarial attitudes with sentiment favoring the well-being of fetuses and against pregnant women (Gustavsson, 1991). The following excerpts offer three perspectives toward perinatal drug abuse that have primary emphasis on unborn fetuses: The first comment reflects the attitudes of some drug dealers; the second statement is a common reaction of partners of pregnant women; and the third depicts the attitude of society at large (Irwin, 1995).

> They [crack dealers] tell me that I shouldn't be doing this in the first place, but I'm gonna do it anyway. And they go, "You know it. I shouldn't even really sell you anything. I shouldn't sell you anything cause you're pregnant. I'm not gonna contribute to that."

> My baby came home with crack in her system, and he [baby's father who is himself a crack dealer] don't want to claim her now.

> I know one girl. She just smokes [crack] and doesn't give a damn. Her stomach is way out there, so she shouldn't be out there [using crack] anyway, cause people be like, "man, look, a pregnant woman!" (pp. 616–617)

Negative attitudes like the ones in the vignettes above are pervasive and often based on assumed medical and developmental consequences of drugs on fetuses (Coles, 1991). The concerns are both supported and refuted by research. Studies of the effects of drug use on fetal development cite problems such as low birthweight, small head size, prematurity, and small size for gestational age (LaFrance et al., 1994). A study of 11,000 infants conducted by the Brown University School of Medicine, however, showed no increase in abnormalities at birth among children who had been exposed to cocaine in utero (Marwick, 1998). Although the latter study has not followed the children into school age and is therefore inconclusive, other studies of adjustment among drug-exposed children also challenge the notion of devastating effects resulting from cocaine use during pregnancy (Carten, 1996; Frank, Augustyn, Knight, Pell, & Zuckerman, 2001). Coles (1991, 1992) concluded that the effects of the social environment are too often ignored in studies of perinatal drug abuse.

In addition to the pejorative attitudes toward women who abuse drugs during pregnancy based on ideas about adverse fetal development is the belief that drug use compromises the reproductive and caregiver roles of women (Chavkin, 1990). It is believed that women who abuse substances are unfit mothers undeserving of their children (Carter, 1997). Society sanctions women for failing to live up to preconceived gender-role expectations by using legal interventions, particularly against poor women of color who use drugs while they are pregnant (Lieb & Sterk-Elifson, 1995).

LEGAL INTERVENTIONS

Legal interventions for perinatal drug abuse may be increasing in the United States. Since 1985, 240 women in 35 states have been prosecuted for using alcohol or illegal drugs while pregnant (Marwick, 1998). Eleven states have developed specific gestational-abuse statutes. The most comprehensive reporting system is in Minnesota and includes toxicological screening (Lieb & Sterk-Elifson, 1995) and "involuntary civil commitment" to drug rehabilitation of pregnant women who have used drugs. Before March 2001, eight states mandated that health care workers report neonates' positive drug toxicology as evidence of child abuse and neglect (Marwick), thus paving the way for court proceedings and actions affecting the parental rights of mothers. On March 21, 2001, the U.S. Supreme Court ruled that it is unlawful to involuntarily test pregnant women who are suspected of drug abuse. In *Ferguson v. City of Charleston* (2001), Charleston, South Carolina, was a litigant in the Supreme Court case and, along with Florida, enforced the greatest number of legal interventions (American Civil Liberties Union, 1992).

Public hospitals were more likely to have mandatory drug screenings and protocols that included reporting positive toxicology to CPS.

It is informative to place the legal interventions that occurred before the March 2001 judicial ruling within a sociocultural context. In doing so, it becomes clear that although illegal drug use is similar across class and racial lines, poor and ethnic minority women were more likely to be criminalized (Carten, 1996; Lieb & Sterk-Elifson, 1995). The manner in which drug screening occurred is an example. Screenings commonly occurred during routine prenatal care (Lieb & Sterk-Elifson), and the stated purpose was protecting fetuses. However, drug screenings were often limited to facilities that served low socioeconomic populations and populations of color (Harrison, 1991; Lieb & Sterk-Elifson), thus making screenings more detrimental for poor and pregnant women from ethnic minority groups.

Reports to CPS were disparate across cultural groups as well. A review of mandatory reporting of perinatal drug addiction in Florida showed that positive drug screening rates were almost equal among white and African American women and among women seen in clinics and private offices. Yet, reporting rates were much higher for African American women than for white women (Harrison, 1991).

The procedures for prosecuting pregnant women for substance use were discretionary and reflected disparities across demographic groups. A 1987 review of court-ordered obstetrical interventions showed that 81 percent of the women were African American, Hispanic, or Asian and 24 percent did not speak English as a primary language (Harrison, 1991). More recent study results indicate that pregnant African American women were nine times more likely to be prosecuted for substance use than pregnant white women (Lieb & Sterk-Elifson, 1995).

Incarceration, like other legal approaches to perinatal drug abuse, also discriminated against poor women and women of color. Women with low incomes generally gave birth in public health settings. Delivering in these facilities increased their chances of incarceration compared with middle- and upper-income women who gave birth in private hospitals that rarely screened for illicit drugs. Public hospitals were more likely to have mandatory drug screenings and protocols that included reporting positive toxicology to CPS. Disclosing positive toxicology to CPS could result in incarceration. Disparities in the rate of incarceration extended to ethnic minority groups, with African American women facing the greatest burden of being imprisoned. Of the 41 pregnant women arrested for abusing drugs in South Carolina from 1989 to 1993, 40 were African American.

The American Medical Association (AMA) stated that drug addiction was an illness that required medical rather than legal intervention, and prosecution did not prevent harm to infants but it often resulted in harm (AMA, 1988). For example, fear of reprisal was a barrier to outreach and often deterred addicted pregnant women from receiving medical care. Avoiding medical care increased the risk of drug exposure before birth and ineffective parenting later (Marwick, 1998). Also, women who abused drugs were more likely to physically abuse their children (Stevens & Arbiter, 1995).

Legal interventions disregarded the treatment and advocacy roles of health care providers (Chavkin, 1990; Marwick, 1998). For example, medical personnel often performed drug screenings without the informed consent of female patients, and the results were then used as evidence during criminal prosecutions (Lieb & Sterk-Elifson, 1995). Addressing perinatal drug abuse through legal intervention was punitive. In large part, it operated on the assumption that although drug treatment programs for women were available in sufficient numbers, women had not made use of the services, and the research conclusively attested to the effectiveness of current drug programs for women with children (Carten, 1996). In fact, drug programs for women, and particularly pregnant women, were largely unavailable (Lieb & Sterk-Elifson). Less than 1 percent of the federal anti-drug budget was targeted for women, yet this minimal amount was expected to include women who were pregnant (Child Welfare League of America, 1992). Also, most drug interventions were designed with men in mind and overlooked the needs of women (Azzi-Lessing & Olsen, 1996; Carter, 1997). Residential treatment programs, for example, rarely provided child care even though 80 percent of the women entering residential drug rehabilitation had children and half had their children living with them at the time they entered treatment (Stevens & Arbiter, 1995). Consequently, mothers who were addicted to drugs, had other children for whom they provided primary care, and had no familial support risked losing custody of their children by entering treatment.

Interventions based on legal ideology distorted client-worker relationships. Salient features of ethical client-helper relationships are establishing trust and respecting the confidentiality, dignity, and uniqueness of individuals (Hepworth, Rooney, & Larsen, 1997). Women entering perinatal care could not be assured of these aspects of treatment. In the following scenarios involving two African American woman who were addicted to drugs, the clients' dignity and confidentiality were each violated while they received perinatal services (Irwin, 1995):

> They [health care providers] look at you, they look at you foul and they tell me [sarcastic voice], "Oh, you're a crack user." And then they want to look at your record, and then this nurse look at it and this other nurse look at it, then this other nurse look at it, then... They talking all loud, everybody around.(p. 617)

> I know a lot of mothers say that they don't get prenatal care cause they feel like as soon as they walk through the door, they will be judged. "Oh you're a crack head. So why... did you get pregnant anyway?" So they don't get prenatal care... they are thinking how they gonna be looked at when they walk in the hospital

door, like they are not good enough to be pregnant. (p. 618)

Experiences such as the ones above not only diminished the quality of services, but also restricted access by causing women to retreat before obtaining the care they sought (Irwin, 1995).

The strained client-worker relationships precipitated by legal interventions also created parallel care systems that were not in the best interest of clients (Lieb & Sterk-Elifson, 1995). Prototypes were nontraditional birthing methods. Parallel care also delayed registering the birth of children and reduced opportunities for health care providers to assist women in obtaining required immunizations and other follow-up care for their infants. In these ways, parallel systems for perinatal care placed both mothers who are addicted and infants at risk.

I'm gonna have my baby at home and then I'm gonna register the birth at three or four months. (Irwin, 1995, p. 626)

HEALTH-RELATED INTERVENTIONS

Health-related approaches to perinatal drug abuse are notably unlike legal interventions. As the Healthy People 2010 plan states, useful approaches to improving health build community partnerships and are systemic, multidisciplinary, absent of disparities across population groups, and attuned to the reciprocal relationship between individual health and community health. Reciprocal means community health is affected by the beliefs, attitudes, and behaviors of everyone in a given community and vice versa (DHHS, 2000).

Components of Healthy People 2010—the national plan for improving public health in the United States—include two discrete goals, 467 objectives, and 28 focal areas. Among the focal areas of the plan are maternal, infant, and child health and substance abuse. Healthy People 2010 proposes to improve maternal, infant, and child health by decreasing maternal drug abuse. Because of the relevant focal areas and strategies of Healthy People 2010 and because the plan creates opportunities for individuals to make healthy lifestyle choices for themselves and their families, it has implications for developing empowerment strategies in perinatal care settings.

IMPLICATIONS FOR EMPOWERMENT

Of concern to social workers is that perinatal drug abuse, a health-related issue of families and children, is often criminalized. Basing perinatal approaches on empowerment strategies that target women who are addicted and health care providers promises to overcome legal interventions and address disparaging attitudes toward perinatal drug abuse.

Empowerment refers to increasing clients' personal, social, and political power so that they can change their situations and prevent reoccurrence of problems (Gutierrez et al., 1995). Because empowerment theory emerged from efforts to develop more effective and responsive services for women and people of color, it is highly relevant to perinatal drug abuse (Gutierrez, 1990).

The empowerment practice goals are helping client systems achieve a sense of personal power, become more aware of the connection between individual and community problems, develop helpful skills, and work toward social change (Gutierrez et al., 1995). Studies cite the usefulness of empowerment practice in improving the contexts of human services organizations in ethnically diverse metropolitan areas (Gutierrez et al.) and helping women of color in oppressed neighborhoods overcome unequal access to resources (Gutierrez, 1990). Empowerment strategies include role playing as a technique for skills training, raising self-esteem, and helping women see the impact of the political environment on issues in their own lives (Gutierrez et al.). In empowerment practice, power is shared, clients are helped to "experience a sense of power" within helping relationships, and professionals are collaborators rather than superiors.

Perhaps the most empowering perinatal service about which social workers and their clients who are addicted can collaborate is helping women become alcohol and drug free. The specific strategies for motivating clients to seek drug rehabilitation (van Wormer, 1995), attain sobriety (Daugherty & Leukefeld, 1998; Levin, 1995; Stevens, & Arbiter, 1995; Wallace, 1992), and use relapse prevention measures (Wallace) are documented in the literature but are not a focus of this article. This article is concerned with empowering strategies for addressing the adverse attitudes and practices to which pregnant women who are addicted are often subjected. Examples include

- teaching pregnant women who are addicted to make formal complaints when they receive unprofessional services in perinatal care settings
- improving access by overcoming scheduling issues and advocating for adequate resources
- enhancing communication skills among women who are pregnant and addicted to drugs
- conducting culturally sensitive in-service training for health care providers
- addressing the unique issues of women of color
- overcoming systemic factors that create barriers to health care
- promoting gender-sensitive programs
- developing community partnerships with relevant groups
- recommending national policies that redefine perinatal drug abuse as a health issue.

Addressing Professional Attitudes and Practices

Two of the most insurmountable barriers for low-income women seeking perinatal care are (1) the pejorative attitudes of providers and (2) the distrust of the health care system (Cook et al., 1999). Stressful interactions with health care providers can adversely affect the drug abuse recovery of women in perinatal care (Azzi-Lessing & Olsen, 1996), further damage their self-esteem (Levin, 1995), and be intimidating as well.

Social workers can help addicted women become empowered in perinatal care settings in which existing professional attitudes and practices are esteem lowering and potentially disempowering by conveying their own positive regard for the worth and dignity of individuals (Hepworth et al., 1997). This includes validating with clients that rude, judgmental, and other unethical practices are oppressive and unacceptable in health care settings (Carter, 2002). Collaborating with women about the best ways to file formal complaints against perinatal care personnel who fail to meet professional standards enhances women's personal power and is a model for social change.

The health of individuals and communities depends on access to quality health care (DHHS, 2000). Case management approaches in which social workers appropriately assist in referring women who require perinatal care are potentially empowering because they facilitate access to services. Social workers can enhance their referrals by becoming knowledgeable about the practices and expectations for clients in perinatal care agencies and using the increased knowledge to improve clients' involvement in their own perinatal care regime (Hepworth et al., 1997). Examples are raising clients' general awareness of an agency's intake procedures and working collaboratively to overcome access barriers that are common in some perinatal care facilities. Access barriers include long waiting periods in facilities and scheduling problems—for example, consistently busy telephone lines and too few available appointments (Cook et al., 1999). Short-term strategies for overcoming barriers could involve scheduling appointments far in advance and adequately planning for such support services as extended child care, transportation, and meals when clients are scheduled for appointments. Long-term strategies should include advocating for increased resources.

By means of role playing or related techniques, addicted clients who require perinatal care can be taught more assertive, and thus personally empowering, means of communicating in health care settings. For instance, it is more useful for both clients and services professionals if a women states, "Hello, I am [name] and I am here for my 3:00 appointment or the results of my lab work" than for her to say, "Hello, I am here for my appointment." Improved client communication may increase access and signal to providers that clients expect dignified, respectful services (Carter, 2002).

Health-related approaches to perinatal care have informed views on diversity. In-service training in which social workers help providers become more culturally sensitive to poor and ethnic minority clients is empowering because it can improve the overall environment of perinatal care settings (Carter, 2002). Our knowledge of human diversity (Council on Social Work Education [CSWE], 1992) and ethical commitment to ethnic-sensitive practice (Devore & Schlesinger, 1996) can enhance our role as trainers. Social workers understand, for instance, the usefulness of community intervention (Rivera & Erlich, 1992) and how to use natural helping networks (Daly, Jennings, Beckett, & Leashore, 1995) and extended families (Billingsley, 1992) when working with poor families and families of color. Natural helpers, such as neighbors who can offer transportation or child care, are invaluable to perinatal drug abuse services. Lack of child care and transportation are access barriers that are personally disempowering to many women who require perinatal care (Cook, et al., 1999).

It is also important to address the unique issues of women of color. For example, HIV infections are common among women who abuse intravenous drugs, but African American women are seven times more likely to die from HIV/AIDS (DHHS, 2000). Patient education on preventing HIV infections and other sexually transmitted diseases and planning for loss of parents and other effects of AIDS on families are important topics of discussion during perinatal care to African American women.

Counteracting Legal Interventions

Some experts believe the current political climate produces gender-biased, racist, and classist policies (Gibbs & Blankhead, 2001; Harrison, 1991; Lieb & Sterk-Elifson, 1995). An example is contemporary policy defining perinatal drug abuse as if it were strictly a legal issue and then targeting for prosecution poor women and women of color. Because of social workers' mandate to promote social justice (CSWE, 1992), it is important that we advocate on behalf of vulnerable populations, for example, pregnant women who are addicted and their unborn children.

In recommending policies that foster adequate income, health insurance, and education, we can raise the socioeconomic status of mothers and, in turn, enhance the health status of drug-exposed babies (Lieb & Sterk-Elifson, 1995). Being poor and less educated are linked to systemic issues like restricted access to health care, living in unsafe neighborhoods, inadequate housing, and limited opportunities to engage in health promotion (DHHS, 2000). Many contemporary drug policies, however, blame women and divert attention from systemic forces, such as poverty, that promote substance abuse (Carten, 1996; Perloff & Jaffee, 1999). A study (Walker, 1991) of 1,000 substance abuse cases in four large cities showed that a sizable number of the parents lost their children to custodial care because of inadequate housing and poverty rather than explicit drug abuse. Healthy People 2010 embraces the empowering strategy of focusing on systemic factors that affect the health status of addicted women and their unborn fetuses.

Although it is important that social workers advocate for health-related perinatal care policies, it is even more empowering if the resulting programs are gender sensitive. Gender-sensitive perinatal programs take into account, among other factors, protecting women's physical health, access issues, and the rate of depression among women who are addicted (Carten, 1996; Carter, 1997). Depression, for example, is strongly correlated with high levels of personal stress, inadequate housing, lack of money for basic needs, and other factors associated with poverty (Azzi-Lessing & Olsen, 1996; Cook et al., 1999). Because depressive symptoms are predictable among women who abuse drugs (Carter, 1997) and can deter health-seeking behaviors, assessing depression in perinatal care settings is gender sensitive. Assessing depression is also a biopsychosocial (Oktay, 1998) strategy that favors health promotion. By treating depression, social workers can help clients in perinatal care settings overcome feelings of helplessness and become more available to engage in social change. Therefore, examining depression in perinatal care settings is personally, politically, and socially empowering to clients (Gutierrez et al., 1995).

Social workers can intensify their perinatal advocacy efforts by developing community partnerships with CPS and perinatal care programs that fulfill the programs' missions while also protecting families and children. Perinatal toxicology screenings are allegedly designed to protect children, and CPS's primary mission is protecting children. However, between 1982 and 1989, when the number of substance abuse-related CPS cases doubled (Child Welfare Administration, 1993), child welfare agencies began separating children from their mothers solely on the basis of positive toxicology, without attempts to apply preventive measures or family rehabilitation (Carten, 1996). It is expedient that social workers help CPS and perinatal care providers refocus their dialogue on the needs of families within social and political contexts (Azzi-Lessing & Olsen, 1996). Partnering agencies may then stop relying heavily on legal strategies and instead advocate for financial and other resources that can improve the health status of all family members—for example, by locating medical facilities in local communities and providing culturally specific health education. Because advocating community partnerships highlights the relatedness of individuals' problems and environmental conditions, it fulfills tenets of empowerment practice and Healthy People 2010.

Community partnerships that reach out to nontraditional partners can be among the most effective tools for improving health in communities (DHHS, 2000). Social workers can further strengthen their campaigns to eliminate legal interventions for perinatal drug abuse by broadening their community partnerships with CPS and perinatal care programs to incorporate women, private companies, and community-based organizations such as criminal justice agencies, legal clinics, employment agencies, and churches (Carter, 2002). By providing research data, social workers can demonstrate to partners how legal means of "protecting" families and children are, in fact, injurious to them. Incarceration, for example, complicates birth outcomes in various ways. When women are released from prison, their own as well as their children's Medicaid eligibility is compromised for at least a month or more. If women and their children have chronic illnesses such as diabetes, HIV/AIDS, or hypertension, treatment adherence is essential, but health care is inaccessible without medical coverage. Women with low incomes, already at the highest risk of poor birth outcomes, are at greater risk of incarceration (Marwick, 1998).

Once community partners are better informed, they can then educate politicians and other policymakers and thereafter solicit their help in adopting national policies that redefine perinatal drug abuse as a health-related issue. One example of such a policy is greater incentives for private corporations to develop partnerships with community-based drug rehabilitation organizations that accommodate mothers who are addicted as well as their children. Another is a policy that rewards medical schools for teaching students how to identify risk factors for substance use during pregnancy. In a survey of primary care physicians, only 17 percent could diagnose illicit drug use, a mere 30 percent were prepared to diagnose misuse of prescription drugs, and only 20 percent could confidently diagnose alcoholism. On the other hand, 82 percent of the physicians could identify patients with diabetes, and 83 percent could diagnose patients with hypertension (National Center on Addiction and Substance Abuse, 2000). Increasing physicians' ability to identify risk factors for drug use during pregnancy is not only a preventive measure for improving maternal, infant, and child health, but a means of reinforcing among physicians and other health care providers the health-related definition of perinatal drug abuse.

CONCLUSION

Health care professionals and society at large exhibit negative attitudes toward women who abuse drugs. By means of empowerment strategies, social workers can potentially help clients who are addicted and pregnant to seek and complete perinatal treatment programs, improve the environment in which perinatal care services are provided, and advocate for policies that define perinatal drug abuse more as a health problem than a legal issue. Desired outcomes of these efforts are improved health care access and quality of life for families in which perinatal drug abuse is an issue.

REFERENCES

American Civil Liberties Union. (1992). *Criminal prosecutions against pregnant women, national update and overview* (Reproductive Freedom Project). New York: Author.

American Medical Association. (1988). *Drug abuse in the United States: A policy report*. In Proceedings of the House of Delegates, 137th Annual Meeting of the American Medical Association, Chicago.

Azzi-Lessing, L., & Olsen, L. J. (1996). Substance abuse-affected families in the child welfare system: New challenges, new alliances, *Social Work, 41,* 15–23.

Billingsley, A. (1992). *Climbing Jacob's ladder*. New York: Simon & Schuster.

Carten, A. J. (1996). Mothers in recovery: Rebuilding families in the aftermath of addiction. *Social Work, 41,* 214–223.

Carter, C. (1997). Ladies don't: A historical perspective on attitudes toward alcoholic women. *Affilia, 12,* 471–485.

Carter, C. (2002). Prenatal care to women who are addicted: Implications for gender-sensitive practice. *Affilia, 17,* 299–313.

Chavkin, W. (1990). Drug addiction and pregnancy: Policy crossroads. *American Journal of Public Health, 80,* 483–487.

Child Welfare Administration. (1993). *Foster care overview, fiscal years 1992–1993*. New York: Author.

Child Welfare League of America, North American Commission on Chemical Dependency and Child Welfare. (1992). *Children at the front: A different view of the war on drugs*. Washington, DC: Author.

Coles, C. (1991, May). *Substance abuse in pregnancy. The infant's risk: How great?* Paper presented at the annual meeting of the American Psychiatric Association, New Orleans.

Coles, C. (1992). Prenatal alcohol exposure and human development. In M. Miller (Ed.), *Development of the central nervous system: Effects of alcohol and opiates* (pp. 9–36). New York: John Wiley & Sons.

Cook, C. A., Selig, K. L., Wedge, B. J., & Gohn-Baube, E. A. (1999). Access barriers and the use of prenatal care by low-income, inner-city women. *Social Work, 44,* 129–139.

Council on Social Work Education. (1992). *Curriculum policy statement for baccalaureate and master's degree programs in social work education*. Alexandria, VA: Author.

Daly, A. Jennings, J., Beckett, J. O., & Leashore, B. R. (1995). Effective coping strategies in African Americans. *Social Work, 40,* 240–248.

Daugherty, R. P., & Leukefeld, C. G. (1998). *Reducing risks for substance abuse: A lifespan approach.* New York: Plenum Press.

Devore, W., & Schlesinger, E. G. (1996). *Ethnic-sensitive practice* (4th ed.). Boston: Allyn & Bacon.

Ferguson v. City of Charleston, 532 U.S. 1–3 (2001).

Frank, D. A., Augustyn, M., Knight, W. G., Pell, T., & Zuckerman, B. (2001). Growth, development, and behavior in early childhood following prenatal care cocaine exposure: A systematic review. *JAMA, 285,* 1613–1625.

Gibbs, J. T., & Blankhead, T. (2001). *Preserving privilege: California politics, propositions, and people of color.* Westport, CT: Praeger.

Gutierrez, L. (1990). Working with women of color: An empowerment perspective. *Social Work, 35,* 149–153.

Gutierrez, L., DeLois, K. A., & GlenMaye, L. (1995). Understanding empowerment practice: Building on practitioner-based knowledge. *Families in Society, 76,* 534–542.

Gustavsson, N. S. (1991). Chemically exposed children: The child welfare response. *Child and Adolescent Social Work, 8,* 297–307.

Harrison, M. (1991). Drug addiction in pregnancy: The interface of science, emotion, and social policy. *Journal of Substance Abuse Treatment, 8,* 261–268.

Hepworth, D., Rooney, R. H., & Larsen, J. A. (1997). *Direct social work practice: Theory and skills.* Pacific Grove, CA: Brooks/Cole.

Irwin, K. (1995). Ideology, pregnancy and drugs: Differences between crack-cocaine, heroin and methamphetamine users. *Contemporary Drug Problems, 22,* 611–637.

Kearny, M., Murphy, S., & Rosenbaum, M. (1994). Mothering on crack cocaine: A grounded theory analysis. *Social Science and Medicine, 18,* 351–361.

Keigher, S. M. (1999). Including "mental" in mental health and social work [Editorial]. *Health & Social Work, 24,* 85–90.

LaFrance, S. V., Mitchell, J., Damus, K., Driver, C., Roman, G., Graham, E., & Schwartz, L. (1994). Community-based services for pregnant substance-abusing women. *American Journal of Public Health, 84,* 1688–1689.

Levin, D. J. (1995). *Introduction to alcoholism counseling: A bio-psycho-social approach.* New York: Taylor & Francis.

Lieb, J. J., & Sterk-Elifson, C. (1995, Winter). Crack in the cradle: Social policy and reproductive rights among crack-using females. *Contemporary Drug Problems,* 687–705.

Marwick, C. (1998). Challenging report on pregnancy and drug abuse. *JAMA, 280,* 1039–1040.

National Center on Addiction and Substance Abuse. (2000). *Missed opportunity: National survey of primary care physicians on substance abuse.* New York: Columbia University Press.

Oktay, J. S. (1998). Genetics cultural lag. What can social workers do to help? [National Health Line]. *Health & Social Work, 23,* 310–315.

Perloff, J. D., & Jaffee, K. D. (1999). Late entry into prenatal care: The neighborhood context. *Social Work, 44,* 116–128.

Rivera, F. G., & Erlich, J. L. (1992). *Community organization in a diverse society.* Boston: Allyn & Bacon.

Stevens, S. J., & Arbiter, N. (1995). A therapeutic community for substance-abusing pregnant women and women with children: Process and outcome. *Journal of Psychoactive Drugs, 27,* 49–57.

U.S. Department of Health and Human Services. (2000, November). *Healthy people 2010: With understanding and improving health and objectives for improving health.* Washington, DC: U.S. Government Printing Office.

van Wormer, K. (1995). *Alcoholism treatment: A social work perspective.* Chicago: Brunner/Mazel.

Walker, C. (1991). *Parental drug abuse and African American children in foster care* (DHHS No. SA–90–2233–1). Washington, DC: U.S. Department of Health and Human Services, Division of Children and Youth Policy.

Wallace, B. C. (Ed.). (1992). *The chemically dependent: Phases of treatment and recovery.* New York: Nelson Hall.

Carolyn S. Carter, PhD, LCSW, *is associate professor, School of Social Work, Howard University, 601 Howard Place NW, Washington, DC 20059; e-mail: cscarter@at@;howard.edu. The author thanks Natalie Woodman, associate professor emerita, Arizona State University, for her help in reviewing the draft of this article.*

From *Health and Social Work,* Vol. 27, No. 3, August 2002, pp. 166-174. © 2002 by the National Association of Social Workers, Inc. Reprinted by permission.

The Road to Recovery:
A Gender-Responsive Program For
CONVICTED DUI FEMALES

By Lawrence M. Sideman and Ellen Kirschbaum

Like many correctional systems, the Arizona Department of Corrections (ADC) has experienced significant growth in the female inmate population. Of the nearly 29,000 inmates committed to ADC, more than 2,200 are females. The general profile of ADC's female inmates shows that many have been victims of some form of physical or sexual abuse or domestic violence, most are mothers with an average of two children; many are unemployed at the time of arrest; and more than 80 percent have a substance abuse problem.

Because of these unique characteristics, ADC recognized the need to examine its policies and practices regarding female inmates. This brought about a system-wide mission change that called for the relocation of female inmates to a single complex dedicated to housing only women. All female inmates, except those housed at the 160-bed Southern Arizona Correctional Release Center in Tucson, are housed at the Arizona State Prison Complex-Perryville (ASPC-PV), approximately 30 miles west of Phoenix.

Creating gender-responsive programming is a critical part of ADC's goals. Recent changes in Arizona's driving under the influence (DUI) laws placed special focus on females convicted of DUI. Until recently, only males convicted of DUI had dedicated housing and programming. A comparison between the number of female inmates convicted of DUI violations in 1995 (51) and 2001 (119) revealed a 133 percent increase versus a 16 percent increase for male inmates during the same period. ADC needed to create a specialized DUI treatment program for women; ASPC-PV's Santa Maria Unit was designated to house these female inmates. As of April, the number of convicted DUI female inmates had reached 150 this year.

In summer 2001, ADC released a request for proposal (RFP) to obtain a provider that could deliver a gender-responsive program for convicted DUI female inmates. The RFP called for a DUI education and treatment program with aftercare/relapse prevention planning. A contract was awarded to Treatment Assessment Screening Center (TASC) of Arizona, a private, non-profit behavioral health outpatient treatment agency. TASC is a nationally recognized innovator in working collaboratively with the criminal justice system in developing and implementing behavioral health treatment programs.

In January, the Road to Recovery, a licensed, gender-responsive alcohol and other drug abuse/dependence education and treatment program for adult female DUI inmates was implemented. The program's primary goal is to provide programming that addresses the unique needs of women and enables participants to understand their addiction and assist them with their recovery.

Gender-Responsive Programming

The literature on gender-responsive approaches identifies differences between men and women and divides them into two categories: sex differences and gender differences (Belknap, 2001). Sex differences are biological differences, including body size, reproductive organs, muscle development and hormones. Gender differences are ascribed by society and relate to expected social roles. When providing treatment and case management services to females, it is important to understand the differences between sex and gender (the latter is about the reality of women's lives and the context in which they live).

If substance abuse treatment programs are to be effective, they must meet women's unique needs. Behavioral health professionals can understand their female clients better if viewed from a holistic biopsychosocial paradigm, which includes behavioral, cognitive, spiritual and emotional components. Women need connection and by incorporating gender-appropriate elements into treatment and case management, it can be achieved.

During the many years of providing services to criminal justice-involved clients, TASC has recognized and acknowledged the differences between men and women and incorporated unique approaches to each population. For example, men and women develop psychologically in different ways. Traditional (patriarchal) theories of human development describe a climb from childlike dependence to mature independence (Miller, 1976). Autonomy, self-sufficiency and a differentiated self are the goals. However, Miller and others challenge the assumption that separation is the route to maturity. Instead, she suggests that those theories describe men's experience and that women's primary motivation is to build a sense of connection to others. Women develop a sense of self-worth when their actions arise out of, and lead back to, connections with others. Connection, not separation, is the guiding principle of growth for women.

Women at high risk for drug abuse are frequently socially isolated. They are single parents, under- or unemployed, and/or recently separated, divorced or widowed. They often are abuse victims. Alcoholic women are likely to have been abused sexually, physically and emotionally more often, by more perpetrators, and for longer periods of time than their nonalcoholic counterparts (Covington and Surrey, 1997). Women are prone to feel personally responsible for problematic relationships and often feel ashamed or condemned. Psychological isolation occurs when the people in a woman's life fail to validate and respond to her experience or her attempts at connection, reports Miller. Covington emphasized the need to provide a supportive environment that is characterized by safety, connection and empowerment. Road to Recovery staff strive to develop relationships with clients that are safe and mutually respectful, empowering and compassionate. Relationships are empathetic and aimed at "power with others" rather than "power over others."

The Road to Recovery program model addresses four areas recovering women have identified as most critical to recovery and avoiding relapse: self, relationships, sexuality and spirituality.

Three Intervention Levels. Because of the multiple and unique factors involved in female substance abusers, the Road to Recovery uses gender-responsive interventions that impact women on three levels:

- **The Affective Level.** Female substance abusers must learn to express their feelings appropriately and to contain them in healthy ways through self-soothing techniques. Because women often become dependent on drugs to seek relief from painful emotional states, they need an environment that helps them understand and work through their feelings.
- **The Cognitive Level.** Education helps correct the women's misperceptions and distorted thinking. They learn a process of critical thinking in which they first consider their thoughts and feelings and then make decisions.
- **The Behavioral Level.** Women must make changes in their drinking and/or drug-use behaviors. For addicted women, the goal is abstinence. For women who are not addicted, success can be increased functioning levels in every aspect of their lives.

Single-Gender Groups. Research suggests that, although men may benefit from mixed-gender groups, women benefit more from all-female groups. In mixed groups, men reveal much more about themselves and their feelings, while women reveal much less. Conversely, in all-female groups, women share a great deal about themselves, their feelings and their relationships.

The Confrontational Approach. The confrontational approach traditionally used in therapeutic communities has not

proved effective with women. Women require a different basis on which to build community: respect, mutuality, empathy, compassion and empowerment, as opposed to confrontation. An emphasis on assets and strengths, rather than tearing down the ego, has proved most effective with women.

Cultural Context and Gender. Although this program is designed to be gender-specific, it is important to realize that, just as women's lives are different from men's lives, women's lives are not all the same. Although there are common threads in all women's lives because of their gender, it is important to be sensitive to cultural and other differences. For example, there are differences in the lives of African-American, Hispanic and Asian women; among heterosexual, bisexual, lesbian and transgendered women; between older and younger women; and between women who reside in urban settings and rural settings. Road to Recovery clinical staff remain aware of and sensitive to these diversity issues and incorporate them into individualized treatment plans, group treatment processes and aftercare release plans.

Program Components

Comprehensive Assessment. The Road to Recovery uses TASC-Automated Assessment Protocol (TAAP), a comprehensive biopsychosocial clinical needs assessment and case planning instrument that takes a holistic approach to substance abuse treatment and assesses the following areas:

- Employment/education;
- Family/social;
- Medical;
- Legal;
- Psychiatric; and
- Drugs and alcohol.

TAAP uses ASI-type (Addiction Severity Index) need severity ratings to determine the recovery dimensions and level of functioning recognized by the American Society of Addiction Medicine-Patient Placement Criteria-2 (ASAM-PPC-2). Included in the assessment are client ratings that indicate how they see their life circumstances. This helps determine women's motivation for change. An individualized needs assessment that describes specific life issues for each woman, along with recommended interventions and rationales for those interventions, is then developed.

DUI Education and Treatment. The Road to Recovery is designed and delivered with consideration for ASP-PV security issues and existing programs and activities. The average length of incarceration at the Santa Maria unit of ASP-PV is four months. Each program participant receives a minimum of six hours per week of direct services with the core curriculum of 16 hours of DUI education and 20 hours of DUI treatment. Program participants are able to complete the education and treatment components in seven weeks. Completion of this portion of the program satisfies Arizona's requirement for a Level-1 treatment intervention. Each woman who successfully completes the program receives a certificate and becomes eligible for driver's license reinstatement.

DUI education is conducted in a large group format of 16 to 40 inmates. The objectives are to:

- Inform about physical and mental impairment caused by alcohol and drug use;
- Inform and educate about the hazards and consequences of impaired driving;
- Promote safe and responsible decision-making about driving;
- Examine drinking behavior; and
- Assist in changing behavior related to alcohol/drug use and driving.

DUI treatment is conducted in a small group of fewer than 16 that provides women with the opportunity to progress to the important point of a lifestyle change by learning new ways to deal with circumstances impinging on their optimal functioning, and to learn more effective ways of coping with these issues. The goals of this format are for inmates to:

- Learn how to break into their alcohol/other drug use and behavior patterns at the earliest possible moment;
- Learn how to implement skills gained in the treatment process to suppress, control and eliminate inappropriate destructive behaviors;
- Learn to identify specific high-risk situations for their individual lapse/relapse to substance use and/or criminal activity;
- Experience alternative coping responses using cognitive-behavioral and cognitive restructuring techniques;
- Experience re-education and re-socialization in order to use new, more adaptive social skills to cultivate satisfying personal/interpersonal situational and functional behavior; and
- Acquire a positive self-concept and develop new attitudes and self-expectations.

The Road to Recovery uses a cognitive-behavioral substance abuse treatment approach, which places a strong emphasis on establishing personal involvement with the women while intervening on cognitive, affective and behavioral levels. DUI treatment includes skill building and enhancement, including relaxation training, anger and stress management, and management of compulsive behaviors.

If an inmate is incarcerated for more than four months and remains in the Santa Maria Unit, she continues in treatment and enters aftercare/relapse prevention treatment. This component consists of a gender-responsive, small group format, which meets five hours per week for the length of time the inmate remains in the DUI treatment unit. It involves developing a workable relapse prevention plan, focusing on individualized, gender-specific issues.

Prerelease treatment focuses on strengthening the knowledge, attitudes and skills obtained in the previous DUI components by using such cognitive-behavior therapeutic techniques as role-playing, behavior rehearsal, modeling, vicarious learning, corrective feedback, etc. Post-release aftercare begins at release. If the inmate is on supervised release status in the community, af-

tercare services are coordinated in conjunction with the supervising parole officer. Services are provided by the existing statewide coordinated case management and counseling that TASC maintains. Aftercare referrals are identified and indicate the inmate's case manager and how to make contact.

TASC's Post-Release Aftercare model emphasizes a skills-building approach to empowerment and the development of life area competencies. The goals of the post-release aftercare component are to provide each woman with the opportunity to:

- Improve educational and employment opportunities;
- Improve familial/social experiences and mental functioning;
- Reduce the harmful consequences/dysfunction related to alcohol and other drug use and addiction-associated behaviors;
- Reduce recidivism; and
- Decrease involvement and exposure to interpersonal domestic violence and child and sexual abuse.

Case Management Services

At the heart of the Road to Recovery aftercare model is the case management function. Case management is primarily a collaborative-helping relationship involving a trained professional, a client (inmate), whose needs are such that she requires assistance in identifying, securing and sustaining the resources (internal and external) necessary to make positive lifestyle changes, and her family.

A relapse prevention/release preparation plan is developed collaboratively with staff that can be used to help each woman effectively transition into the community. This transition plan includes:

- The inmate's goals;
- The inmate's relapse triggers;
- The inmate's general education regarding pharmacological interventions to treat symptoms and/or cravings, and stress reduction techniques;
- Community social service resources;
- Pro-social activities;
- General needs such as housing, transportation, vocation, education, child care, health care, community-based relapse prevention/aftercare programming and self-help/mutual help support groups; and
- Names, phone numbers and other information to remove barriers for the inmate to be successful in the community.

Independent Evaluation. A program's success is based on evaluation and ADC incorporated this component into the program design. Evaluation component funding has been obtained through the assistance of the Arizona Practice Improvement Collaborative, which provides funding for conducting small-scale pilot studies and activities that facilitate treatment providers' capabilities to conduct evaluations and research on the treatment services they provide. Beginning in October, an independent evaluator will furnish a formative evaluation strategy that will provide data necessary to make informed programmatic and policy decisions. Qualitative as well as quantitative measures to assess the process and impact of the program will be investigated during a 12-month period. The evaluation will involve collection of information on several different issues—knowledge, motivation and attitude change, and outcome.

The Road to Recovery program is based on the belief that people are capable of learning and changing their behaviors related to impaired driving. Society no longer ignores or denies that drinking and driving is a serious problem. In the future, consequences for repeat DUI offenses undoubtedly will be more severe than they currently are. Therefore, this program may be one of the best investments ADC can make and the best investment of time and energy an inmate can make. What is learned here may help females with alcohol or other drug-related difficulties avoid future legal problems, additional incarceration and loss of their driver's license. But more important, the information provided here may save their lives or the life of a loved one.

REFERENCES

Belknap, J. 2001. *The invisible woman: Gender, crime and justice, second edition*. Belmont. Calif.: Wadsworth.

Bureau of Justice Assistance. 1991. *Implications of the drug use forecasting data for TASC programs: Female arrestees*. Washington, D.C.: U.S. Department of Justice.

Covington, S. 1999. *Helping women recover: A program for treating substance abuse*. San Francisco: Jossey-Bass.

Covington, S. and J. Surrey. 1997. The relational model of women's psychological development: Implications for substance abuse. In *Gender and alcohol: Individual and social perspectives*, eds. S. Wilsnack, and R. Wilsnack, 335–351, New Brunswick, N.J.: Rutgers University Press.

Miller, J. 1976. *Toward a new psychology of women*. Boston: Beacon Press.

Miller, J. 1990. *Connections, disconnections and violations*. Working paper series, no. 33. Wellesley, Mass.: Stone Center.

U.S. Department of Health and Human Services. *Substance abuse treatment for women offenders: Guide to promising practices*, Technical Assistance Publication, Series 23.

Wellisch, J., M. Prendergast and M. Anglin. 1993. Number and characteristics of drug-using women in the criminal justice system: Implications for treatment. *Journal of Drug Issues*, 23(1):7–30.

Lawrence M. Sideman, Ph.D., is a licensed psychologist and assistant director/clinical director for TASC Inc. in Arizona and is a faculty member at the University of Phoenix. Ellen Kirschbaum is administrator for the Arizona Department of Corrections' Office of Substance Abuse Services.

Addicted, Neglectful Moms Offered Treatment, Custody

By Henri E. Cauvin
Washington Post Staff Writer

For many of the drug-dependent mothers who end up in D.C. Superior Court, charged with neglecting their children, the choices are rarely good.

Going into residential treatment might be their best hope for curing their destructive addictions, but it would often leave their children languishing for months in foster care, far from the one person they depend on.

A program launched yesterday by the D.C. courts and the city's social services agencies aims to give at least a few troubled mothers a better choice.

Instead of being forced to choose between treatment and their children, a few dozen mothers will enter a six-month drug rehabilitation program with their children, under the supervision of the District's new Family Treatment Court.

In a city with just 100 District-funded residential treatment slots for an estimated 60,000 addicts, the 18 beds that the new program will add will be precious.

By housing the children with their mothers and keeping them in the schools they were attending, officials hope to avoid the anxiety and depression that young children frequently feel when they are separated from the people and places they know best.

At the facility, the mothers will have help caring for the children but still will be expected to feed and dress them.

Anita Josey-Herring, the Family Court judge who will preside over Family Treatment Court, said she was skeptical about the proposal at first. "I actually had to be convinced that having kids accompany the parent into residential treatment was a good idea," she said.

The initiative, a pilot project, is modeled after efforts in Virginia, Florida and elsewhere. Seeing those programs at work persuaded Josey-Herring that they can give parents "an incentive to stop using drugs. They could see their child. They could hold their child."

Krista Evans, coordinator of women's programs at the city's Addiction Prevention and Recovery Administration, said that children and their mothers typically benefit from the new setting.

"In most cases, it's a better environment, because it's highly structured and there's a lot of support," Evans said.

"The child was probably, in most cases, parenting themselves, and now, being in a safe environment, they are able to react as children," she said.

The District's child welfare system has long been criticized as among the country's most dysfunctional. For years, it has struggled, often unsuccessfully, to deal effectively with a large caseload.

With more than 2,000 neglect cases in the court system as of Jan. 1 and more than half of those affected by drug use, the Family Treatment Court for now will reach a small number of mothers.

In all, 36 women will be chosen to participate, 18 of them in the next few days and 18 more six months from now, after the first group has completed its treatment program and moved into aftercare. Officials declined to say where the privately run residential facility will be located, saying they need to protect the privacy and ensure the safety of participants.

At the center of the new initiative is Family Court, created by Congress in 2001 after reform. The court faces new local and federal mandates to resolve a child's fate in abuse and neglect cases within 18 months.

Josey-Herring said the Family Treatment Court will give judges an important tool. Finding stable, permanent homes for the children in these cases is the overriding goal, she and others said.

If a mother overcomes her drug habit, completes the program and demonstrates progress toward becoming a good parent, her chances of being reunited with her children are good. But a parent who fails to do so, in spite of the intensive support and supervision, risks having her child or children put up for adoption and other consequences.

"We're not guaranteeing that the children will be returned to the parents," Josey-Herring said. "What we're saying is: If you are successful, it enhances your chances. But it does not guarantee it."

The project, about a year in the planning, is a collaboration by D.C. Superior Court; the Department of Health; the deputy mayor for children, youth, families and elders; and the Child and Family Services Agency, which will foot the $1.4 million bill for the treatment and supervision of participants.

Officials set up a plan to identify candidates for the program. Once a neglect case has been identified by a police officer or social worker, the city will conduct an initial screening to determine whether a mother and her children might be eligible.

Within a couple of days, a more exhaustive screening by social workers from the court and the Addiction Prevention and Recovery Administration would take place.

A few days later, the candidate could be before Josey-Herring, who will make the final decision on who enters the program, which is voluntary and requires participants to sign a contract.

Not every drug-addicted mother will be a candidate. Only those accused of neglect are eligible; mothers accused of abuse will not participate. Mothers with severe psychiatric problems or histories of violent behavior also will be excluded.

Along with their drug treatment, the women will be counseled on education, health and nutrition, with yoga a planned part of the program.

While in the program, they will appear every two weeks before Josey-Herring for progress reports.

"You're rebuilding people, essentially," she said. "You're helping them to understand that they are valuable and they have a life worth living."

Strategy For Alcohol Abuse Education:
A Service Learning Model Within a Course Curriculum

ABSTRACT

Drug abuse education, particularly on a college level, should involve students with their college and local community to establish a more fundamental understanding of the consequences of drug abuse. Therefore, we proposed a student court monitoring of driving while intoxicated (DWI) cases utilizing a service learning strategy. As a requirement for a chemical and substance abuse class, students took part in court monitoring of DWI cases within a judicial district. Students also provided a reflective paper in which they could share their subjective feelings, opinions, and overall observation of the courtroom environment. The court-monitoring of DWI cases has been implemented by Mothers Against Drunk Driving and has served as an effective tool designed to increase the likelihood of convictions, decrease the likelihood of dismissals, and in the case of a repeat offender, increase the length of jail sentence. This article examines the service learning strategy's initiation, developmental process implementation, specific outcomes, and offers suggests for future implementation and duplication within other college drug abuse courses.

Gerald D. Thompson, Susan Lyman, Kathy Childers, and Patricia Taylor

Since the passage of the 1989 Drug-Free Schools and Communities Act Amendment, many organizations and subsequent programs were developed to promote drug abuse education on the college level. The goal of drug abuse education remains not just to formally educate. Drug abuse education should also be designed to involve students in an interactive way with their local communities to bring about a more fundamental understanding of the consequences of drug abuse. Although many organizations such as the Network of Colleges and Universities Committed to the Elimination of Drug and Alcohol Abuse as well as the National College Student Organizational Network for Drug and Alcohol Education were developed in the early 1990s, many of their programs involved only administrative and student-lead extracurricular activities and programs (Office of Educa-

tional Research and Improvement, 1990). Activities such as mentoring, peer intervention, pledge contracts, and dramatized skits, although partially successful, fail to connect to the real negative consequences of drug abuse (Johnson, Anaretti, Funkwhouser, & Johnson, 1988).

It has been common the past and is still popular today that most substance abuse education programs at the high school and college levels include values clarification, questionnaires, student organization policy development, and the formation of advisory boards. Although very beneficial, these programs do not include specific course content devoted to building a practical and interactive relationship between the community and the student (Eddy, 1992; Werch, Pappas, & Castellon-Vogel, 1996). Higher education has a responsibility to the students and the communities

they serve to promote healthy behaviors. The coordination of prevention messages and activities with other aspects of a college student's life is essential. Colleges and universities need to be actively involved in coordinating community-wide activities (Bosworth, 1997; Johnson et al., 1988).

Until the mid-1990s, student drinking issues were largely the responsibility of alcohol educators and deans of students (Barber, 1992; Wechsler, Dowdall, Maener, Gledhill-Hoyt, & Lee, 1998). Because of this increasing mandate for the university to address drinking behaviors among its students, college presidents often have to get involved (Wechsler, Kelley, Weitzman, San Giovanni, & Seibring, 2000). It is, therefore, reasonable to require that chemical and substance abuse education programs and activities should be consistent with a college or university's mission. These programs should involve, consequently, not only student organizations and counseling departments but also should contain educational components that place and keep the student in close proximity to the issues and consequences of drug abuse.

CURRICULUM-SPECIFIC SERVICE LEARNING OPPORTUNITIES

Once activities and programs are identified and have been proven to have a positive impact on the reduction of drug abuse, a college or university has the responsibility of incorporating them into curriculum-specific service learning opportunities. Across the nation, drug abuse programs continue to suffer because of the lack of a proper conduit through which they can be administered. We proposed that the proper conduit might be one of service learning.

The definition of service learning is simply the integration of real life experiences with textbook facts and theories. It is reasonable to assert that the combination of a drug abuse centered curriculum within a service learning model would have several advantages (Eyler, Giles, & Schmiede, 1996). Service learning has been successfully used within courses to facilitate effective learning, and it creates a long-term commitment and appreciation toward community involvement (Kraft & Swadener, 1994). These advantages are as follows:

- Helps students connect to others—establishes bonds with peers, faculty members, public servants, victims of substance abuse, as well as the drug offender

- Helps students develop commitment to active citizenship—gives them a sense of responsibility to do something about community problems

- Enhances understanding of issues and subject matter—expands their understanding when they experience drug and alcohol abuse ex-

amples in their service learning experience

- Helps students reframe their thinking about the use, misuse, and abuse of drugs and alcohol—when service learning is coupled with reflection

Because of the above mentioned advantages of the service learning model, we have developed a strategy for alcohol education within a drug abuse course on a college campus. This article explores the strategy's initiation, developmental process implementation, specific outcomes, and offers suggestions for future implementation and duplication within other college drug abuse courses.

STRATEGY INITIATION

From an educator's perspective, it is often very difficult to gauge whether students are actually experiencing affective learning. Conventional methods of assessing student comprehension can be used, but usually a question remains, however faint, "Has the student gained a sincere appreciation of concepts and facts that were presented?" and, more important, "Will it change their behavior?" Therefore, as educators we remain constantly in search of new and innovative ways of delivering course information to better assess student understanding. One such idea came into being after inviting the local area president of Mothers Against Drunk Driving (MADD) as a guest speaker to a chemical and substance (drug) abuse class. After the presentation, the area president of MADD commented that the local chapter was having problems with their driving while intoxicated (DWI) court monitoring program. The problem was that only a small number of individual volunteers were doing the work of monitoring the DWI court proceedings. This came as no surprise because most of the MADD volunteer members held full-time jobs, and all of the DWI court cases were heard during the day. Logistically, it was virtually impossible to implement a viable and consistent

program of court monitoring without a large pool of volunteers who had the time and energy to devote to the program. Students could fill the role of court monitors perfectly while satisfying the requirements of a great class project.

The court-monitoring of DWI cases, which is implemented by MADD, serves as an effective tool designed to increase the likelihood of convictions, decrease the likelihood of dismissals, and in the case of a repeat offender, increase the length of jail sentence. The goals of the court-monitoring program are:

- To improve the judicial system by compiling pertinent statistical information on the handling of DWI cases

- To provide feedback to the state legislators on the effectiveness and enforceability of the current DWI laws

- To let those determining the results of criminal cases know of the public's interest in the outcome (MADD, 1993b)

After discussing the court-monitoring program with the Louisiana executive director of MADD, we spoke with the university's office of public relations to verify its position with MADD's DWI court-monitoring program. We also determined the feasibility of administering such a program through one of the university's courses. In other words, it was extremely important that the program being initiated be congruent with or at least not contrary to the university's overall mission and working relationship with the community. The Public Relations Department noted that not only was a court-monitoring program consistent with the university's mission, but it was also inherently consistent with the university's policy on community involvement. Subsequently, the public relations department sent out a press release notifying the media and the public that such a program would be initiated.

Once the program was cleared through the university system, the

---

Figure 1. Driving While Intoxicated (DWI) Court Monitoring Form

Student Name or Assigned Number:_____

Date:_____   **Case Number:**_____

Judge:_____   **Prosecutor:**_____

Defense Attorney:_____   **Charge:**_____

Case Information

Defendant:_____   **Arresting Officer:**_____

BAC Results: _____

Other Evidence: _____

Prior Convictions: _____

Property Damage: _____

Injuries: _____

Death(s): _____

Judgement

Fine: _____   **Suspended:**   ❐ Yes   ❐ No

Jail Time _____ mos/yrs   **Suspended:**   ❐ Yes   ❐ No

License Suspended: ❐ Yes   ❐ No   **If yes, how long?** _____

Revoked: ❐ Yes   ❐ No

Other Action: _____

_____

_____

Treatment

Alcohol Information School: ❐ Yes   ❐ No   **If yes, how long?** _____

Alcohol Inpatient Treatment: ❐ Yes   ❐ No   **If yes, how long?** _____

Probation: ❐ Yes   ❐ No   **If yes, how long?** _____

Conditions of Probation: _____

_____

Follow-up: _____

Charges Reduced: ❐ Yes   ❐ No

If yes, to what charge?_____

Restitution: ❐ Yes   ❐ No   **If yes, provisions?**_____

Community Service: ❐ Yes   ❐ No   **If yes, how long?** _____

---

next step was to ensure the proper scheduling of students to court-monitoring cases. Although seemingly very straightforward, scheduling was one of the most difficult tasks to accomplish. At the time of program's initiation the Louisiana 15th Judicial District and the Lafayette City Court System was in the process of restructuring. As a result of this, there were constant DWI district and city court time changes. However, once both city and district court times were obtained and verified, student scheduling proceeded.

Because both city and district courts in the downtown area were located minutes away from the main campus, transportation problems did not occur. However, for those campuses that are located a distance away from where court proceedings occur, some sort of prearranged transportation schedule should be implemented. At the least there should be car-pooling among students so that costs to students are kept at a minimum.

The last step was to arrange a meeting with the Louisiana Executive Board of MADD to propose that the student court-monitoring program be administered through a curriculum-specific service learning course. After the program was discussed with them, they approved it with the requirement that the information gathered within the classroom experience be made available to both the state and local chapter of MADD.

PROCESS IMPLEMENTATION

Before the implementation of the DWI court-monitoring program, there were a few logistical and administrative problems to be overcome to be most effective and efficient, we needed to maximize the number of times that students would have the opportunity to view DWI court cases. Therefore, the program needed to be initiated as close to the start of the semester as possible. Because of this, we had to reorganize some key features of our chemical and substance abuse course. Information from the chapter titled "Drugs and the Law" was moved to an earlier time so that the students would receive the information on alcohol and the law within the proper context. Consistent with contextual delivery of drug information, the state executive director of MADD also presented information on court monitoring.

This information consisted of the following:

- Introduction to the mission of MADD: The mission of MADD is to stop drunk driving and to support victims of this violent crime. MADD's goal in regard to court monitoring is to observe the system and collect important data concerning DWI cases.
- The purpose of court monitoring: According to the National Highway Traffic Safety Administration (Shihar, 1990), statistics that can be gathered through a court-monitoring program can provide the following information: (1) an analysis of sentences handed down by particular judges for particular offenses, (2) the number of DWI cases heard during a given period in a particular jurisdiction, and (3) the number of DWI cases that actually go to trial in a particular jurisdiction.
- The role of a court monitor: The judicial system needs to know that the public is concerned and wants to know what happens to DWI offenders. A defendant prosecuted to the fullest extent of the law may be deterred from committing another offense. As a courtroom monitor, one must document everything seen and heard. A monitor's presence in court can have a great impact. Judges, prosecutors, defense lawyers, and police quickly learn who is a court monitor, even if no identification is worn.
- Introduction to DWI cases and the criminal justice system

- Familiarization with key courtroom terms and definitions
- Acquainting the student with the DWI court monitoring form (Figure 1)
- Showing a video on the court-monitoring program: The video reviewed important guidelines to follow when court monitoring, such as not wearing any badges; not bringing any reading material, such as a newspaper, into the courtroom; arriving on time; acting professionally; sitting at the front of the courtroom; and a host of other suggestions that enhance the courtroom experience (MADD, 1993a).

All information had to be presented and made available to the students prior to any monitoring of courtroom cases.

OUTCOMES

The court-monitoring program was initiated primarily to provide students with the opportunity to be directly involved with the community. The experience as a court monitor gave the student a chance to be placed within a service learning environment. As a requirement for the chemical and substance abuse class, students took part in court monitoring of DWI cases within a judicial district. This service learning project was considered as mandatory for successful completion of the course. Students were required to fill out a court-monitoring form detailing the specifics of the observed DWI case. Students also were required to write a short summary of the court proceedings. This summary was a reflective paper in which the student could share his or her subjective feelings, opinions, and overall observation of the courtroom environment.

Reflective writing is a very important component of the service learning model. Through the reflective summary of the individual student, one could assess the effective component of learning—the central question being "has the student gained a sincere appreciation of the consequences of DWI offenses"

(Dass & Gorman, 1991). All materials, including both the court monitoring form and the subjective summary report, were subsequently made available to the Louisiana state chapter of MADD.

Summaries written by individual students were very interesting and thought provoking. From this service learning experience most students came away with an overall positive practical experience. One student wrote:

I am really glad I got an opportunity to sit in court and watch DWI cases. This was very interesting to me. I am a criminal justice major and I have sat in on court sessions many times. But before this assignment I had never witnessed DWI cases. I always wondered what went on and if it was the same thing I have always seen. Even though many things were similar to my previous experiences, it was also very different. I have to say it was very compelling.

First of all, I could not believe how many people were there waiting to get called up by the judge. They had a huge docket the day that I went. I was expecting the court to be filled with people my age (around 21 or 22). I always thought people my age got millions of DWI's [as a result of] coming from clubs or parties. Actually, there was only one guy who looked about my age. All the other people, men and women, were of older ages maybe late fifties or early sixties.

Another thing that amazed me was how fast the judge moved through the docket. It was almost like he was trying to hurry up as fast as he could. He would call the person up, talk to them for about 2 minutes and then give them their sentence. It seems to me that he should have given them a lecture of some sort. Overall, I am very glad I got to experience this. It was very entertaining and informative in many ways.

Clearly, this service learning experience had an impact on this student regardless of her previous court observation experience. Another student wrote:

On October __, 1999, I went to the District Courthouse in Lafayette, to sit in on a Driving While Intoxicated (DWI) case. It presented a young woman, ____, this was her second DWI offense. In fact, this was about all the information I received due to the amount of time the judge takes to hear all the other small cases. These were many small offenses of driving with no license, and running stop signs, all those were paid off. I went at about 9:00 a.m. and the big case of the second offense DWI was delayed to be heard at 10:45, everything was so unorganized and people walking around in the courtroom. The judge took about two recesses in order to let the prosecutor and defense attorneys get ready and organize them in the proper way. Actually the judge was ready to start the case, asking the young woman questions about, "Was this your first offense? What was her blood alcohol level?" And before she could answer the judge requested that she recess to let everyone get ready. So the judge went to her office. I even went to try and find the judges office but was unable to find her in her office. In conclusion, this court monitoring exercise took a lot of time and was difficult to fit between my class schedule and the judge's schedule.

Although this student obviously did not have a positive experience, the summary report presented very interesting but alarming information about the courtroom monitoring experience. Still another student wrote:

This court experience was of my very own. My attorney is _____. The prosecutor in this case was _____. The judge presiding this case was Judge _____. The police officer that pulled me over was _____. In this case he testified that he gave the field sobriety test and that I failed to perform them correctly. His main argument was that I was supposed to have my hands at my side, and I placed them on my hips. My attorney tried to explain to him that the

tests were performed correctly, and that it may have been my nerves, because my hands were on my hips the entire video. And not only that, but [also] indeed that my hands, being on my hips, were in fact by my side. It was quite obvious after viewing the tapes that I was only "legally intoxicated." Another issue was that a police officer must read all (rights) before asking to give the breathalyzer, and this police officer failed to do so. Although a technicality, the Judge warned the police officer that she would not rule with my attorney's plea to throw the results of the breathalyzer out on account that he did not read all parts, but in the future she would have to because of my size and the time I drank them. At the end the Judge basically told me that there was not a doubt in her mind that she would have found me innocent, but because of my BAC she had to find me guilty. My attorney has appealed to another judge and my sentencing day is December __. 1999. He thinks I have a good chance because of what the judge said at the end. When I was leaving, the prosecutor, the police officer, and a professor, who was just witnessing, all wished me luck and said they thought I performed all of the tests great. This just goes to show that you can only have a few beers and can be considered legally drunk. Unfortunately, I got caught. I don't intend for this to happen to me again, but I was told by a cop, "always refuse the breathalyzer." I learned my lesson the hard way.

This young student's experience was unique because at the time of participation in this court-monitoring project, the student had also been charged with DWI. It seems that the two previous student statements show more effective learning taking place, however. This student was just sorry about getting caught and learned a way to beat the system by simply refusing to take the breathalyzer test. This student's experience was a self-serving one, and the student cannot be considered to have gained a sincere appreciation of the

consequences of alcohol abuse. However, through this service learning experience the student did get a chance at a learning opportunity, and the judicial system benefited by her participation, nonetheless.

SUGGESTIONS FOR FUTURE IMPLEMENTATION

Initially, it was difficult to obtain correct information on the exact times and dates of DWI court proceedings from city and district court officials. It is recommended that before visiting your local city and district courthouses, the most efficient means of acquiring correct information would be through a liaison. Preferably this liaison would be someone from the clerk of court's office. Therefore, any information obtained from any other source can be given to that individual for confirmation.

The number of days that a judicial district actually holds court is an important aspect to this project. In our case there were only 2 days in which DWI court cases were heard. This made scheduling for students extremely difficult, allowing for only 2 days during which to perform their court-monitoring assignments. Although students have more flexible time than full-time MADD volunteers have, students still had logistical problems scheduling court-monitoring times around their regularly scheduled courses. It is possible that if the court were so informed of the logistical difficulties that stem from such a restricted time frame, the court might be willing to rearrange court dates and times to better accommodate student DWI court monitors. It is also possible that with future court-monitoring programs more than one city and judicial district could be involved.

Consistent with one of the tenets of the service learning model, it is suggested that the judge, prosecutor, and defense attorney make themselves available to colleges, instructors, and students. Perhaps through classroom presentations, university seminars, and individual appointment, both professional and personal relationships could be established. Ultimately, through this process the student will gain a better understanding of the various roles that professionals play within the criminal justice system and the consequences of alcohol and drug abuse.

REFERENCES

Barber, B. R. (1992). *An aristocracy of everyone, the politics of education and the future of America*. New York: Oxford University Press.

Bosworth, K. (1997). *Drug abuse prevention: School based strategies that work* (Report No. EDO-SP-96-4) Washington, DC: ERIC Clearinghouse on Teaching and Teacher Education. (ERIC Document Reproduction Service No. ED 409 316).

Dass, R., & Gorman, P. (1991). *How can I help? Stories and reflections on service*. New York: Knopf.

Eddy, M. S. (1992). *College alcohol and drug abuse prevention programs: An update* (Report No. BBB27915). George Washington University, Washington, DC: ERIC Clearinghouse on Higher Education (ERIC Document Reproduction Service No. ED 347 960).

Eyler, J., Giles, D. E. Jr., & Schmiede, A. (1996). *A Practitioner's guide to reflection in service-learning*. Nashville: Vanderbilt University.

Johnson, E. M., Anaretti, S., Funkwhouser, J. E., & Johnson, S. (1988). Theories and models supporting prevention approaches to alcohol problems among youth. *Public Health Reports*, 578–586.

Kraft, R. J., & Swadener, M. (Eds.). (1994). *Building community: Service learning in the academic disciplines*. Denver: Colorado Campus Compact.

Mothers Against Drunk Driving (MADD). (1993a). *Court-monitoring in non-victim cases* [Video]. National Office Programs Department. (Available from Mothers Against Drunk Driving, 2401 Bristol Court SW, Olympia, WA 98502).

Mothers Against Drunk Driving (MADD). (1993b). *Court-monitoring reference guide*. National Office Programs Department. (Available from Mothers Against Drunk Driving, 2401 Bristol Court SW, Olympia, WA 98502).

Shinar, D. (1990). *Impact of Court Monitoring on DWI Adjudication*. Washington, DC: National Highway Traffic Safety Administration (DOT HSS807678).

Office of Educational Research and Improvement. (1990). *Standards of the network of colleges and universities committed to the elimination of drug and alcohol abuse*. Washington, DC: ERIC Clearinghouse on Higher Education (Eric Document Reproduction Service No. ED 297 661).

Wechsler, H., Dowdall, G. W., Maener, G., Gledhill-Hoyt, J., & Lee, H. (1998). Changes in binge drinking and related problems among American college students between 1993 and 1997. Results of the Harvard School of Public Health College Alcohol Study. *Journal of American College of Health*, 47, 57–68.

Wechsler, H., Kelley, K., Weitzman, E. R., San Giovanni, J. P., & Seibring, M. (2000). What colleges are doing about student binge drinking. Survey of College Administrators. *Journal of American College of Health*, 48, 219–226.

Werch, C. E., Pappas, D. M., & Castellon-Vogel, E. A. (1996). Drug use prevention efforts at colleges and universities in the United States. *Substance Use and Misuse*, 31, 65–80.

Gerald D. Thompson, PhD, and Susan Lyman, PhD, are assistant professors at the University of Louisiana at Lafayette, Department of Kinesiology, 225 Cajundome Blvd, Lafayette, LA 70506; E-mail: gdt3053@louisiana.edu. Kathy Childers and Patricia Taylor are the executive director and local president, respectively, of the Louisiana Affiliate of Mothers Against Drunk Driving.

From *American Journal of Health Education*, March/April 2002, pp. 88-93. © 2002 by AAHPERD. Reprinted by permission.

HIV/Hepatitis Prevention in Drug Abuse Treatment Programs: Guidance From Research

A large body of research examines the relationship between HIV and drug dependence, but considerably less information is available on viral hepatitis and drug dependence. This article summarizes research indicating what drug abuse treatment programs can do to prevent their patients from acquiring HIV or hepatitis infection and to limit the consequences for patients who are already infected. Drug treatment programs can play a pivotal role in preventing, detecting, and treating HIV and hepatitis. Some activities can be accomplished by providers' simply becoming aware of the issues; others will require significant infusion of leadership, education, and fiscal support.

James L. Sorensen, Ph.D.
Carmen L. Masson, Ph.D.
David C. Perlman, M.D.

In the United States, drug users have been disproportionately affected by the AIDS epidemic. As a result, the substance abuse research community has developed substantial knowledge about how to prevent HIV infection and systems to facilitate the management of those already infected. Yet, the drug treatment practitioner's current knowledge of hepatitis, particularly hepatitis C, is similar to what was known about AIDS a decade ago. There is a growing, but still incomplete, understanding of the transmission of hepatitis C, its acute presentation, and how it behaves as a chronic infection. Treatment is available for chronic hepatitis C. While treatment effectiveness may be limited, the importance of detecting hepatitis C infection, particularly acute (new-onset) infection, has been bolstered by recent evidence that treatment during the acute stage may prevent the establishment of chronic infection (Jaeckel et al., 2001).

In drug treatment programs, addressing medical issues such as infectious diseases may be secondary to the goal of reducing patients' drug abuse. Staff members in drug treatment programs may wonder how much attention they should give to these problems, particularly if they feel they have little to offer clients by way of prevention or treatment. Nevertheless, by decreasing drug use and HIV risk behaviors and by educating patients about

HIV, drug abuse treatment has become one of the most powerful AIDS prevention techniques in our public health arsenal. With adequate funding and public health support, drug abuse treatment programs can play a central role in preventing and detecting hepatitis as well.

Drug abuse treatment providers have unequaled opportunity to reach drug abusers with health information and interventions. This article presents a number of suggestions, based on research, about what a drug treatment program can do to address HIV and hepatitis infections. First we review the extent of these infections among drug users. Then we discuss techniques for using research-developed assessment and diagnostic tools. Finally, we suggest primary and secondary preventive activities that a treatment program can implement to limit the spread and consequences of infection.

PREVALENCE OF HIV AND HEPATITIS AMONG DRUG USERS

The prevalence of HIV among drug users entering treatment varies across different settings, ranging from 0 to 35 percent. Some transmission of HIV continues among those in drug abuse treatment, especially younger injecting drug users (IDUs) (Murrill et al., 2001). IDUs are at high risk of infection with HIV and hepatitis A, B, and C viruses through unsterile injection practices and unsafe sexual behaviors. Injection drug use is a factor in one-third of all AIDS cases in the United States, more than one-half of new HIV infections, and one-half of new hepatitis C infections. IDUs as a group have high prevalence of viral hepatitis: Approximately 40 to 70 percent develop hepatitis A infection at some time in their injection careers, while their prevalence rates for hepatitis B and C are 50 to 90 percent. Some noninjecting users of illicit drugs, such as crack smokers, are also at risk of contracting viral hepatitis.

There is significant overlap between modes of transmission and hence between risk factors for HIV and hepatitis A, B, and C.

Hepatitis is an inflammation of the liver, most often caused by alcohol or a virus. In the past, health providers often assumed that nearly all drug users were infected with hepatitis A and B by the time they entered drug abuse treatment, but today significant numbers of drug users in the community are free of these viruses. Thus, many patients entering treatment could benefit from vaccines to protect against hepatitis A and B. Although many or most IDUs become infected with hepatitis C during their first year of injecting, some patients entering treatment programs are still uninfected and susceptible.

TRANSMISSION OF HIV AND HEPATITIS

HIV is transmitted through sharing of unsterile syringes and through unprotected sexual activity. The virus may also be transmitted from mother to child during birth and the weeks before and after—the perinatal period. New data suggest that sexual transmission of HIV is also an important mode among IDUs: Male IDUs who have sex with men and female IDUs who trade sex for money are more likely to become HIV-infected than IDUs who do not engage in those behaviors (Kral et al., 2001).

There is significant overlap between modes of transmission and hence between risk factors for HIV and hepatitis A, B, and C. Because HIV and hepatitis are transmitted by many of the same routes, risk-reduction efforts aimed at HIV transmission have also reduced the spread of hepatitis. However, hepatitis can be transmitted in more ways than HIV. Hepatitis A and B may be transmitted to household members and other close contacts who are not sexual partners.

Hepatitis A is spread through unsanitary living conditions, inadequate personal hygiene, and direct or indirect anal-oral contact, including sexual behaviors. Transmission of the virus in feces predominates, but hepatitis A is also transmitted via contact with contaminated drug injection equipment. Use of contaminated water to prepare drugs and contamination of drugs hidden in the rectum may play a role. Hepatitis A causes acute, not chronic, inflammation of the liver.

Hepatitis B virus is found in the semen, blood, and saliva of infected persons and is usually spread by contaminated syringes and unprotected sexual contact. From 1 to 10 percent of patients develop chronic liver inflammation, which may progress to cirrhosis and liver cancer.

Hepatitis C virus is transmitted through contaminated blood (for example, during syringe sharing) and through needle-stick injuries and unprotected sexual contact. In addition, recent research shows hepatitis C transmission associated with the sharing of unsterile injection equipment other than syringes (cookers, filtration cotton, rinse water) (NIDA, 2000). Hepatitis C appears to spread more rapidly among IDUs than does HIV, because of higher prevalence of hepatitis C among injection partners and a higher infectivity of hepatitis C once it gets into the bloodstream (Garfein et al., 1996; Hagan and Des Jarlais, 2000). From 10 to 60 percent of individuals infected with hepatitis C virus develop some form of chronic liver inflammation.

Drug abuse treatment and interventions such as syringe exchange and outreach, which have focused on reducing the use of contaminated syringes, have been associated with lower incidence of HIV infection but have had less consistent or no effects on new cases of hepatitis C. To affect the transmission of hepatitis C, risk-reduction interventions are needed that address not only syringe use, but also sexual behaviors and the use of injection paraphernalia in addition to syringes (such as filtration cottons, cookers, and rinse water).

STAFF ASSESSING PATIENTS' RISKS

Tools Available

Drug abuse treatment programs can incorporate risk assessment and educational messages about HIV risks into their intake and counseling protocols. The assessment must be done with an instrument that can reliably measure both drug-related and sex-related risk behaviors. Several self-report measures have been designed to assess drug use, injection practices, and sexual behaviors associated with HIV risk. Among the most widely used instruments are three that have demonstrated high reliability and validity: the Risk Behavior Assessment Questionnaire (NIDA, 1991), the Risk Assessment Battery (Treatment Research Institute, *www.tresearch.org/Assessment% 20Inst /Assess_inst.html*), and the Texas Christian University (TCU) AIDS Risk Assessment (Camacho et al., 1997; *www.ibr.tcu.edu*).

The Risk Assessment Battery Questionnaire and TCU AIDS Risk Assessment may be particularly useful in clinical settings because they can be administered in 15 minutes or less and require minimal staff training. A computerized version of the Rick Assessment Battery is as accurate as the paper-and-pencil version (Navaline et al., 1994). To maximize the accuracy of assessments, counselors can establish a non-judgmental context; explicitly assure patients of privacy and confidentiality; explain why questions are being asked (when the purpose of questions is not obvious to a patient); consider the impact of related problems (such as psychiatric or legal difficulties) on assessment of risk behaviors; and, where appropriate and feasible, use self-administered or computerized tests to eliminate the need for patients to report socially sensitive information face to face.

Laboratory Testing and Counseling

Given the demonstrated clinical value of medical and psychosocial interventions to treat and prevent HIV, drug abuse treatment programs should offer HIV testing and counseling. The only exceptions would be programs that see patients for shorter periods than the time needed to obtain test results and provide feedback. In general, IDUs who know they are infected engage in high-risk activities less frequently than those who are not infected or do not know their HIV status. While patients newly diagnosed with HIV occasionally develop stress reactions and inject drugs more frequently, such responses are generally transient and not usually associated with the increases in risky injection behaviors that can lead to further HIV transmission. Supportive pretest and post-test counseling, which can anticipate such reactions and reduce their impact, are an indispensable part of the testing process.

The rates of false positive reactions among HIV tests (which routinely include both ELISA and Western Blot assays) are extremely low; hence, any confirmed positive test should be taken as evidence of HIV infection. In the rare circumstances in which HIV Western Blot results are indeterminate, individuals should be referred for expert evaluation.

Blood tests can indicate whether a patient is susceptible to hepatitis A or B (and thus should receive vaccine) or has antibodies that reflect previous exposure and immunity (in which case vaccination is not needed). The tests can also reveal whether a patient has active or resolved hepatitis B infection. For the hepatitis C virus, an antibody test reveals only prior exposure to the virus and does not indicate whether the infection is new (acute), chronic (long-term), or resolved. Findings indicating chronic active hepatitis B infection or evidence of exposure to hepatitis C infection should prompt referral for clinical evaluation and possible treatment. Screening for hepatitis B has been recommended as a routine part of care in drug abuse treatment programs (Center for Substance Abuse Treatment, 1995; *www.health.org/govpubs/bkd131/*), and these programs are valuable settings for hepatitis A and C screenings, as well. For more specific guidance in the interpretation of hepatitis tests, see box, "How To Interpret Hepatitis Test Results."

PRIMARY PREVENTION OF INFECTION

We use "primary prevention" to describe strategies to limit the drug abuse patient's exposure to infectious agents and to minimize the impact of such exposure. Primary preven-

---

How To Interpret Hepatitis Test Results

Hepatitis B

- The absence of any hepatitis B markers demonstrates susceptibility to hepatitis B; vaccination is indicated.

- The presence of hepatitis B surface antigen demonstrates active hepatitis B infection, which may progress to chronic liver disease. False positive tests are extremely uncommon.

- The presence of hepatitis B surface antibody demonstrates immunity to hepatitis b, either from prior vaccination (in which case the hepatitis B core antibody would be negative) or from prior naturally acquired but resolved disease (in which case hepatitis B core antibody would be positive).

- Some individuals may have isolated hepatitis B core IgG antibody reactivity. This may be due to either low-level active infection (in which case a hepatitis B DNA test would be positive) or very remote resolved hepatitis B infection with loss of hepatitis B surface antibody over many years (the development of hepatitis B surface antibody in response to a dose of vaccine confirms this) or to a false positive hepatitis core antibody test. In the latter instance, hepatitis B vaccination is indicated.

Hepatitis C

- Hepatitis C antibody reactivity means that hepatitis C infection is likely. Referral for clinical evaluation is indicated

  to confirm active hepatitis C infection by documenting detectable hepatitis C virus by a viral load assay,

  to assess for liver disease with liver function tests, and

  possibly, to conduct a liver biopsy to consider treatment of hepatitis C.

---

tion efforts include education and counseling, vaccination, and outreach to bring IDUs into treatment.

Risk Education

To address the problem of HIV/AIDS among patients and their contacts, drug abuse treatment programs have incorporated education about reducing risky behavior as part of drug counseling protocols. Gibson and colleagues (1998; also *http://hivinsite.ucsf.edu/InSite.jsp?page–kb–07&doc=kb–07–04–01–01*) reviewed the controlled research evaluations of a range of counseling interventions aimed at preventing IDUs from acquiring HIV/AIDS. They found that more intensive interventions—that is, those with more patient contact—seemed to reduce risky injection drug use practices and sexual behaviors more than did less intensive interventions. Components of successful programs include individual or group counseling sessions focused on skill-building, relapse prevention, and HIV counseling and testing.

What a Drug Treatment Program Can Do To Incorporate HIV/Hepatitis Prevention

Assessment and Diagnosis

Assess risks of acquiring or transmitting infection
Obtain history of prior hepatitis disease and/or vaccination
Conduct serologic screening for HIV and hepatitis
Identify candidates for HIV treatment and for hepatitis A and B vaccines

Preventing Infection (Primary Prevention)

Engage patient in drug abuse treatment
Provide pre- and post-test counseling when screening for HIV and hepatitis
Educate and provide counseling about risky needle use and sexual risk behaviors
Deliver hepatitis A and B vaccines
Build ties to outreach agencies

- Syringe exchange programs
- HIV counseling and testing centers
- Community outreach agencies

For IDUs who continue to inject, refer to reliable sources of sterile syringes

Limiting the Consequences of Disease (Secondary Prevention)

Link patients to or provide primary medical care (active referral strategies, on-site care)
Link patients with agencies that address their problems with retention in medical care and drug abuse treatment
Promote medication adherence: reminder systems, social support, incentive strategies

General Information and Communications

Keep abreast of changing research, ethical and legal issues
Educate staff and community about medical complications of drug abuse and treatment options
Join community leaders and patient representatives in providing information about how to address HIV and hepatitis more effectively

Drug abuse treatment programs and syringe exchange programs (SEPs) can improve, however, at providing hepatitis prevention education and interventions. In a recent survey of two New York City SEPs, the majority of IDUs had previously been in drug abuse treatment. Although most were concerned about hepatitis, most had not been tested for hepatitis C virus, were not aware that vaccines were available to prevent hepatitis A and B, and did not know that hepatitis C therapy existed (Perlman et al., 2001).

While there is debate about the optimal approach to hepatitis C treatment for active drug users (Edlin et al., 2001), few would argue against providing education about how to reduce risks for hepatitis as part of drug abuse counseling. Those entering drug abuse treatment should be provided with education about viral hepatitis and offered hepatitis testing. Counseling can help prevent new infection among those who are still susceptible

and help those already infected to avoid transmitting the disease to others. The content of counseling should reflect emerging evidence that sharing of cottons and cookers transmits hepatitis C, that risk-reduction strategies applied to HIV prevention can also help to prevent hepatitis transmission, and that vaccination for hepatitis A and B may be important if the patient is susceptible.

Patients with chronic hepatitis B infection or recent or chronic hepatitis C infection should be advised that treatment exists that can help prevent progression of the disease, and they should be referred for evaluation for therapy. Chronic hepatitis B infection or other liver disease may be treated with lamivudine, which is associated with improvement in liver function in more than 50 percent of patients treated. Treatment of chronic hepatitis C infection with alpha interferon agents alone (either alpha interferon or PEG-alpha interferon) or in combination with ribavirin may prevent progression of, or even reverse, liver disease in infected patients. Overall, about 30 to 40 percent of all patients can expect to have sustained viral clearance with the combination of an interferon agent and ribavirin. Recent data suggest that the treatment of acute hepatitis C can prevent the establishment of chronic hepatitis C infection (Jaeckel et al., 2001).

Vaccines

Although there is not yet any vaccine against hepatitis C, vaccination can prevent hepatitis A and B. For those with chronic hepatitis C infection who are susceptible to hepatitis A or B, vaccination is important, since infection with other forms of hepatitis may lead to liver failure. The rates of vaccination for hepatitis A and B are low among IDUs, however, suggesting lost opportunities for prevention. The most successful vaccine delivery systems to date are those that either administer vaccines at the drug abuse treatment site or use incentives to encourage patients to follow through on being vaccinated elsewhere. Models based solely on providing vouchers for free vaccines have produced less impressive rates of completed immunization (Des Jarlais et al., 2001).

Two vaccines for hepatitis A and two for hepatitis B have been approved for use in the United States. They should not be given to patients with prior hypersensitivity to the vaccines or their components. Hepatitis A and hepatitis B vaccines may be used together, generally minimizing inconvenience to patients without increasing adverse effects or decreasing effectiveness. Providing the two vaccines at the same time may also increase the likelihood that patients will complete the vaccine series. The hepatitis A vaccine is given at month 0 (the start of hepatitis treatment) and 6 months; the hepatitis B vaccine is given at 0, 1, and 4 to 6 months. Alternatively, for patients who need immunization against both hepatitis A and B, a recently approved combination vaccine may be used (at 0, 1, and 4 to 6 months) to reduce the number of injections.

Although complete courses of each vaccine are needed for optimal benefit, there is significant clinical value to patients who receive incomplete courses or even single doses; therefore, there is no need to guarantee that a patient will complete the series before initiating vaccination. To ensure that susceptible drug abusers receive at least one vaccine dose, the usual practice is to obtain a blood sample for testing and administer a first dose of vaccine at the initial visit.

Hepatitis B vaccination in SEPs has been a useful component of the public health response to a hepatitis B outbreak among IDUs in Pierce County, Washington. A pilot study of SEP-based hepatitis B vaccination in New York City had an 83-percent rate of completed vaccine series (Des Jarlais et al., 2001).

Outreach to IDUs

Drug abuse treatment programs can build ties to other community-based programs for cooperative efforts in HIV and hepatitis prevention. Some SEPs offer HIV counseling and testing, flu and pneumonia vaccines, and other medical services either at the program site or by referral elsewhere. Many SEPs provide prevention services in neighborhoods where drug users live to reach those who are unwilling or unable to use conventional services elsewhere. SEPs can also promote prevention by linking IDUs—including those contacted through outreach efforts such as field workers' visits to homes and shooting galleries—with drug abuse treatment. In one study, Heimer (1998) found that both SEP and non-SEP clients used the SEP to obtain referrals to drug abuse treatment, and of those requesting treatment, 60 percent started therapy. Moreover, compared with clients referred by other sources, drug users referred by SEPs have comparably good short-term drug abuse treatment outcomes.

HIV counseling and testing centers where drug users present for confidential or anonymous HIV testing have the potential to serve as sources of referral to drug abuse treatment, medical care, and other prevention services. The advantage of this approach is that the initial contact may afford the provider an opportunity to engage the patient in ongoing prevention and drug abuse treatment services.

Community outreach, which relies on peers and community residents to identify out-of-treatment drug users and initiate risk-reduction counseling, may also serve as a conduit to prevention services. Basic risk-reduction activities usually include raising awareness about HIV and other blood-borne diseases, teaching skills to reduce risky drug use and sexual behaviors, providing materials for protection (for example, condoms and bleach), and counseling and testing for HIV. Studies show that outreach interventions are effective in reducing risky injection drug use practices and increasing protective behaviors, including entry into drug abuse treatment, needle disinfection, and condom use (Coyle et al., 1998). Drug treatment personnel could benefit from reading NIDA's manual on how to conduct effective community outreach (NIDA, 2000).

In summary, linkages between drug abuse treatment programs and community-based prevention services, such as SEPs and HIV counseling and testing centers, have the potential to reduce the risk of both HIV and hepatitis. Creating formal agreements or linkages between drug abuse treatment programs and these referral sources may assist drug users in accessing drug abuse treatment, prevention, and health care services.

SECONDARY PREVENTION: LIMITING DISEASE CONSEQUENCES

The term "secondary prevention" here refers to interventions for people who are already infected with HIV or hepatitis. The goals of secondary prevention are to limit the medical consequences of infection and diminish the further spread of the disease. An excellent manual for drug abuse treatment providers offers a range of tips and suggestions (Center for Substance Abuse Treatment, 2000), including ways to incorporate primary medical care, mental health, and social services into drug abuse treatment programs; to link with other "wrap-around" services such as case management; and to keep abreast of changing legal and ethical issues of treating people who have HIV infection.

Links to Primary Care

Patients in drug abuse treatment may encounter substantial barriers to receiving health care, such as lack of insurance or transportation, perceived attitudes of providers, social disorganization, and competing priorities. Patients generally receive few medical services while in drug abuse treatment, yet drug treatment programs can play a critical role in determining outcomes such as acceptance of therapy, appointment-keeping, and adherence to medication schedules.

Drug treatment programs are in a pivotal position to reach a population that is at risk for HIV and hepatitis and has high prevalence of those diseases.

Research has provided a growing body of evidence that delivering medical and psychosocial services at drug abuse treatment sites increases patients' utilization of primary medical care, medical screening, and mental health services; improves medication compliance and medical outcomes, retention in treatment, and substance use outcomes; and reduces emergency room visits (e.g., Selwyn et al., 1989). Moreover, HIV-related medical care programs incorporated into drug abuse treatment settings show high rates of utilization and medication compliance and have the potential to deliver hepatitis prevention services to drug users (Selwyn et al., 1989).

Service delivery models that provide medical care onsite at drug abuse treatment programs (or nearby) have several advantages, including attention to multiple service needs during a single visit, enhanced communica-

RESPONSE: APPLYING HIV STRATEGIES TO HEPATITIS PREVENTION

Eric Ennis, director of adult outpatient services for Addiction Research and Treatment Services, University of Colorado Health Sciences Center, Denver, led five ARTS clinicians in a roundtable discussion.

Janelle Blake: In the past year or two, our clients who have died were lost to liver diseases and not HIV-related diseases. This is a very important article.

Marla Corwin: It's written clearly and simply. I feel that I could give it directly to clients and say, 'Read this,' and they would understand what they're reading.

The HIV analogy

Eric Ennis: I was struck by the fact that the article suggests the same strategies and techniques that we have used for years to counsel HIV-positive clients can also be applied to counseling hepatitis C patients and for use in prevention. It seems so obvious and yet it had never crossed my mind to use HIV prevention techniques as hepatitis B and C prevention techniques.

Counseling is important because of clients' resistance to testing and their shock when they test positive.

Corwin: The HIV prevention strategies that we use, talking to our clients and screening and education, those techniques could be incorporated and applied for free. This is the kind of counseling that we already do.

Ennis: As a general rule, injection drug users who know they are infected engage in high-risk drug and sexual activities less frequently than those who are uninfected or unaware of their HIV status. In applying this to hepatitis C, we could perhaps appeal to our hepatitis C-positive clients to reduce these same high-risk practices using the same appeals we make to our HIV-positive clients—to be considerate of others, to not spread the virus, respect themselves, respect others. I just never applied this to hepatitis C clients.

Client resistance

Ennis: As an administrator, I find this article minimizes the importance of client resistance.

Corwin: The counseling is important because of the client's resistance to testing and their shock when they test positive. They don't think, 'Oh my God; I'm going to die,' like they do when they hear they are HIV positive. But they might think, 'Oh my gosh; I have a serious illness.' They are focused on 'I have this illness,' so it takes several more sessions to explain, 'This is what it means. Have you come up with questions since the last time we talked? What are your concerns? Here, I have gathered some information for you to read. It might help you formulate some questions.'

Olivia Estep: Where I struggle with my hepatitis C clients is getting them the care they need for blood work. Even though we have all these resources, they still tend to fall through the cracks.

Daria Leslea: There has been some resistance to that initial testing, because it is also our responsibility to inform the health department that we have such-and-such numbers of positive HIV cases and such-and-such numbers of positive hepatitis cases. I've come across patients saying they didn't want to be tested because they don't want this knowledge to be shared. We tell hepatitis patients that this information is confidential; we would just like to have some numbers about the pathology of a particular disease. I've had a hard time getting this across to patients.

Even if you have testing and vaccinations available for clients, there are still some problems. Some clients are concerned about the risks of vaccinations and the side effects of medicines, some do not want to take the time, others don't want to know whether they have HIV or hepatitis. Resistance is really high, especially in the African-American community and males.

Resource constraints and strategies

Blake: My understanding is that the insured clients are tested for all the hepatitis viruses and given vaccinations, but that there isn't funding available to do that for our clients who aren't insured.

Leslea: That's true. Where is the money coming from for hepatitis A counseling or vaccinations? It seems to me that there should be a protocol, and admission to the program would ensure that these things happen.

Ennis: The article says, 'Many of these activities (for instance, educating the staff about hepatitis) do not require additional resources, and some, such as building linkages to potential affiliate programs, make good sense for any organization.' While that may be true, it's a dismissal of the time and energy it takes to incorporate extra things into treatment. Even one additional risk assessment form adds 10 minutes. We all know how hard it is to get done what we currently are supposed to do.

Imagine if we had a half-time nurse whose job it was just to meet with new patients, to talk about infections related to drug use, and to screen them, test them, and then offer vaccines. And then if we had the money for the nurse and the vaccines, think about the huge impact that would have, even if we caught one person a month who hadn't been vaccinated yet and prevented that person from getting hepatitis C. It wouldn't cost that much. The funding out there is so piecemeal and so small. It's hard to keep consistent funding. It's hard to implement this kind of prevention activity in a consistent, long-term fashion because of the scramble to get the resources.

Scott Powers: There is an organization not mentioned in the article that provides a newsletter that is a good resource for clinicians and clients on the subject of hepatitis C. It's the Hep C Connection. Their newsletter is available online at no cost at *www.hepc-connection.org*.

tion between drug treatment and primary care providers, and the ability to accommodate patients who at times visit without appointments. Combining drug abuse treatment with regular medical care is associated with fewer subsequent hospitalizations. Therefore, averting costs of inpatient stays by promoting continuity of medical and drug abuse treatment either onsite or through linkage mechanisms may prove to be a cost-effective model of care for drug abusers.

Links to Other Services

Relatively few studies have examined the effectiveness of various linkage mechanisms to promote use of medical services among individuals enrolled in drug abuse treatment programs. Linkage strategies that have been used to improve drug abuse patients' access to medical care include case management and transportation. Findings on the utility of case management to increase access to medical care have been mixed, however, and successful case management may not be possible without funding initiatives to support such programs. Although few studies have examined the influence of transportation on utilization of drug abuse treatment services, some evidence suggests that transportation may be an important linkage mechanism (Friedmann et al., 2000).

Promoting Medication Adherence

By helping patients take needed medications, drug abuse treatment programs can play an important role in the delivery of HIV/hepatitis preventive and medical services. Any hepatitis vaccination program must consider issues of adherence, as completion of the vaccine series affords optimal protection. Specific data on factors affecting retention of IDUs in hepatitis prevention programs are sparse, but a number of drug use, demographic, and behavioral factors have been associated with patients' failure to comply with treatment for drug abuse, TB, and HIV and with other medical interventions. Hence, programs designed to deliver HIV and hepatitis prevention interventions to IDUs in treatment settings should make use of strategies demonstrated or likely to promote greater adherence, such as positive reinforcement, incentives, and other strategies (see box, "What a Drug Treatment Program Can Do To Incorporate HIV/Hepatitis Prevention").

CONCLUSION

Staffs in drug abuse treatment programs have considerable ability to prevent, detect, and diminish the adverse consequences of HIV and hepatitis A, B, and C viruses. The boxed text summarizes the evidence-based interventions that we recommend. Many of these activities (for instance, educating the staff about hepatitis) do not require additional resources, and some, such as building linkages to potential affiliate programs, make good sense for any organization. Other potentially valuable interventions

may not be feasible within a treatment program's current budget; for example, vaccinating patients for hepatitis A and B may be beyond the services usually provided. Many of these interventions require the involvement of the community's public health leadership. Combining drug abuse treatment with both hepatitis vaccination and interventions to reduce risk behaviors has the potential to be a highly efficient, synergistic approach to hepatitis prevention for IDUs and their contacts.

Drug treatment programs are in a pivotal position to reach a population that is at risk for HIV and hepatitis and has high prevalence of those diseases. Researchers and practitioners can be a powerful team, especially working with policymakers, to determine how drug abuse treatment programs can prevent HIV and hepatitis in their communities, to further disseminate research-based interventions, and to bring many of the new HIV and hepatitis strategies into local treatment settings.

ACKNOWLEDGMENTS

Support was provided in part by grants from the National Institutes of Health (K01–DA–0–0408, P50–DA–0–9253, R01–DA–1–2221, R01–DA–0–8753, R01–DA–0–9005, and R01–DA–1–1344), Center for Substance Abuse Treatment Task Order 282–98–0026, and the National Alliance for Research in Schizophrenia and Affective Disorders.

CORRESPONDENCE

James L. Sorensen, Ph.D., University of California, San Francisco, San Francisco General Hospital, Building 20, Room 2117, 1000 Potrero Avenue, San Francisco, CA 94110; tel.: (415) 206–3969; fax: (415) 206–5233; e-mail: james@itsa.ucsf.edu.

REFERENCES

Camacho, L.M.; Bartholomew, N.G.; Joe, G.W.; and Simpson, D.D., 1997. Maintenance of HIV risk reduction among injection opioid users: A 12-month posttreatment followup. *Drug and Alcohol Dependence* 47(1):11–18.

Center for Substance Abuse Treatment, 1995. "Screening for Infectious Diseases Among Substance Abusers." Treatment Improvement Protocol (TIP) Series 6. DHHS Publication No. (SMA) 95–3060. Rockville, MD: U.S. Department of Health and Human Services, Substance Abuse and Mental Health Services Administration.

Center for Substance Abuse Treatment, 2000. "Substance Abuse Treatment for Persons With HIV/AIDS." Treatment Improvement Protocol (TIP) Series 37. U.S. DHHS Publication No. (SMA) 00–3410. Rockville, MD: U.S. Department of Health and Human Services, Substance Abuse and Mental Health Services Administration.

Coyle, S.L.; Needle, R.H.; and Normand, J., 1998. Outreach-based HIV prevention for injecting drug users: A review of published outcome data. *Public Health Reports* 113 (Supp 1):19–30.

Des Jarlais, D.C., et al., 2001. Providing hepatitis B vaccination to injecting drug users through referral to health clinics vs. on-site at a syringe exchange program. *American Journal of Public Health* 91(11):1791–1792.

Edlin, B.R., et al., 2001. Is it justifiable to withhold treatment for hepatitis C from illicit-drug users? *New England Journal of Medicine* 345(3):211–215.

Friedmann, P.D.; D'Aunno, T.A.; Jin, L.; and Alexander, J.A., 2000. Medical and psychosocial services in drug abuse treatment: Do stronger linkages promote client utilization? *Health Services Research* 35(2):443–465.

Garfein, R.S., et al., 1996. Viral infections in short-term injection drug users: The prevalence of the hepatitis C, hepatitis B, human immunodeficiency, and human T-lymphotropic viruses. *American Journal of Public Health* 86(5):655–661.

Gibson, D.R.; McCusker, J.; and Chesney, M., 1998. Effectiveness of psychosocial interventions in preventing HIV risk behavior in injecting drug users. *AIDS* 12(8):919–929.

Hagan, H., and Des Jarlais, D.C., 2000. HIV and HCV infection among injection drug users. *Mount Sinai Journal of Medicine* 67:423–428.

Heimer, R., 1998. Can a syringe exchange serve as a conduit to substance abuse treatment? *Journal of Substance Abuse Treatment* 15(3):183–191.

Jaeckel, E., et al., 2001. Treatment of acute hepatitis C with interferon alfa–2b. *New England Journal of Medicine* 345(20):1452–1457.

Kral, A.H., et al., 2001 Sexual transmission of HIV–1 among injection drug users in San Francisco, USA: Risk-factor analysis. *Lancet* 357(9266):1397–1401.

Murrill, C.D., et al., 2001. Incidence of HIV among injection drug users entering drug treatment programs in four U.S. cities. *Journal of Urban Health* 78(1):152–161.

National Institute on Drug Abuse, 1991. Risk Behavior Assessment Questionnaire. October edition. Rockville, MD: NIDA Community Research Branch.

National Institute on Drug Abuse, 2000. *The NIDA Community-Based Outreach Model: A Manual To Reduce the Risk of HIV and Other Blood-Borne Infections in Drug Users*. NIH Publication No. 00–4812. Rockville, MD: NIDA.

Navaline, H.A., et al., 1994. Preparation for AIDS vaccine trials. An automated version of the Risk Assessment Battery: Enhancing the assessment of risk behaviors. *AIDS Research and Human Retroviruses* 10(Supp. 2):S281–S283.

Perlman, D.C., et al., 2001. Knowledge of hepatitis among IDUs at NYC syringe exchange programs (SEPs) (abstract). *Drug and Alcohol Dependence* 63(Suppl 1):S121.

Selwyn, P.A., et al., 1989. Primary care for patients with human immunodeficiency virus (HIV) infection in a methadone maintenance program. *Annals of Internal Medicine* 111(9):761–763.

James L. Sorenson, Ph.D. and **Carmen L. Masson, Ph.D.**, University of California, San Francisco and San Francisco General Hospital, San Francisco, California.

David C. Perlman, M.D., Beth Israel Medical Center, New York, New York.

Index

Test Your Knowledge Form

We encourage you to photocopy and use this page as a tool to assess how the articles in *Annual Editions* expand on the information in your textbook. By reflecting on the articles you will gain enhanced text information. You can also access this useful form on a product's book support Web site at *http://www.dushkin.com/online/*.

NAME: _____   DATE: _____

TITLE AND NUMBER OF ARTICLE: _____

BRIEFLY STATE THE MAIN IDEA OF THIS ARTICLE: _____

_____

LIST THREE IMPORTANT FACTS THAT THE AUTHOR USES TO SUPPORT THE MAIN IDEA:

_____

WHAT INFORMATION OR IDEAS DISCUSSED IN THIS ARTICLE ARE ALSO DISCUSSED IN YOUR TEXTBOOK OR OTHER READINGS THAT YOU HAVE DONE? LIST THE TEXTBOOK CHAPTERS AND PAGE NUMBERS:

_____

LIST ANY EXAMPLES OF BIAS OR FAULTY REASONING THAT YOU FOUND IN THE ARTICLE:

_____

LIST ANY NEW TERMS/CONCEPTS THAT WERE DISCUSSED IN THE ARTICLE, AND WRITE A SHORT DEFINITION:

We Want Your Advice

ANNUAL EDITIONS revisions depend on two major opinion sources: one is our Advisory Board, listed in the front of this volume, which works with us in scanning the thousands of articles published in the public press each year; the other is you—the person actually using the book. Please help us and the users of the next edition by completing the prepaid article rating form on this page and returning it to us. Thank you for your help!

ANNUAL EDITIONS: Drugs, Society, and Behavior 04/05

ARTICLE RATING FORM

Here is an opportunity for you to have direct input into the next revision of this volume.
We would like you to rate each of the articles listed below, using the following scale:

1. **Excellent: should definitely be retained**
2. **Above average: should probably be retained**
3. **Below average: should probably be deleted**
4. **Poor: should definitely be deleted**

Your ratings will play a vital part in the next revision.
Please mail this prepaid form to us as soon as possible.
Thanks for your help!

RATING	ARTICLE	RATING	ARTICLE
	1. Drug Research and Children		34. GHB's Deadly Allure
	2. Tobacco		35. Ban Ephedra Now!
	3. Is the Drug War Over? The Declining Proportion of Drug Offenders		36. Prescription Drug Abuse: FDA and SAMHSA Join Forces
	4. Prescription Drug Abuse Deadlier Than Use of Illegal Drugs		37. 'The Perfect Crime'
	5. American Banks and the War on Drugs		38. Harder Times for Meth Makers
	6. Survival of the Druggies		39. Combating Methamphetamine Laboratories and Abuse: Strategies for Success
	7. Beyond the Pleasure Principle		40. About Face Program Turns Lives Around
	8. It's a Hard Habit to Break		41. Congress Stiffens Requirements for Drug Treatment in Prisons and Jails
	9. The End of Craving		42. As Drug Use Drops in Big Cities, Small Towns Confront Upsurge
	10. Hungry for the Next Fix		43. Beware the Dark Side of Pharmacy Life
	11. A New Treatment for Addiction		44. Drug Arrests at the Millennium
	12. Finding the Future Alcoholic		45. Fetal Alcohol Syndrome Prevention Research
	13. Drug Abuse in the Balance		46. Campus Boozing Toll
	14. In the Grip of a Deeper Pain		47. Drug Treatment Programs
	15. Is Pot Good for You?		48. Higher Learning
	16. The Dangers of Diet Pills		49. U.S., Canada Clash on Pot Laws
	17. Why Rx May Spell Danger: 'Do You Know the Difference Between Use and Abuse of Prescription Medicines?'		50. Washington's Unsavory Antidrug Partners
	18. Addicted to Anti-Depressants?		51. Illegal Drug Use and Public Policy
	19. When Drinking Helps		52. How to Win the Drug War
	20. Binge Drinking Holds Steady: College Students Continue to Drink Despite Programs		53. A New Weapon in the War on Drugs: Family
	21. More Than a Kick		54. Harm Reduction: A Promising Approach for College Health
	22. The Agony of Ecstasy		55. Smoking Cessation
	23. Afghanistan's Opium: A Bumper Crop		56. Perinatal Care for Women Who Are Addicted: Implications for Empowerment
	24. Appalachia's New Cottage Industry: Meth		57. The Road to Recovery: A Gender-Responsive Program for Convicted DUI 'Females'
	25. Heroin Hits Small-Town America		58. Addicted, Neglectful Moms Offered Treatment, Custody
	26. Life or Meth?		59. Strategy for Alcohol Abuse Education: A Service Learning Model Within a Course Curriculum
	27. Ecstacy Use Declines as More Teens Recognize Risks of Drug		60. HIV/Hepatitis Prevention in Drug Abuse Treatment Programs: Guidance From Research
	28. A Worry for Ravers		
	29. New Coke		
	30. Clicking for a Fix: Drugs Online		
	31. The Orphan Drug Backlash		
	32. Use Caution With Pain Relievers		
	33. 'I Felt Like I Wanted to Hurt People'		

(Continued on next page)

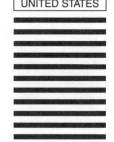

**NO POSTAGE
NECESSARY
IF MAILED
IN THE
UNITED STATES**

BUSINESS REPLY MAIL
FIRST CLASS MAIL PERMIT NO. 551 DUBUQUE IA

POSTAGE WILL BE PAID BY ADDRESEE

McGraw-Hill/Dushkin
2460 KERPER BLVD
DUBUQUE, IA 52001-9902

ABOUT YOU

Name   Date

_____

Are you a teacher? ❏   A student? ❏
Your school's name

_____

Department

_____

Address   City   State   Zip

_____

School telephone #

_____

YOUR COMMENTS ARE IMPORTANT TO US!

Please fill in the following information:
For which course did you use this book?

_____

Did you use a text with this ANNUAL EDITION?   ❏ yes ❏ no
What was the title of the text?

_____

What are your general reactions to the *Annual Editions* concept?

_____

Have you read any pertinent articles recently that you think should be included in the next edition? Explain.

_____

Are there any articles that you feel should be replaced in the next edition? Why?

_____

Are there any World Wide Web sites that you feel should be included in the next edition? Please annotate.

_____

May we contact you for editorial input?   ❏ yes ❏ no
May we quote your comments?   ❏ yes ❏ no